DIAGNOSIS, CONCEPTUALIZATION, AND TREATMENT PLANNING FOR ADULTS

A Step-by-Step Guide

DIAGNOSIS, CONCEPTUALIZATION, AND TREATMENT PLANNING FOR ADULTS
A Step-by-Step Guide

Edited by

Michel Hersen
Pacific University

Linda Krug Porzelius
St. Charles Medical Center

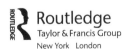

Routledge
Taylor & Francis Group
New York London

Routledge
Taylor & Francis Group
711 Third Avenue
New York, NY 10017

Routledge
Taylor & Francis Group
2 Park Square
Milton Park, Abingdon
Oxon OX14 4RN

International Standard Book Number-13: 978-0-8058-3492-5 (Softcover)
Library of Congress catalog number: 2001040312

Library of Congress Cataloging-in-Publication Data

Catalog record is available from the Library of Congress

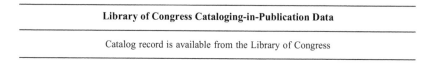

Visit the Taylor & Francis Web site at
http://www.taylorandfrancis.com

and the Routledge Web site at
http://www.routledge.com

To the memories of Leon Hersen,
Herman Whitmore, and Jean Whitmore

Contents

Preface

After working with graduate students in clinical psychology for many years, it has become apparent to us that there is a major transfer gap between the knowledge they acquire in the classroom and how they apply it to thorny client problems. Although most graduate programs teach how to 1) diagnose and assess cases, 2) conceptualize them, and 3) treat them effectively, the relationship among the three processes is frequently unclear to students when they reach the doors of the clinic. Thus, this book had its genesis in our frustration and need as clinical supervisors.

Our text is planned to teach students, in pragmatic fashion, the strategies used by experts to diagnose adults seen in outpatient settings and to present and conceptualize cases for the purpose of selecting targets and treatments. It bridges the transition from the theoretical knowledge of the classroom to the ability to operationalize procedures in the clinic. It is organized so as to answer clearly the questions most frequently posed by students to supervisors when they begin their clinical apprenticeships. We believe the text will facilitate the work of clinical supervisors and elucidate the issues for their students and trainees.

The reader will note that the book contains 15 chapters and is divided into two parts. Part I, General Issues, discusses concepts that are prerequisite to understanding the material in Part II. Part II, Specific Disorders, presents the kinds of disorders and problems typically seen in outpatient clinics for adults. Contributors to the book were asked to follow a standard outline to facilitate the instructor's work when using this text. To the extent possible, in some instances with minor modifications, this outline has been adhered to by our contributors:

1. Description of the disorder
2. Methods to determine diagnosis
3. Additional assessments required

Many people have contributed to the fruition of this text. First, we thank our friends at Lawrence Erlbaum, including Larry Erlbaum, Susan Milmoe, Kate Graetzer, and Jason Planer for valuing this project. Second, we are grateful to our eminent contributors for taking time out from the busy schedules to share with us their expertise; and third, we thank Carole Londerée, Alex Duncan, and Angelina Marchand for their gracious technical help.

Michel Hersen
Linda Krug Porzelius

Part I

General Issues

1

Overview

Linda Krug Porzelius
St. Charles Medical Center

This textbook is designed to teach beginning therapists the applied process of using the results of assessments to formulate a diagnosis, develop a conceptualization, and make plans for treatment. Excellent textbooks teach practical aspects of assessment, diagnosis, and treatment planning, but few walk students through the entire process. In addition, few offer specifics on how to develop a case conceptualization, although conceptualization plays a pivotal role in moving from assessment to treatment planning. Therefore, the text presents a general model of conceptualization (Table 1.1) and demonstrates use of the model through case examples. Students learn not only a clear method for developing case conceptualizations, but also important differences in conceptualizations across different diagnostic groups. The enormous body of research on the characteristics and etiology of each diagnostic group, such as depression, cannot be ignored in developing an individual case conceptualization. Although all clients have unique presentations and stories, knowledge about their diagnostic group can provide important guidelines for viewing each.

WHAT IS CASE CONCEPTUALIZATION?

Case conceptualization explains the nature of a client's problems and how he or she came to have them. As Berman (1997) states, you must explain *"what the client is like* as well as theoretical hypotheses for *why the client is like this"* (p. xi). Other terms used for this concept are *formulation* or *working hypothesis*.

3

TABLE 1.1
Case Conceptualization Model

a. Modeling and learning
b. Life events
c. Genetics and temperament
d. Physical conditions
e. Drugs
f. Socioeconomic and cultural factors

Weerasekera (1996) defines *formulation* as a "hypothesis of how an individual comes to present with a certain disorder or circumstance at a particular point in time" (p. 5).

Thus, the case conceptualization organizes assessment data into a meaningful outline, applying research and theory to make sense of a client's current presentation. Although the diagnosis summarizes a client's symptoms, it is not enough. Therapists must know more about their clients than symptoms and diagnosis. Therapists must go beyond diagnosis, developing hypotheses to explain how the clients came to have a particular set of psychological and interpersonal problems. Therapists review all potential contributors to the problem, examining distal and proximal factors; causal, maintaining, and precipitating factors; and internal and environmental factors. Therapists then identify the most central contributors, develop explicit hypotheses about clients' problems, develop treatment plans based on the hypotheses, and intentionally test the hypotheses during treatment.

HISTORY OF THE CONCEPT

Historically, little attention was paid to conceptualization. Although psychodynamic approaches rely on formulation in treatment, most other theoretical approaches addressed conceptualization to a much lesser extent. For reviews of the history of conceptualization and formulation in psychotherapy, see Eels (1997) or Weerasekera (1996). The usefulness of a thoughtful case conceptualization is increasingly recognized among therapists with diverse theoretical backgrounds. Indeed, case conceptualization may be even more helpful given the increasing demands from managed care for short-term treatments, for clear justification of treatment need, and for explicit treatment goals and plans. The 1990s saw the publication of several books on conceptualization, considerably more than in previous decades. Similarly, the number of articles written on conceptualization increased during the same time period. A small body of research is beginning to develop concerning the process and utility of case conceptualization, most of which is focused on psychodynamic formulation (for a review, see Weerasekera, 1996). Although the proposition that case conceptualization leads to better treatment planning seems reasonable, research has not yet documented the utility of particular conceptualization models. It is greatly needed to document the reliability and utility of conceptualization methods.

DEVELOPING A CASE CONCEPTUALIZATION

A major purpose of this text is to provide the student with a tool for constructions coherent case conceptualizations. To construct a conceptualization, you will use material from all types of assessments: client interviews, collateral interviews, medical records, psychological tests, behavioral observations, self-monitoring, and so on. You will summarize symptoms, but you must go beyond a reiteration of symptoms, derive meaning from the client's current presentation, and explain how he or she developed the symptoms. Steps 1 through 3 are detailed as follows. In Step 1, the therapist reviews potential contributing factors to the problem. In Step 2, he or she synthesizes material from this review of contributing factors into a meaningful narrative, including hypotheses about how the client came to have his or her problem. In Step 3, the therapist uses the hypotheses to develop treatment targets and identify appropriate interventions.

The conceptualization model presented here provides useful categories for sorting all of the available information about a client after the assessment process. The length of the assessment process as well as the thoroughness of the assessment vary depending on time and resources available to the therapist. However, regardless of how much information we obtain about the client, we always end up knowing only a limited amount about each individual. Although not all information is known, the therapist should develop a preliminary case conceptualization early in the therapy process, striving to find a balance between the immediate and pressing needs of the client and the ideal of a comprehensive assessment (Eels, 1997).

Step 1: Review and Organize Information

The first step in developing a conceptualization is to organize information in the categories listed in Table 1.1 and described in the following paragraphs. For each client, some factors contribute to the problem whereas other factors do not. You attempt to explain the client's presentation in terms of causal factors as well as vulnerability factors, maintaining factors, and precipitating factors. As part of the process, you apply your knowledge about the client's symptoms and diagnosis, etiology of disorders, normal and abnormal development, and social and cultural influences on behavior. In short, you apply all you have learned to make sense of your client's current presentation.

A diverse array of theoretical constructs may need to be considered. One of the primary difficulties in teaching students how to conceptualize client problems is that they often have experience with a limited number of theoretical constructs. Obviously, we must be familiar with a construct before we can apply the construct to a particular case. Without a thorough consideration of causal and maintaining factors in a client's problems, therapists may have a tendency to view only one or two aspects, leaving out information important to developing an effective treatment plan. Furthermore, without explicit, systematic consideration of all possible contributing factors, clinicians tend to jump quickly to one hypothesis, raising the potential for biases in clinical judgment (Garb, 1998). Using the conceptualization model described later, the beginning therapist explicitly considers many categories of causal and maintaining factors.

As an example of an incomplete evaluation of contributors, a therapist evaluates a woman who is depressed and recommends a combination of cognitive–behavioral therapy and antidepressants. The woman came into therapy after an argument with her boss and talked about her feelings of inadequacy in her work. Work problems clearly seemed related to her depression. The therapist begins working with the client on self-monitoring of automatic thoughts related to situations at work. It is likely that this therapist will be somewhat helpful by focusing on treatment of work problems and by teaching the cognitive model. However, did the therapist choose the most central or most important target? In order to provide the best cognitive behavioral treatment for this woman, the therapist must understand the combination of factors that contributed to this woman becoming depressed at this time in her life, as well as any factors that may be maintaining her depression. To what extent do communication problems with her husband contribute to her feeling helpless, frustrated, and depressed? Might role conflicts contribute to her problem? For example, she wants to begin having children, but fears that her work and career will stop progressing. Are physical factors contributing to her depression, such as mood changes with perimenopause or onset of a physical illness? Failure to consider diverse physical, interpersonal, or cultural contributing factors may lead the therapist to miss important treatment targets.

A brief description of each category is given in the following to provide students with a general understanding of the categories. The contributing and maintaining factors described here cut across theoretical boundaries to explain who the client is, rather than using information from only one or two theoretical orientations. The model presented previously provides a short list of broad factors that can easily be used in practice.

Modeling and Learning.   Across theoretical schools the relative emphasis on early childhood experiences differs, but all suggest some assessment of important developmental influences. It is important to know something about who raised the client and who the important role models were across the lifespan. Modeling and learning experiences may contribute to a client's problems through their impact on personality, interpersonal and coping skills, cognitive schemas, or other characteristics. Although the therapist strives to conduct a thorough assessment of modeling and learning experiences, the conceptualization does not include all material from the assessment. Rather, the therapist sorts through assessment information, looking for events or themes that seem to have played a significant role in the client's current problems. For example, a prominent theme for Mary is that she has never felt that she "fit in," being shy and moving frequently during childhood. In attempting to explain how the current presentation developed, the therapist may draw on general developmental theories or on theory specific to a particular disorder. For example, for the adolescent girl who has Anorexia Nervosa, family structure and communication may be important contributing factors.

Life Events. Most theoretical orientations posit some role for the impact of a person's life experiences on who we are. Powerful life experiences, such as serious illness, divorce, rape, or assault, cause serious psychological problems for some individuals. More universal life experiences, such as leaving home, getting married, becoming a parent, or retiring, also contribute to psychological problems for some individuals. Chronic long-term stress from ongoing stressful experiences, such as ongoing marital or job difficulties, may contribute to difficulties. For example, cognitive–behavioral theories of anxiety disorders propose that individuals exposed to highly stressful environments develop core schemas in which the world is viewed as dangerous, leading to hypervigilance and misinterpretations of nondangerous experiences.

Genetics and Temperament. Through studies of twins and adopted children, research identifies genetic factors as important contributing factors to most psychological disorders, although the mechanisms of transmission are often not understood. Vulnerability to a disorder is believed to be inherited, but is also modified by life experiences. We may inherit a tendency for problematic modulation of hormonal levels or neurotransmitter activity, as theories of schizophrenia or obsessive compulsive disorder, for example, suggest. We may inherit a general disposition or temperament that makes us vulnerable to a particular disorder. The therapist draws on research about genetic contributing factors to the client's disorder as well as research on inherited temperaments that increase vulnerability to particular disorders.

Physical Conditions. Therapists too often ignore physical factors, perhaps because training generally emphasizes psychological aspects of problems. Physical factors can affect psychological problems through different pathways. *Brain damage* obviously and sometimes dramatically influences psychological presentation, whether from traumatic head injury, stroke, or a dementia.

Any physical problem that interferes with *sleep, energy, or appetite* may contribute to psychological problems. Physical problems that impede *activity* can also affect psychological functioning. Individuals who struggle with *physical disability or chronic illness* may face obstacles to independent living and participation in enjoyable activities, which could contribute to isolation, feelings of helplessness, and depression. For example, a young man injures his back in an accident on his construction job, which leads to a year of unemployment while he receives medical treatments. Unable to work or provide adequately for his family, he feels increasingly more helpless and depressed.

Physical characteristics also influence people psychologically. For example, girls who are mildly overweight in adolescence are more likely to diet and more likely to develop a serious eating disorder (French, Perry, Leon, & Fulkerson, 1995). People who are unattractive, disfigured, in a wheelchair, or overweight are often exposed to serious discrimination and prejudice, which could contribute to psychological problems. Sometimes, in a misguided attempt to deny any personal prejudice, therapists may simply ignore an undesirable characteristic, such as overweight. However, by simply ignoring the client's weight problem, the therapist may miss important information about how the client is treated by family, friends, or strangers because of being overweight.

Drugs.   Many drugs, including alcohol, caffeine, nicotine, illegal drugs, over-the-counter medications, psychotropic medications, and medications taken for physical problems, whether prescribed by a doctor or obtained through a "natural" food store can have an impact on a person's psychological problems. Therapists generally pay attention to the use of alcohol, illegal drugs, and psychotropic medications, but are less likely to ask about medications taken for physical problems. However, many prescription medications have important side effects that can indirectly affect a person's psychological functioning by causing fatigue, sleep problems, decline in sexual drive, weight gain or loss, or even mood changes. Herbal treatments are becomingly increasingly popular and may have significant side effects, although less is known about these drugs. Although medication is generally only one of many contributors to a problem, treatment is impeded when the impact of medication is ignored. Therapists should be aware of what medications their clients are taking and their potential side effects.

Socioeconomic and Cultural Factors.   Traditionally, psychologists have tended to focus on individual aspects of a problem, but contemporary theoretical models identify the importance of a person's environment including living conditions, type of work, and support from friends and family. These environmental factors are in turn affected by broader socioeconomic and cultural factors. The therapist attempting to explain a client's current presentation must have some knowledge of this research, and should assess the ways in which social factors may contribute to problems. In his book on clinical judgment, Garb (1998) urged clinicians to consider not only the client, but also factors outside him or her that contribute to the problem. Socioeconomic factors include class and economic group. Poverty contributes to inadequate health care and increases stress and exposure to violence.

Cultural factors, such as ethnicity, culture, race, gender, religion, and lifestyle, can affect psychological problems through their impact on values, role expectations, family interactions, social support, or help-seeking behaviors. The majority of psychologists come from middle to upper middle, white, mainstream cultures in the United States. Increasingly, therapists are called on to become more knowledgeable about and sensitive to the cultural issues their clients present. Therapists must acquire knowledge about ethnic and racial groups, gender roles, religious groups, or other relevant cultural factors for their clients. Extensive discussion of diversity issues is beyond the scope of this book, but it is now a requisite component of clinical training and professional competency.

Step 2: Organize Information into a Meaningful Story

In the process of sorting assessment information for the categories mentioned previously, you are applying relevant knowledge and theory about human behavior to your client's problems. After considering a diverse array of explanatory constructs, you must integrate the information to develop a clear and meaningful story or theory about how the client came to have his or her problems. You begin making educated guesses or hypotheses about the central causes and important maintaining factors for your client, choosing only the most relevant information. The overall conceptualization tells a story, using your hypotheses, about how the client's problems developed, why the client is seeking treatment now, and why his or her efforts to overcome the problem have not been successful. The hypotheses can then be tested, and either discarded or used to guide treatment.

How does one go from a list of problems and contributing factors to a brief, coherent story that encompasses all-important points? One of the challenges to developing an effective conceptualization is that a plethora of information must be sorted through to provide a brief summary and explanation of the client's problems. Obviously, not all information can be included. Therapists may tend to make long, inclusive lists of contributing factors that are too cumbersome to put to effective use. Eells, Kendjelic, and Lucas (1998) developed and applied a system for coding case conceptualizations from psychological reports. An analysis of 56 reports found that therapists often gave simple lists of descriptive information without integrating the information or providing hypotheses as to how the individual came to develop his or her problems. When therapists did specify contributors to the clients' problems, psychological factors were hypothesized to be important much more often than were biological, social, or cultural factors. Another study found that beginning as compared to experienced therapists tend to structure client information in a more simplistic manner, with fewer, less complex links between pieces of information (Mayfield, Kardash, & Kivlighan, 1999). Perhaps teaching therapists an explicit conceptualization model will help them to develop more sophisticated ways in which to organize and understand client information. Eels (1997) instructs therapists to develop a conceptualization that is complex enough to provide a reasonable summary of the client's problem yet simple enough to use easily. Meier (1999) recommended using the rule of parsimony, keeping the theory "as simple as possible, without being trivial or simplistic" (p. 857). Practically speaking, the therapist must be able to recall hypotheses during a session in order to test them. In sorting through the information, therapists should rely more on information that is consistently found from multiple sources or types of assessments (Nezu, Nezu, Friedman, & Haynes, 1997). Assessment information that comes from the most reliable and valid sources, such as well-validated psychological inventories, should weigh more strongly than impressionistic information (Nezu et al., 1997).

Step 3: Identify Treatment Targets and Interventions

The conceptualization summarizes problem areas, telling a meaningful story about how the problems developed, which in turn suggests which problems should be treated first, what treatment is the most appropriate, the probable length of treatment, and the prognosis. The therapist who thoroughly reviewed all categories of potential contributing factors should be more likely to consider a diversity of treatment targets and approaches and is better able to make hypotheses about which treatments will be most helpful to a particular client. The hypotheses make up a working model that is used to guide treatment. Treatment may target behavior problems, such as impulsive overspending; painful emotions, such as depression or anxiety; problematic thoughts, such as obsessional thinking; physical problems, such as insomnia; or skill deficits. Treatment may also target the client's environment or interaction with friends, family, or coworkers. In the previous example of the woman seeking treatment for depression, treatment may target beliefs and attitudes about coworkers, the marital relationship, beliefs and values about motherhood and work, or physical aspects of the problem.

As noted previously, hypotheses directly suggest both treatment targets and interventions. However, the therapist's hypotheses about and theory of the client may be wrong. Assessment data never capture all aspects of a client. In addition, biases in clinical judgment may lead to erroneous hypotheses. Garb (1998) described the common problem of confirmatory bias, in which therapists, beginning and experienced, make the mistake of assuming that their explanation is true and proceed to seek information consistent with the hypothesis while discarding conflicting information. Therapists often fail to consider alternative hypotheses or test their hypotheses. You should not treat your conceptualization as reality. Rather, you make hypotheses based on your theory and then test them during sessions, looking for information to confirm or disconfirm your hypotheses. The conceptualization should be considered a tentative best guess that is continually revised as new information is obtained. When the clinician faces a treatment that is not working, the case conceptualization may help him or her more systematically consider alternative hypotheses and treatment plans (Tompkins, 1999). Meier (1999) described the process as a "feedback loop" in which the therapist assesses, conceptualizes, develops, and implements an intervention; assesses the success of the intervention; then revises the conceptualization as needed to develop a more effective treatment.

SUMMARY

The model presented here provides the beginning therapist with an applied method of learning how to develop useful case conceptualizations. Students first review and organize client information into the categories listed in Table 1.1, then summarize the information into a meaningful theory about how the client came to have his or her problem at this particular time. Specific hypotheses about contributing, maintaining, and protective factors are developed that directly suggest appropriate treatment targets and interventions. The therapist continues to look for evidence to confirm or disconfirm the hypotheses. The conceptualization is revised as needed to more accurately identify hypotheses and effective treatments.

The development of a case conceptualization provides therapists with a way to move from diagnosis to treatment plan. The conceptual model presented here cuts across theoretical boundaries to help beginning therapists identify broad factors that contribute to client problems.

Chapters 2 and 3 describe general concepts in involved diagnosis, behavioral assessment, and treatment planning. Chapters 3 through 15 focus on one problem area or diagnostic group seen by therapists in outpatient settings. The authors of each chapter illustrate the process of assessment, diagnosis, conceptualization, and treatment planning through case examples.

REFERENCES

Berman, P. S. (1997). *Case conceptualization and treatment planning: Exercises for integrating theory with clinical practice*. Thousand Oaks, CA: Sage Publications.

Eels, T. D. (1997). *Handbook of psychotherapy case formulation*. New York: Guilford Press.

Eells, T. D., Kendjelic, E. M., & Lucas, C. P. (1998). What's in a case formulation? Development and use of a content coding manual. *The Journal of Psychotherapy Practice and Research, 7,* 144–153.

Garb, H. N. (1998). *Studying the clinician: Judgment research and psychological assessment.* Washington, DC: American Psychological Association.

French, S. A., Perry, C. L., Leon, G. R., & Fulkerson, J. A. (1995). Changes in psychological variables and health behaviors by dieting status over a three-year period in a cohort of adolescent females. *Journal of Adolescent Health, 16,* 438–447.

Mayfield, W. A., Kardash, C. M., & Kivlighan, D. M., Jr. (1999). Differences in experienced and novice counselors' knowledge structures about clients: Implications for case conceptualization. *Journal of Counseling Psychology, 46,* 504–514.

Meier, S. T. (1999). Training the practitioner–scientist: Bridging case conceptualization, assessment, and intervention. *The Counseling Psychologist, 27,* 846–869.

Nezu, A. M., Nezu, C. M., Friedman, S. H., & Haynes, S. N. (1997). Case formulation in behavior therapy: Problem-solving and functional analytic strategies. In Tracy D. Eels (Ed.), *Handbook of psychotherapy case formulation* (pp. 368–401). New York: The Guilford Press.

Tompkins, M. A. (1999). Using a case formulation to manage treatment nonresponse. *Journal of Cognitive Psychotherapy, 13,* 317–330.

Weerasekera, P. (1996). *Multiperspective Case Formulation: A step towards treatment integration.* Malabar, FL: Krieger Publishing Company.

2

Diagnosis, Differential Diagnosis, and the SCID

Daniel L. Segal, Jessica Corcoran,
and Alicia Coughlin
University of Colorado at Colorado Springs

Diagnosis and differential diagnosis can be likened to detective work among mental health professionals: A person in distress presents for evaluation or treatment and clinicians must use all their professional skills to "solve" the diagnostic mystery and formulate some initial clinical impressions. An important part of the diagnostic process is differentiating or discriminating one disorder from other disorders and is called *differential diagnosis*. Structured interviews have been developed largely to assist clinicians in solving difficult differential diagnostic puzzles. In this chapter, the major issues and strategies regarding psychiatric diagnosis and differential diagnosis are analyzed. The chapter concludes with an in-depth discussion of a popular structured interview, the Structured Clinical Interview for *DSM–IV* (SCID).

DIAGNOSIS

Diagnosis can be defined as the identification and labeling of a psychiatric disorder by examination and analysis. Clinicians diagnose clients based on the symptoms that the client experiences. Clinicians typically consult the primary diagnostic guide (in the Western world) called the *Diagnostic and Statistical Manual of Mental Disorders*, 4th edition (*DSM–IV*; American Psychiatric Association, 1994), which classifies psychopathology according to 17 basic diagnostic categories, including personality disorders. The *DSM–IV* increases the accuracy of diagnosis because the manual explicitly lists the criteria necessary to diagnose each specific mental disorder. Extensive literature reviews were used to extract the most significant clinical symptoms in order to achieve an appropriate diagnosis. Although far from perfect, the *DSM–IV* functions as one of the most accurate manuals used to diagnose mental disorders. The only major competitor to the *DSM–IV* is the World Health Organization's *International Classification of Diseases*, 10th edition (*ICD–10*), which is widely compatible with the *DSM–IV*.

According to the *DSM–IV*, persons with a particular diagnosis (e.g., major depression) need not exhibit identical features, although they should present with certain cardinal symptoms (e.g., either depressed mood or anhedonia). Notably, the criteria for many disorders (according to the *DSM–IV*) are *polythetic*, which means that an individual must exhibit a minimum number of symptoms to be diagnosed, but not all symptoms need be present (e.g., five of nine symptoms must be present for a diagnosis of major depression). Use of polythetic criteria allows for some variation among people with the same disorder. However, individuals with the same disorder should have a similar history in some areas; for example, a typical age of onset, prognosis, and common comorbid conditions. Other important information about a diagnosis includes prevalence and course data; the extent of its genetic loading (i.e., whether it consistently runs in families; the concordance rates among twins); the extent to which it is affected by psychosocial forces; the extent to which the disorder varies according to gender, age, and culture; the subtypes and specifiers of the disorder; associated laboratory findings, physical examination findings, and general medical conditions; and information about differential diagnosis. Fortunately, information about many of these areas for each mental disorder is provided in the text of *DSM–IV*.

The *DSM–IV* is much improved compared to earlier editions of the manual regarding its attention to multicultural and diversity awareness, which is necessary to diagnose individuals outside the majority culture. International experts were involved to ensure a wide pool of information on cultural factors in psychopathology and diagnosis. It includes information about cultural factors that may influence some disorders. For example, cultural considerations for conduct disorder include immigrant youth who exhibit aggressive behavior necessary for survival. Perhaps most importantly, a glossary of many culture-bound disorders are described in Appendix I (pp. 843–849) of the *DSM–IV*: Outline for Cultural Formulation and Glossary of Culture-Bound Syndromes. In this section, information is provided about the names of culture-bound syndromes, the cultures in which it occurs, and a description of the main psychopathological features. As an example, a disorder called *susto* occurs mainly in South and Central America and is an illness in which a traumatic event purportedly causes the soul to leave the body. Another example is *brain fag*, which occurs mainly in West African students in response to stress and includes such symptoms as impaired concentration, blurred vision, and head and neck pain. In all, 25 conditions are discussed, which is an important beginning to increasing the cross-cultural validity of the *DSM–IV*.

The *DSM–IV* Multiaxial System

A major innovation in the *DSM* is the application of a *multiaxial approach*. In the multiaxial system, each person is rated on five distinct dimensions or axes, with each axis referring to a different domain of the person's functioning. Although only Axis I and Axis II cover the diagnosis of abnormal behavior, the inclusion of axes III–V indicates awareness that factors other than a person's symptoms should be considered in a thorough assessment. Indeed, each domain is important in that it can help the clinician understand the experience of the person more fully, plan treatment, and predict outcome. The multiaxial system also provides a convenient and standard format for organizing and communicating clinical information, captures the complexity of clinical phenomena, and describes potentially important differences in functioning among persons with the same diagnosis. Each axis is briefly described next.

Axis I: Clinical Disorders and Other Conditions That May Be a Focus of Clinical Attention.
All disorders and conditions experienced by the client are reported on Axis I with the exception of personality disorders and mental retardation which are coded on Axis II. Axis I comprises 16 broad categories under which specific disorders are subsumed. Fifteen of the 16 categories describe diagnosable mental disorders. The final category, Other Conditions That May Be a Focus of Clinical Attention, denotes conditions that are not mental disorders but may prompt the need for psychological intervention. Examples include parent–child relational problem, malingering, bereavement, and phase-of-life problems.

Axis II: Personality Disorders and Mental Retardation.
Personality disorders are inflexible and maladaptive patterns of behavior reflecting extreme variants of normal personality traits that have become rigid and dysfunctional. Ten personality disorders are standard in the *DSM–IV*: paranoid, schizoid, schizotypal, antisocial, borderline, histrionic, narcissistic, avoidant, dependent, and obsessive–compulsive personality disorder. *Personality disorder not otherwise specified* is also included as an option. *Depressive personality disorder* and *passive–aggressive personality disorder* are included in Appendix B for Further Study. The evolution of the personality disorder diagnosis across versions of the *DSM* reveals a rich and sometimes ironic history (see Coolidge & Segal, 1998, for a complete analysis). Interestingly, prominent dysfunctional personality traits can also be listed in Axis II when symptoms are noteworthy

but below diagnostic threshold. Significant uses of various defense mechanisms can also be noted on Axis II, although this technique appears uncommon in clinical practice.

Axis III: General Medical Conditions. On this axis, the clinician lists any current physical disorders (e.g., epilepsy, cirrhosis of the liver, diabetes) that could be relevant to the understanding or management of the client's psychological problems. It is advisable to list all important medical conditions experienced by the client and to be inclusive rather than exclusive.

Axis IV: Psychosocial and Environmental Problems. All social and environmental stressors experienced by the client are reported on Axis IV. The clinician should note as many stressors as are judged relevant. Examples include recently divorced, inadequate finances, illiteracy, recent death of parent (or loved one), and lives in a high-crime neighborhood. The possibilities for stressors are endless, and all that affect the client should be reported. According to *DSM–IV* convention, it is typical to note only those stressors that have been present during the year preceding the current evaluation. However, the clinician can note stressors occurring prior to the previous year if they contribute significantly to the mental disorder or have become a focus of treatment. For example, childhood sexual abuse may be an important factor in the development of Posttraumatic Stress Disorder and should be noted as a current stressor.

Axis V: Global Assessment of Functioning (GAF). GAF scale ratings are recorded on Axis V. Here, the clinician's judgment of the client's overall level of functioning is described on a 0–100 scale, with higher numbers indicative of better functioning. Explicit descriptions of functioning in 10-point increments are provided in the *DSM–IV*. For example, a GAF range from 31 to 40 indicates "some impairment in reality testing or communication," scores ranging from 51 to 60 suggest "moderate symptoms or moderate difficulty in social, occupational, or school functioning," and scores from 71 to 80 denote mild symptoms that are "transient and expectable reactions to psychosocial stressors" with slight functional impairment (APA, 1994, p. 32). Typically, current GAF ratings are provided. Sometimes clinicians include the client's highest GAF within the previous year or at some other relevant time, such as at discharge from an inpatient unit. GAF scale ratings (albeit subjective) are useful in describing the overall level of impairment of a client, tracking clinical progress of a client over time, and predicting prognosis.

Purposes and Bene ts of Diagnosis

The application of formal diagnostic labels to clinical phenomena results in a number of important benefits. Diagnosis is helpful because it increases communication among clinicians and researchers. Communication is facilitated when professionals share an understanding of disorders and their symptoms. For example, a clinician may state that a person has paranoid schizophrenia. Other professionals who are familiar with this diagnostic terminology understand that this person may experience persecutory delusions, auditory hallucinations, as well as disorganized speech, catatonic behavior, and flat affect (APA, 1994). A wordy explanation of symptomatology is unnecessary among professionals who are familiar with the *DSM–IV*.

Knowledge of disorders and symptoms also helps clinicians organize information elicited from clients. For example, if an individual presents with intense crying spells, feelings of worthlessness, and difficulty sleeping, a clinician may probe about presence or absence of other symptoms of major depression (e.g., anhedonia, appetite disturbance, concentration problems, lethargy, suicidal impulses) to confirm or rule out the diagnosis.

Diagnosis also plays an important role in the legal arena. For example, mental health professionals are sometimes called to testify whether a defendant is competent to stand trial or has a mental disorder that may have impaired the defendant's judgment. Diagnosis can help a seriously mentally ill person be placed in a mental health facility instead of a prison. Also, neuropsychological evaluations are often conducted to determine the competency or ability of a person to make medical and financial decisions.

Another important aspect of diagnosis is that diagnosis should determine treatment. Similar to the medical model in which a diagnosis of strep throat implies the successful treatment by a course of antibiotic medications, diagnosis in mental health can influence the type of psychotherapy provided. In recent years, the field has provided many empirically validated psychological treatments of specific mental disorders (see excellent review by DeRubeis & Crits-Cristoph, 1998). For example, efficacious treatments for major depression include cognitive therapy, behavior therapy, and interpersonal therapy. Unfortunately, empirically validated psychological treatments are not available for many disorders (e.g., bipolar disorder, dissociative identity disorder), although evaluation of treatments for many psychological disorders is an active area of funding and research.

Diagnosis is also important with regard to the clinician's ability to receive payment for mental health services by insurance companies. It is a sad reality that many insurance companies require a diagnosis before paying for treatment. Moreover, some insurance companies pay for services for some disorders whereas other companies refuse to pay for services for the same disorder.

A final purpose of diagnosis is that it can be used to enhance research about causes and treatments of psychiatric disorders. Indeed, if researchers can group similar people together accurately, researchers can study environmental and biological similarities among such persons to discover potential causes of the disorder. Researchers can also compare the efficacy of various treatment modalities for different disorders. Basically, the *DSM–IV* can be used as a diagnostic tool as well as a guide for treatment, especially when research has demonstrated the validity of a particular treatment empirically.

Criticisms and Limitations of Diagnosis

Although the *DSM–IV* system arguably is the most sophisticated and comprehensive diagnostic manual ever created, diagnosis and classification remain far from perfect. Criticisms of diagnosis are discussed next.

Problems with Reliability and Validity of Diagnosis. *Reliability* refers to consistency, stability, and dependability of measurement. Reliability of psychiatric diagnosis is a fundamental prerequisite for a valid or meaningful psychiatric classification scheme. The most relevant type of reliability regarding psychiatric diagnosis is *interrater reliability*, which refers to extent of agreement between two or more clinicians who examine the same client. Imagine the not-so-uncommon dilemma in clinical practice when different clinicians arrive at a different diagnosis for the same client. That unfortunate individual likely would not feel confident in either clinician or their recommended treatment plans.

Until only recently, reliability of diagnosis in clinical practice and research was typically poor, even for popular mental disorders such as major depression and schizophrenia. In many cases, poorly defined diagnostic criteria negatively affected reliability. Another contributing factor was the lack of standardization of questions that were asked of clients to evaluate symptoms and ultimately to arrive at a psychiatric diagnosis. Notably, these problems have been addressed and ameliorated since the 1980s. Recent versions of the *DSM* have introduced and refined the use of operationalized, specified, empirically derived, and standardized criteria for mental disorders. The problem of unstandardized questioning was addressed by the development of structured interviews that provide standardized questions as well as guidelines for categorizing or coding responses. These developments have revolutionized the diagnostic process and improved reliability to the extent that reliability for most major diagnoses is presently good.

Validity refers to the extent to which a diagnosis is meaningful (i.e., the extent to which it tells us something important about the typical symptom presentation, etiology, pathogenesis, course, and response to treatment for a particular diagnosis). Validity is strongly related to reliability: acceptable levels of reliability must be confirmed before conclusions about validity can be drawn. Without adequate reliability, the issue of validity becomes moot; by definition, the diagnosis is worthless if it cannot be measured accurately. Strong reliability, however, does not guarantee validity, as it is possible for clinicians to have perfect agreement but be incorrect about all cases. Compared with reliability, validity is more difficult to gauge and document accurately, and thus represents a formidable challenge for our field. Indeed, concerns about the validity of diagnosis is considered presently to be among the most serious issues facing the mental health community. Consequently, research on validity of diagnosis is a top priority. The interested reader is referred to Segal (1997) for a more complete discussion of the issues surrounding reliability and validity.

The Categorical Model. The *DSM–IV* acknowledges that diagnosis is based on a categorical model, which assumes a "Yes/No" or "Sick/Well" approach in which individuals either have the disorder (i.e., they meet criteria, they are diagnosable) or they do not (despite possibly having several symptoms but not enough to meet formal criteria). In contrast, the dimensional approach classifies clinical presentations based on quantitative descriptions of various domains of functioning, such as the degree of mania or body image distortion. In this approach, disordered behaviors fall on the same continuum with normal behaviors and are not something entirely different as the categorical approach would suggest. The dimensional approach also allows for a description of clinical presentations that do not have clear boundaries.

In a thoughtful critique of the categorical model, Widiger (1997) notes that justification for this model comes from several sources: medicine uses a categorical model, categorical diagnosis is simple to understand, and clinical decisions are often categorical (e.g., the need to hospitalize a suicidal person). However, there are many problems with the categorical model. For instance, mental disorders result from a complex interaction of biological, psychological, and social factors, and thus do not lend themselves to the simplicity of categories. A distinct boundary between each category is difficult to determine, and applying such definite categories to mental disorders implies a uniformity that does not exist (Widiger, 1997). In addition, individuals diagnosed with the same disorder do not necessarily share the same features because criteria are polythetic and various combinations of symptoms meet the diagnosis. Thus, variability within each disorder continues to be a problem that plagues the categorical approach to diagnosis. Another problem with the categorical model is the substantial comorbidity of mental disorders, which raises the question of whether a single disorder is actually present instead of the co-occurrence of several distinct disorders (Widiger, 1997). For example, among those with personality disorders, comorbidity with additional personality disorders and clinical disorders (such as depression) is the rule rather than the exception.

Another inadequacy of the categorical model is the clinical reality that some clients do not fit neatly into any of the categories, suggesting poor clinical utility of some diagnoses. The cutoff between meeting and falling below the criteria for a mental disorder is not always obvious. Consequently, a high prevalence of boundary clients (individuals who do not meet the full criteria for a disorder) is seen in practice. Therefore, "boundary categories" are created to diagnose these clients (Widiger, 1997). An example of a boundary category is substance abuse, which requires fewer and less severe symptoms to reach a diagnosis than does substance dependence (APA, 1994). Another example is *cyclothymia*, which is a fluctuating mood disturbance with episodes of hypomania and depression that are not of the severity or frequency to meet the full criteria for a manic or depressive episode, respectively. Clinicians may fail to diagnose many individuals because of the rigid requirements established by a categorical diagnostic manual. For example, a diagnosis of a major depressive episode requires that a client have five of nine symptoms. A client who is unable to concentrate, feels worthless, has lost interest in pleasure, and expresses suicidal thoughts but reports no other symptoms would not meet the necessary criteria for a major depressive episode. A dimensional system, which would place individuals on a continuum, would communicate more clinical information because it would report attributes that are subthreshold in a categorical system.

Whereas the *DSM–IV* provides a classification system, it states that, "although this manual provides a classification of mental disorders, it must be admitted that no definition adequately specifies precise boundaries for the concept of 'mental disorder.' The concept of mental disorder, like many other concepts in medicine and science, lacks a consistent operational definition that covers all situations" (APA, 1994, p. xxi).

Accordingly, one must not assume homogeneity even among individuals with the same diagnosis, as these diagnostic categories minimize the uniqueness of the person. In the future, it is possible that a combination of categorical and dimensional models may coexist that would draw on the benefits of both approaches. (For a complete discussion of this issue, see Widiger, 1997.) One empirical question to be addressed is whether some disorders truly are exclusively categorical; that is, do some types of psychiatric illnesses represent something completely and qualitatively different from normal functioning? The opposite question is whether all forms of mental illness are extreme variants of normal behaviors. In any case, serious research should address this important issue in diagnosis.

Limited Role of Etiology in Diagnosis.   Another shortcoming of the *DSM–IV* is that it is a classification system based primarily on descriptive syndromes and largely ignores etiological factors. Inclusion of a disorder in a classification does not require that there be knowledge about its etiology. An individual may meet the criteria for a *DSM–IV* diagnosis; however, it does not provide any information regarding the cause of the disorder, nor the degree of control that a person may have over the associated behaviors.

Negative Effects of Labeling. Another controversy involves the labeling of people with a psychiatric diagnosis. Labeling clients with a diagnosis can cause harm by stereotyping and stigmatizing them. The label may also act as a self-fulfilling prophecy, in which the client assumes that he or she is doomed. For example, a client may be given the diagnosis of schizophrenia, which is typically regarded as a chronic, lifelong disorder that generally requires medications that can cause negative side effects. The diagnostic label of schizophrenia may overwhelm a client who may believe that there is little chance for significant recovery. Because the emphasis of the *DSM–IV* is on pathology, deficits, limitations, and symptoms, it is possible that some individuals are not encouraged to use their own strengths, abilities, and natural capacity for self-healing.

Limited Cultural Relevance of the DSM–IV. A lofty goal of the *DSM–IV* was that it would be relevant in a wide variety of contexts and to individuals with diverse cultural and ethnic backgrounds. Clearly, many efforts were made in this regard during preparation of the *DSM–IV* and it is an improvement over earlier editions (as discussed earlier). Despite some advances, several criticisms of the *DSM–IV* in this area are legitimate. The *DSM–IV* still appears to have a false assumption that its primary syndromes represent universal disorders. The underlying thesis of the universality of disorders is based on Western conceptions of disease that are inherently problematic and have limited cross-cultural relevance (Thakker & Ward, 1998). As a case in point, it is clear that some mental disorders are rarely found outside the West (e.g., anorexia nervosa, dissociative identity disorder). Evidence also suggests that some disorders, particularly schizophrenia and depression, do have significant cross-cultural variations, contrary to earlier views. In diagnosing individuals from cultures outside the mainstream United States, the accuracy of assessment may, in fact, decrease because the cultural background of a person could affect the content and form of the symptom presentation. For example, Native Americans might discuss having visions during religious ceremonies. Taken out of context, the person might be considered to be experiencing psychotic symptoms. It is likely that in some clinical situations, the cultural context of the presenting symptoms are not considered, and certain behaviors may be labeled deviant simply because they are not characteristic of the dominant culture (Corey, Corey, & Callanan, 1998).

Even when a clinician exercises careful clinical judgment in diagnosing a minority, the *DSM–IV* may not offer enough valid information to diagnose the individual accurately. Clinicians must be careful when diagnosing across cultures to not misunderstand or misdiagnose symptoms that may be accounted for by cultural differences. Thus, it would be prudent for clinicians to receive formal training in multicultural issues. Further research on the impact of culture on abnormal behavior is also warranted so that refinements can be made in future editions of the *DSM*.

DIFFERENTIAL DIAGNOSIS

What exactly is differential diagnosis? According to the *DSM–IV*, *differential diagnosis* is defined as the process of differentiating one disorder from other disorders that have some similar presenting characteristics. It often takes a bit of detective work and careful interviewing. The process is dependent on several levels of observation, each of which reinforces the others to build a comprehensive framework.

When presented with one or several symptoms, it is the clinician's job to choose the condition that best accounts for an individual's symptoms from a vast array of *DSM–IV* conditions. Consequently, clinicians must have a good understanding of the primary psychiatric disorders. This understanding includes such factors as typical age of onset, gender ratio, typical course of the disorder, family involvement, and the likelihood of treatment response. For example, major depressive disorder is more frequent in women, has an average onset during the mid-20s, typically runs a recurrent course, has a higher incidence in other members of the family, has few residual symptoms between episodes, and has a good response to psychotherapy and antidepressants. Therefore, if a client presents for the first time in his or her 70s, has no history of emotional problems, has no other family members with a history of affective disturbances, and the symptoms are reported with other unusual complaints, then causes other than depression must be considered. Differential diagnosis is one of the most important jobs faced by the clinician, as the narrowing down of possible contenders leads to an initial diagnosis that then determines the appropriate treatment plan.

In this section, we discuss the role of *DSM–IV* in differential diagnosis and present other strategies to assist in this process. First, however, we discuss the important issue of differentiating normal from abnormal behavior.

Differentiating Normal from Abnormal Behavior

How does a clinician differentiate between normal and abnormal functioning? The *DSM–IV* offers some advice: "each of the mental disorders is conceptualized as a clinically significant behavioral or psychological syndrome or pattern that occurs in an individual and is associated with present distress or disability or with a significantly increased risk of suffering death, pain, disability, or an important loss of freedom" (APA, 1994, p. xxi).

Two major symptoms, namely impairment and dyscontrol, can be used to distinguish normal from abnormal behavior. Regarding impairment, most disorders require that the presenting symptoms "cause clinically significant . . . impairment in social, occupational, or other important areas of functioning" (APA, 1994, p. 7). If a client does not experience impairment in one or more of these areas, he or she generally does not have a mental disorder as defined by the *DSM–IV*. The *DSM–IV* acknowledges, however, that it can be difficult to distinguish normal from abnormal behavior, and clinicians must exercise discretion when evaluating impairment. If it is unclear whether a client possesses the criteria for impairment, family members and significant others can be questioned to differentiate between small daily living problems and significant impairment. Also, clients from different cultures may express impairment in different ways than the majority culture. The *DSM–IV* does offer clinical guidance for most disorders and acknowledges some cultural considerations that may influence the course of the disorders.

One important indicator of significant impairment is the need for clinical intervention. Thus, if a client enters therapy for a specific problem, it is likely that the individual is clinically impaired. Clients also may not reach the threshold for a disorder but may indeed be clinically impaired. For example, a client may be significantly impaired but may not meet a specified time frame requirement for a particular disorder. As such, clinicians may diagnose the client as having one of the nine major categories not otherwise specified (NOS) (e.g., mood disorder NOS, anxiety disorder NOS).

Another major symptom that can differentiate normal from abnormal behavior is lack of control (*dyscontrol*), which can be defined as thoughts or actions that are not under the control of the individual (Widiger, 1997). Again, clinical discretion must be used when differentiating normal from abnormal levels of dyscontrol because individuals vary in the amount of control over their thoughts and behaviors. Consider the case of a client who lacks control in a specific area but demonstrates adequate control in other domains of life. Does this person have a mental disorder? The answer is "yes" if the lack of control in one life area or context affects other areas of control or functioning. For example, an alcoholic may be unable to control his or her drinking behavior, and thus be unable to fulfill obligations to career and family.

The Role of *DSM–IV* in Differential Diagnosis

The *DSM–IV* provides a great deal of help to clinicians regarding the difficult process of differential diagnosis because it is critical to consider all possible alternative disorders. When placed in the position of diagnosing individuals, it is imperative that a clinician have a considerable working knowledge of the *DSM–IV*. Clinicians must be aware that the multiaxial classification considers not only clinical and personality disorders, but also includes medical conditions, environmental influences, and an assessment of the individual's overall functioning. Equally important is the knowledge concerning the diagnostic criteria of specific disorders under each general class of illness. Many disorders possess similar symptoms, but differ only on the severity and duration of their symptoms. For example, schizophreniform disorder is characterized by the same presenting symptoms as schizophrenia, but differs only on the duration of the presenting symptoms.

Appendix A of the *DSM–IV* (pp. 689–701) provides decision trees for six classes of disorders. These trees include Mental Disorder Due to a General Medical Condition, Substance-Induced Disorders, Psychotic Disorders, Mood Disorders, Anxiety Disorders, and Somatoform Disorders. The trees are meant to aid the clinician in understanding the organization and hierarchical structure of the *DSM–IV*. In order to use the decision trees, a clinician must first decide on the appropriate class of disorder that best fits the nature of the client's presenting problem. For example, if a client presents with euphoria and rapid speech, the clinician would select the Mood Disorder Decision Tree. Similarly, if the client presents with bizarre mannerisms and delusions, the Psychotic Decision Tree should be consulted.

Each tree begins with a set of clinical symptoms. From there, the clinician answers a series of yes/no questions that follow the diagnostic criteria of the *DSM–IV* to rule out possible alternatives. For example, the Mood Disorder Decision Tree begins by ruling out general medical conditions and mood problems caused directly by substance intoxication or withdrawal. Next, the tree guides the clinician in determining the type of past and present mood episodes in an attempt to better identify the most appropriate diagnosis for the presenting symptoms.

In addition to decision trees, clinicians should be aware that the *DSM–IV* provides a section on differential diagnosis for each specific disorder. Included in these sections are a list and description of the most closely related disorders that may be possible alternatives for an individual's presenting symptoms. Possible alternative disorders are not only described, but an explanation regarding how these disorders differ from the one being considered is also given. This ensures that the clinician has made the most accurate and appropriate diagnosis. As mentioned, oftentimes the difference between two disorders depends solely on duration and severity of symptoms.

Another important differential diagnosis issue concerns differentiating a psychological cause from a Mental Disorder Due to a General Medical Condition (GMC) and a Substance-Induced Mental Disorder. A mental disorder that is due to a GMC is characterized by the presence of psychiatric symptoms that are judged to be the direct physiological effect of a medical condition. For example, a client with depressive symptoms could have a thyroid condition that actually causes symptoms of depression. Conversely, a Substance-Induced Mental Disorder is characterized by psychiatric symptoms that are judged to be caused directly by the ingestion or exposure to a psychoactive substance. In fact, ruling out an organic etiology is a vital first step in the differential diagnosis process.

It is not always easy to understand the role that medical conditions may play in a client's psychological problems. Psychiatric disorders can be influenced by medical conditions and vice versa. The clinician should record on Axis III any organic disorders that are related to or exacerbated by the psychiatric condition. Be aware that numerous medical disorders (e.g., multiple sclerosis, hyperthyroidism, hypothyroidism, stroke, hypoglycemia, congestive heart failure, hepatitis, brain tumors) may be "disguised" as psychological disorders. If a mental health clinician suspects a client has a medical condition, it would be prudent to refer the client for a medical work-up. It is important to keep these guidelines in mind whenever you are placed in the position of diagnosing someone, as the guidelines help ensure that the individual's symptoms could not be better accounted for by a different disorder with a potentially different treatment.

Other Guidelines for Differential Diagnosis

An important and thoughtful rationale for psychiatric differential diagnosis is provided in the *DSM–IV Handbook of Differential Diagnosis* (First, Frances, & Pincus, 1995). In this book, the authors attempt to simplify the complex task of differential diagnosis, and they provide three different methods to accomplish the task: Differential Diagnosis by Steps, Differential Diagnosis by Decision Trees, and Differential Diagnosis by Tables. The Differential Diagnosis by Steps guide addresses the differential diagnostic concerns that must by considered in every client. The Differential Diagnosis by Decision Trees guide outlines the process involved in choosing from among potential *DSM–IV* diagnoses. Finally, the Differential Diagnosis by Tables guide is useful after a preliminary diagnosis has been made to ensure that adequate consideration of all relevant alternatives has been completed.

Differential Diagnosis by Steps. This strategy breaks down the process of differential diagnosis into six steps (First et al., 1995). First and foremost is the task of deciding if the presenting symptoms are truly valid and not an attempt to deceive the clinician. Thus, Step 1 involves ruling out Malingering and Factitious Disorder. Step 2 calls for the clinician to rule out whether the presenting symptoms are directly caused by substance intoxication or withdrawal. For example, the effects of hallucinogenic drugs can mimic the symptoms of schizophrenia. Withdrawal from highly addicting substances (e.g., heroin, alcohol) can produce highly anxious, agitated, and confused mental states. According to First et al. (1995), overlooking a substance etiology is the single most common diagnostic error made in clinical practice, and thus clinicians should be thorough in their assessment here. After determining that the individual has been using a substance, it is crucial to establish a causal relationship between the substance and the presenting symptoms. The substance may be a direct cause of the symptoms, a consequence of having a mental disorder, or independent of the symptoms. If it is decided that the client's symptoms are due to the direct effects of a substance, a *DSM–IV* Substance-Induced Disorder must be diagnosed.

If a substance-induced etiology has been ruled out, Step 3 is designed to rule out a General Medical Condition (GMC). Almost any presentation of psychiatric symptoms can be caused by the direct physiological effects of a GMC. As such, this is an important and difficult distinction in diagnosis (First et al., 1995). For example, tumors have been known to cause any number of psychiatric symptoms, hypothyroidism can mimic the symptoms of depression, and head injuries can cause symptoms similar to substance withdrawal. Not only can psychiatric symptoms appear identical to many GMCs, but their relationships are often complexly interwoven. If a GMC is present, an etiological relationship must then be established and a *DSM–IV* diagnosis of Mental Disorder Due to a General Medical Condition must be given.

If a GMC has been ruled out as an etiology, Step 4 involves determining which primary *DSM–IV* diagnosis best accounts for the presenting symptoms. To facilitate differential diagnosis, the *DSM–IV* is divided into classes of disorders based on common presenting symptoms. The decision trees discussed in the next section are helpful in providing decision points among the primary classes of mental disorders.

Step 5 in the guide to differential diagnosis is distinguishing an adjustment disorder from the not otherwise specified (NOS) category. An *adjustment disorder* is defined as the development of clinically significant emotional or behavioral symptoms that are in response to a psychosocial stressor. There are many specific types of adjustment disorder. Each type is based on the predominant symptoms, such as adjustment disorder with depressed mood; with anxiety; with disturbance of conduct; and with mixed disturbance of emotions and conduct. The NOS denotation is used when a client has an atypical or unusual presentation and does not fit neatly into a specific diagnosis. In fact, unusual or atypical presentations are common in clinical practice. The sixth and final step involves establishing whether the presenting symptoms fall within the realm of a disorder or can be considered normal. Consideration of cultural context, clinician and client bias, and an assessment of functional impairment is required during this step.

Differential Diagnosis by Decision Trees. Decision trees are another guide to differential diagnosis that provide an overview of the diagnostic system. The first step in using a decision tree is to decide which tree(s) apply to the individual's presenting symptoms. In the *DSM–IV Handbook of Differential Diagnosis*, the decision trees are divided into two sections. The first section includes 24 trees based on presenting symptoms (e.g., delusions, memory impairment, impulsivity), whereas the second includes three etiology-based trees (i.e., GMC, substance induced, and stress induced).

Accompanying the 24 symptom-based decision trees are a brief overview of the possible causes of the presenting symptom, the types of behavior that characterize the particular symptom, and the likely disorders for which the symptom may be appropriate. In using these trees, the clinician must answer a series of yes/no questions that follow the stepwise guide to making a differential diagnosis discussed in the previous section.

Similarly, the three etiology-based trees are supplemented with a section that includes guidance on how to best determine the source of the presenting symptoms as well as information regarding different etiologies and the possible interaction of multiple etiologies. In using these trees, clinicians again answer a series of yes/no questions that facilitate the narrowing down of possible causes of the presenting symptoms.

Differential Diagnosis by Tables. The use of differential diagnosis tables helps to ensure that the process of diagnosing mental disorders is systematic and comprehensive (First et al., 1995). There are 62 tables provided in this handbook that include the most common and important *DSM–IV* disorders.

The left column of each table consists of the disorders that must be ruled out as part of the differential diagnosis for a particular disorder. The distinguishing symptoms that may be helpful in ruling out possible alternative disorders are listed in the right column. For example, differential diagnosis for Mental Retardation involves ruling out Learning Disorders, Communication Disorders, Pervasive Developmental Disorders, Dementia, and Borderline Intellectual Functioning. For the five disorders just mentioned, the features that differentiate them from Mental Retardation are also provided.

Differential Diagnosis and Dual Diagnosis

Many clients seen in practice meet criteria for more than one psychiatric disorder. *Dual diagnosis* generally refers to the comorbidity of a substance use disorder and a psychiatric disorder (First & Gladis, 1993). It is essential to evaluate dual diagnosis because of high prevalence rates and important treatment implications. If a client is diagnosed with an Axis I condition and also has a substance abuse problem that is ignored, the client may not progress because one half of the "problem" remains unaddressed. In order to assess for a possible dual diagnosis, a clinician should evaluate substance abuse routinely. Ask about substance use directly and be aware that some clients may minimize the symptoms of substance abuse and focus on other symptoms that are easier for the client to acknowledge. Besides questioning the client, clinicians can have a urine sample screened, ask family and friends about the client's pattern of substance use, examine the case notes to look for symptom patterns that may be indicative of a substance problem, and evaluate the client's substance use throughout treatment. As the therapeutic relationship develops, the client may more readily admit to problems with substances than during the initial intake evaluation.

If a clinician discovers that a client has a dual diagnosis, the etiologic relationship between the two disorders must be established (First & Gladis, 1993). There are three possible outcomes regarding dual diagnosis: (a) there is a primary psychiatric disorder and a secondary substance abuse disorder, (b) there is a primary substance abuse disorder and a secondary psychiatric disorder, and (c) both the substance abuse disorder and the psychiatric disorder are primary.

The psychiatric disorder is considered primary when the psychiatric disorder is present when substances are not abused. If the psychiatric disorder is primary and the substance abuse disorder is secondary, the clinician should evaluate the possibility that the client is using substances to self-medicate. For example, an individual with depression may use stimulants (such as cocaine) to lift their negative emotions. In contrast, a substance abuse disorder may be primary when psychiatric symptoms occur as a result of acute intoxication or withdraw. If the substance abuse disorder is primary, the clinician must determine if the psychiatric symptoms occur within days or several weeks from withdrawal or while the client is intoxicated. Usually psychiatric symptoms become worse with repeated substance abuse. In the case that the substance abuse disorder and the psychiatric condition are both primary, the disorders are considered independent of one another, but each may influence the other.

THE STRUCTURED CLINICAL INTERVIEW FOR *DSM–IV*

The ability to accurately diagnose psychiatric disorders has improved remarkably since the 1980s. During this time, numerous structured diagnostic interviews were developed for clinical, research, and training applications, and these instruments have strongly contributed to the advancement in diagnostic clarity and precision. Structured interviews have been devised to assist in diagnosis of all major Axis I (clinical) and all standard Axis II (personality) disorders. The Structured Clinical Interview for *DSM–IV* Axis I Disorders (SCID–I) is among the most prominent and popular of these instruments.

Overview and History of the SCID–I

The SCID is a flexible, interviewer-administered, semistructured diagnostic interview designed for use by trained clinicians to diagnose most adult Axis I *DSM–IV* mental disorders. The current version is the product of many prior editions that were updated and modified over time. With each revision, the SCID has been reworked to enhance accuracy and ease of use. It is used primarily with adult respondents due to the language, format, coverage, and type of responses needed for administration. Note, however, that it may be modified appropriately for older adolescents. Since its inception, the SCID has enjoyed widespread popularity as an instrument to obtain reliable and valid psychiatric diagnoses for clinical, research, and training purposes.

The original SCID was designed for application in both research and clinical settings. Recently, the SCID has been split into two versions: the Research Version and the Clinician Version. The Research Version covers more disorders, subtypes, and course specifiers than the Clinician Version and therefore takes longer to complete. The benefit, however, is that it provides for a wealth of diagnostic data that is of particular value to clinical researchers. Researchers interested in obtaining a copy of the Research Version should contact Biometrics Research at 212-543-5524 or visit the SCID website at www.scid4.org. The Clinician Version of the SCID (SCID–CV; First, Spitzer, Gibbon, & Williams, 1997a) is designed for use in clinical settings. It has been trimmed down to encompass only those *DSM–IV* disorders that are most typically seen in clinical practice and can further be abbreviated on a module-by-module basis.

Description, Features, and Conventions of the SCID–CV

The SCID–CV contains six self-contained modules of major diagnostic categories (Mood Episodes, Psychotic Symptoms, Psychotic Disorders, Mood Disorders, Substance Use Disorders, and Anxiety and Other Disorders). Specific *DSM–IV* diagnoses covered by the SCID–CV are shown in Table 2.1. The modular design of the SCID–CV is a major innovation because administration can easily be customized to meet the unique needs of the user. For example, the SCID can be shortened or lengthened to include only those categories of interest, and the order of modules can be altered.

The format and sequence of the SCID was designed to approximate the flowchart and decision trees followed by experienced diagnostic interviewers. The SCID begins with an open-ended overview portion during which the development and history of the present psychological disturbance are elicited and tentative diagnostic hypotheses are generated. Then the SCID systematically presents modules that allow for assessment of specific disorders and symptoms. Most disorders are evaluated for two time periods: current (meets criteria for previous month) and lifetime (ever met criteria).

Consistent with its ties to *DSM–IV*, formal diagnostic criteria are included in the SCID booklet, thus permitting interviewers to see the exact criteria to which the SCID questions pertain. This unique feature makes the SCID an excellent training device for clinicians because it facilitates the learning of diagnostic criteria and appropriate probes. The SCID has many open-ended prompts that encourage respondents to elaborate freely about their symptoms. At times, open-ended prompts are followed by closed-ended questions to fully clarify a particular symptom. Although the SCID provides structure to cover criteria for each disorder, its flexible semistructured format provides significant latitude

TABLE 2.1

Diagnoses Covered by the Structured Clinical Interview for *DSM–IV* Axis I
Disorders—Clinician Version

Mood Disorders
    Bipolar I Disorder
    Bipolar II Disorder
    Cyclothymic Disorder
    Bipolar Disorder NOS
    Major Depressive Disorder
    Dysthymic Disorder
    Depressive Disorder NOS
    Mood Disorder Due to a GMC
    Alcohol-Induced Mood Disorder
    Other Substance-Induced Mood Disorder
Schizophrenia and Other Psychotic Disorders
    Schizophrenia
    Schizophreniform Disorder
    Schizoaffective Disorder
    Delusional Disorder
    Brief Psychotic Disorder
    Psychotic Disorder Due to a GMC with Delusions
    Psychotic Disorder Due to a GMC with Hallucinations
    Alcohol-Induced Psychotic Disorder with Delusions
    Alcohol-Induced Psychotic Disorder with Hallucinations
    Other Substance-Induced Psychotic Disorder with Delusions
    Other Substance-Induced Psychotic Disorder with Hallucinations
    Psychotic Disorder NOS
Substance Use Disorders[a]
    Alcohol
    Amphetamine
    Cannabis
    Cocaine
    Hallucinogen
    Inhalant
    Opioid
    Phencyclidine
    Sedative, Hypnotic, or Anxiolytic
    Other (or Unknown) Substance
Anxiety Disorders
    Panic Disorder with Agoraphobia
    Panic Disorder without Agoraphobia
    Obsessive–Compulsive Disorder
    Posttraumatic Stress Disorder
    Anxiety Disorder NOS
    Anxiety Disorder Due to a GMC
    Alcohol-Induced Anxiety Disorder

(*Table continues on next page*)

TABLE 2.1 (*Continued*)

Other Substance-Induced Anxiety Disorder
Agoraphobia without History of Panic Disorder
Social Phobia
Specific Phobia
Generalized Anxiety Disorder
Somatoform Disorders
  Somatization Disorder
  Undifferentiated Somatoform Disorder
  Hypochondriasis
  Body Dysmorphic Disorder
Eating Disorders
  Anorexia Nervosa
  Bulimia Nervosa
Adjustment Disorder
  Adjustment Disorder with Depressed Mood
  Adjustment Disorder with Anxiety
  Adjustment Disorder with Mixed Anxiety and Depressed Mood
  Adjustment Disorder with Disturbance of Conduct
  Adjustment Disorder with Mixed Disturbance of Emotions and Conduct
  Unspecified Adjustment Disorder

Note. NOS = Not Otherwise Specified; GMC = General Medical Condition.
[a] *Note.* "abuse" or "dependence" can be diagnosed for each drug class.

for interviewers to restate questions, ask for further clarification, probe, and challenge if the initial prompt was misunderstood by the interviewee or clarification is needed to fully rate a symptom. SCID interviewers are encouraged to use all sources of information about a respondent, and gentle challenging of the respondent is encouraged if discrepant information is suspected.

Each symptom criterion is rated as "?," "−," or "+." The minus (−) indicates that the criterion was below threshold or false, whereas the plus sign (+) means that the symptom criterion was clearly present and clinically significant. The question mark (?) denotes that inadequate information was obtained to code the criterion. The SCID flowchart instructs interviewers to "skip-out" of a particular diagnostic section when essential symptoms are judged to be below threshold or false. These skip-outs result in decreased time of administration, as well as the passing over of items with no diagnostic significance. Administration of the SCID is typically completed in one session and involves between 45 and 90 minutes, although application with a respondent manifesting extensive current and past psychopathology can add considerable length. Once administration is completed, all current and past disorders for which criteria are met are listed on a Diagnostic Summary sheet.

The SCID is optimally administered by trained clinicians who have knowledge about psychopathology, *DSM–IV* criteria, and diagnostic interviewing.

Indeed, with its semistructured format, proper administration often requires that interviewers restate or clarify questions in ways that are sometimes not clearly outlined in the manual in order to judge accurately if a particular symptom criterion has been met. The task requires that SCID assessors have a working knowledge of psychopathology and *DSM–IV* as well as basic interviewing skills. Standard procedures for training to use the SCID include carefully reading the SCID *User's Guide* (First, Spitzer, Gibbon, & Williams, 1997b), reviewing the SCID administration booklet and score sheet, viewing SCID videotape training materials that are available from the SCID authors, and conducting many role-playing practice administrations with extensive feedback discussions. Next, trainees may administer the SCID to representative participants who are jointly rated so that a discussion about sources of disagreements can ensue. In research settings, a formal test–retest reliability study may also be done.

The Structured Clinical Interview for *DSM–IV* Axis II (SCID–II)

To complement the Axis I version of the SCID, a version focusing on Axis II personality disorders according to *DSM–IV* has been developed and is called the *Structured Clinical Interview for DSM–IV Axis II Personality Disorders* (SCID–II; First, Gibbon, Spitzer, Williams, & Benjamin, 1997). The SCID–II has a similar semistructured format as the Axis I version, but it covers the 10 standard *DSM–IV* personality disorders as well as personality disorder NOS, depressive personality disorder, and passive–aggressive personality disorder from *DSM–IV* Appendix B.

The SCID–II is usually used in conjunction with the SCID–I, which typically is administered prior to personality assessment. This is encouraged so that the respondent's present mental state can be considered when judging accuracy of self-reported personality traits. The basic structure and conventions of the SCID–II closely resemble those of the SCID–I. One unique feature of the SCID–II is that it includes a Personality Questionnaire, which is a brief, self-reporting, forced-choice yes/no screening component that can be administered prior to the interview portion. The purpose of the questionnaire is to reduce overall administration time because only those items that are scored in the pathological direction are further evaluated in the structured interview portion.

During the structured interview component, the pathologically endorsed screening responses are further pursued to ascertain whether the symptom criteria is actually at clinically significant levels. Here, the respondent is asked to elaborate about each suspected personality disorder criteria and specified prompts are provided. Like the Axis I SCID, the *DSM–IV* diagnostic criteria are printed on the interview page for easy review and responses are coded similarly (? = inadequate information, 1 = absent or false, 2 = subthreshold, and 3 = threshold or true). Each personality disorder is assessed completely, and diagnoses are made before proceeding to the next disorder. The modular format permits researchers and clinicians to tailor the SCID–II to their specific needs and reduce administration time. Clinicians who administer the SCID–II are expected to use their clinical judgment to clarify responses, gently challenge inconsistencies, and ask for additional information as required to rate each criterion and disorder accurately. Collection of diagnostic information from ancillary sources is permitted. Complete administration of the SCID–II typically takes less than 1 hour. Training requirements and interviewer qualifications are similar to that of the SCID–I.

The psychometric properties of the SCID–I and SCID–II have been evaluated in numerous investigations with encouraging results. The interested reader is referred to Segal (1997) for a full discussion of reliability and validity data for the SCID–I and SCID–II. Continued studies are needed to carefully evaluate and document the psychometric properties of the SCID, especially as new versions are published. Overall, the SCID instruments have proved to be popular and useful diagnostic assessment tools. They are available in several foreign languages and have been applied successfully in cross-cultural investigations. The SCID can be expected to enjoy widespread application in psychiatric research, service, and training for many years to come. Its continued evolution will likely make it a popular and effective instrument for psychiatric diagnosis in the 21st century.

SUMMARY

In this chapter we discuss the central issues regarding diagnosis and differential diagnosis, including a description of the *DSM–IV* system, a critical examination of the benefits and limitations of diagnosis, and an analysis of several models of differential diagnosis to guide mental health professionals. We then describe and review a popular structured interview that aids in the diagnostic process. Throughout, we emphasize the critical importance of accurate psychiatric diagnosis. We hope that the information in this chapter guides you in your "detective" work as a clinician, helps you unravel the diagnostic mysteries with which so many clients present, and assists you in your therapeutic work.

REFERENCES

American Psychiatric Association. (1994). *Diagnostic and statistical manual of mental disorders* (4th ed.). Washington, DC: Author.

Coolidge, F. L. & Segal, D. L. (1998). Evolution of the personality disorder diagnosis in the *Diagnostic and Statistical Manual of Mental Disorders. Clinical Psychology Review, 18*, 585–599.

Corey, G., Corey, M., & Callanan, P. (1998). *Issues and ethics in the helping professions*. Albany: Brooks/Cole Publishing Company.

DeRubeis, R. J., & Crits-Cristoph, P. (1998). Empirically supported individual and group psychological treatments for adult mental disorders. *Journal of Consulting and Clinical Psychology, 66,* 37–52.

First, M. B., Francis, A., & Pincus, H. A. (1995). *The DSM–IV handbook of differential diagnosis.* Washington, DC: American Psychiatric Press.

First, M. B., Gibbon, M., Spitzer, R. L., Williams, J. B. W., & Benjamin, L. (1997). *Structured Clinical Interview for DSM–IV Axis II Personality Disorders (SCID–II).* Washington, DC: American Psychiatric Press.

First, M. B., & Gladis, M. M. (1993). Diagnosis and differential diagnosis of psychiatric and substance use disorders. In J. Solomon, S. Zimberg, & E. Shollar (Eds.), *Dual diagnosis: Evaluation, treatment, training, and program development* (pp. 23–37). New York: Plenum.

First, M. B., Spitzer, R. L., Gibbon, M., & Williams, J. B. W. (1997a). *Structured Clinical Interview for DSM–IV Axis I Disorders—Clinician Version (SCID–CV).* Washington, DC: American Psychiatric Press.

First, M. B., Spitzer, R. L., Gibbon, M., & Williams, J. B. W. (1997b). *User's guide to the Structured Clinical Interview for DSM–IV Axis I Disorders—Clinician Version (SCID–CV).* Washington, DC: American Psychiatric Press.

Segal, D. L. (1997). Structured interviewing and DSM classification. In S. M. Turner & M. Hersen (Eds.), *Adult psychopathology and diagnosis* (3rd ed., pp. 25–57). New York: Wiley.

Thakker, J., & Ward, T. (1998). Culture and classification: The cross-cultural application of the *DSM–IV. Clinical Psychology Review, 18,* 501–529.

Widiger, T. A. (1997). Mental disorders as discrete clinical conditions: Dimensional versus categorical classification. In S. M. Turner & M. Hersen (Eds.), *Adult psychopathology and diagnosis* (3rd ed., pp. 3–23). New York: Wiley.

3

Outpatient Behavioral Assessment and Treatment Target Selection

Stephen N. Haynes, Karl G. Nelson, Ilisa Thacher,
and Joseph Keaweàimoku Kaholokula
University of Hawai'i at Manoa

Behavioral assessment is an evolving psychological assessment paradigm whose concepts and methods are derived from applied and experimental behavior analysis, learning, and cognitive-behavioral construct systems (Bellack & Hersen, 1998; Haynes & O'Brien, 2000; Mash & Terdal, 1997; Shapiro & Kratochwill, 2000). The behavioral assessment paradigm presumes that judgments about a client, such as identification of the client's most important behavior problems and their causes, are most likely to be valid when the clinician adopts a scholarly, data-based approach to clinical assessment. That is, clinical judgments are most likely to be valid when the clinician uses methods of assessment that have been validated and are relevant for persons similar to the client and when the clinician collects information that might contravene his or her hypotheses about the client (Garb, 1998; Nezu & Nezu, 1989).

Behavioral assessment often involves frequent measures of behavior and environmental events and integrates information from multiple sources, such as parents, spouses, and other health-care professionals. Unlike other assessment paradigms, behavioral assessment focuses on identifying functional relations relevant to behavior problems and the client's goals. It focuses less on diagnosis, descriptions of the client's behavior problems, and the role of personality variables.[1] Behavioral assessment also includes multiple methods, such

---

[1] Two events have a functional relation when they covary. Consequently, a functional relation does not imply a causal relation, but is a relation between two events that can be expressed as an equation (Haynes & O'Brien, 2000). Examples of functional relations include the conditional probability of

as naturalistic and analog observation, self-monitoring, psychophysiological assessment, informant reports, and behavioral interviews and questionnaires.

As with all assessment paradigms, behavioral assessment strategies are guided by assumptions about the causes of a client's behavior problems. The behavioral assessment paradigm assumes that many behavior problems are a result of multiple interacting factors and that the causes of a specific behavior problem can differ across clients. Furthermore, the causal factors that are most important for a client's behavior problems can change across time. Important causal factors often include social settings, a client's learning history, what the client thinks about his or her behavior problems and their causes, and how others respond to the behavior problems. These presumed causal factors often become the targets of assessment and intervention.

Behavioral assessment has been applied in multiple disciplines and settings and for multiple purposes. It is an important methodological and conceptual component of clinical, counseling, and school psychology, applied and experimental behavior analysis, behavioral medicine, rehabilitation, developmental psychology, education, and social work. The behavioral assessment paradigm has been used in inpatient and outpatient psychiatric settings, rehabilitation settings, schools, counseling centers, and hospitals. It has also been used to help children, adults, couples, families, classrooms, communities, and institutions. Information from behavioral assessment can be useful in treatment outcome evaluation, program evaluation, and in screening for treatment and educational placement. It can assist the therapist to identify strengths and weaknesses in family functioning and the applied or experimental researcher to make estimates of functional relations. Of particular relevance for this chapter, the behavioral assessment paradigm guides behavioral clinical case formulation and the selection of targets for treatment (Bellack & Hersen, 1998; Haynes & O'Brien, 2000; Mash & Terdal, 1997; Shapiro & Kratochwill, 2000).

In this chapter, we address a narrow range of applications of behavioral assessment—behavioral clinical case formulation and treatment planning with adults in an outpatient setting. The behavioral clinical case formulation is a synthesis of multiple judgments about a client's behavior problems, goals, and related causal factors. It involves the integration of clinical assessment- and research-based hypotheses about a client's behavior problems for the purpose of designing the most effective treatment program and selecting the targets of treatment.

In the first three sections we review the conceptual foundations, strategies, and methods of behavioral assessment. In the next section, we present an overview of behavioral clinical case formulation and review models of

---

one event (e.g., a critical comment by a spouse) given another event (e.g., a critical comment by the partner), or the correlation between two events (e.g., the correlation between self-reported pain and mood).

behavioral clinical case formulation by Jackie Persons, Art and Christine Nezu, Marsha Linehan, and Junko Tanaka-Matsumi. In the last section, we describe a model of behavioral clinical case formulation that is guided by the functional analysis and functional analytic clinical case models.

We offer several tenets about the conceptual foundations, strategies, and methods of behavioral clinical case formulation and treatment target selection.

1. Many clients have multiple, functionally interrelated behavior problems.

2. The importance of, and functional relations among, the same behavior problems can differ across clients.

3. A client's behavior problem can be a result of multiple causal variables, and the causal relations relevant to a particular behavior problem can differ across clients and settings.

4. Contemporaneous, socioenvironmental causal variables, particularly those with a *reciprocal causal relation* with behavior problems (causal relations in which the behavior affects the environment, which, in turn, affects the behavior in a reverberating fashion), are especially important in behavioral clinical case formulation.

5. A client's behavior problems and the causal relations relevant to those behavior problems are dynamic—they can vary across time.

6. Given the conditional and dynamic nature of causal relations for a client's behavior problems, behavioral assessment emphasizes the measurement of important behaviors and events in multiple settings, using multiple sources and time-series measurement strategies.

7. Several models of clinical case formulation can help the clinician select treatment foci.

8. The *functional analysis* is an approach to behavioral clinical case formulation that emphasizes the identification of functional relations relevant to a client's behavior problems and important, controllable causal variables that affect those behavior problems.

9. The Functional Analytic Clinical Case Model is a vector diagram of a functional analysis, designed to help the clinician make decisions about treatment foci.

INTRODUCTION TO THE CONCEPTS, STRATEGIES, AND METHODS OF BEHAVIORAL ASSESSMENT

The behavioral assessment paradigm includes many assumptions about behavior and its causes, about the best strategies for understanding persons with behavior problems, and about the best strategies for selecting treatment targets and formulating treatment goals. The paradigm also includes multiple methods of measuring behavior and relevant events. These assumptions and methods shape the content and form of the behavioral clinical case formulation.

The following sections present an overview of the concepts and methods of the behavioral assessment paradigm with an emphasis on the assessment of adults in outpatient psychiatric settings. The first two sections discuss the characteristics of behavior problems and causal relations. The subsequent sections discuss the strategies and methods of behavioral assessment. More detailed discussions of these topics can be found in Haynes and O'Brien (2000), Bellack and Hersen (1998), Mash and Terdal (1997), and O'Brien and Haynes (1993).

Assumptions About the Nature of Behavior Problems

Most persons come to the attention of mental health professionals because they have behavior problems that are distressing to themselves or others. Consequently, the description and specification of a client's behavior problems are important components of the behavioral clinical case formulation. This description can be complex—there can be more than one behavior problem, multiple behavior problems can affect each other or be correlated, each behavior problem can have multiple dimensions, and the characteristics of a behavior problem can vary across settings (such as home and work) and time. The specification of a client's behavior problems is important because it affects decisions about which treatment is most likely to be effective for a particular behavior problem.

Clients often have multiple behavior problems. In order to select those problems upon which to focus treatment, a behavioral clinical case formulation should include estimates of the relative importance of each problem. For example, a client may report having diabetes, depressed mood, marital problems, and alcohol abuse. However, the problems may differ in the degree to which they affect the quality of life for the client or harms the client or others. Estimates of the relative importance of behavior problems are central components of the behavioral clinical case formulation because they help the clinician estimate the relative impacts of potential treatments that address different problems: Treatments that affect important behavior problems have a greater impact on the client's quality of life than treatments that have a similar magnitude of effect but on less important behavior problems.

A client's behavior problems can be functionally related in several ways. First, several behavior problems can covary because they are affected by the same causal variable. For example, chronic pain can account for covariance between a client's poor sleep and depressed mood. Second, behavior problems can covary when one serves as the causal variable for the other. For example, marital arguments may affect the likelihood that a client will drink excessively). Finally, behavior problems may have no functional relation because they are not affected by the same causal variable and do not affect each other (Haynes, Kaholokula, & Nelson, 2000).

Behavior problems may also have reciprocal (bidirectional) causal relations. For example, marital conflict can affect a client's mood. When depressed, the client may interact with his or her partner in a more irritating and less supportive manner, thereby increasing marital conflict. Reciprocal causal relations may involve more than two problems, such as when marital conflict and mood have reciprocal relations with substance use and parent–adolescent conflict.

It is often useful to describe the *response modes* (i.e., "motor," "cognitive," and "physiological" modes) and the *dimensions* (e.g., rate, magnitude, duration) of a client's behavior problems in behavioral clinical case formulation because they can be differentially important across clients and they often do not covary strongly across time. For example, social anxiety may be most strongly manifested in avoidance of social situations for one client, whereas for another client it may be manifested in subjective distress and dysfunctional thoughts in social situations. Also, one client may experience frequent but short bouts of depressed mood, whereas another client may experience infrequent but severe episodes of depressed mood. In these examples, the target of treatment would differ across clients with the same behavior problem.

Behavior problems (more specifically, their modes and dimensions) are often conditional. They seldom occur randomly. Rather, behavior problems are more or less likely to occur in some environments or in some states (such as under the influence of alcohol or after sleep loss) than in others. The magnitude and duration of a behavior problem can also vary across environments and states. A client may report a high level of anxious thoughts when around familiar people or places, but experience only mild levels of anxious thoughts when around familiar people and places or under the influence of alcohol.

Specification of modes of, dimensions of, and conditions affecting a behavior problem is also important in behavioral clinical case formulation because they can be associated with different causal relations. What causes onset of episodes of depressed mood may be different from what causes maintenance of depressed mood episodes once the episode has begun. As we discuss later, behavioral interventions often select as targets those causal variables that most strongly act to maintain a behavior problem or affect the acquisition of alternative behaviors.

In addition, all aspects of behavior problems can change over time. This dynamic aspect of behavior problems has implications for the selection of behavioral assessment strategies and methods, which are discussed later in this section.

Causal Variables and Relations for Behavior Problems

In behavioral assessment, specification of the client's behavior problems is an important but insufficient basis on which to select treatment targets and focus and plan treatment. We want to know the causal variables and causal relations that affect a client's behavior problems. Causal variables are particularly important in behavioral case formulation because they are often the immediate targets of treatment—we presume that if we can affect a causal variable, the behavior problems that are affected by the causal variable will also change.

A *causal variable* is any variable (e.g., a particular class of response contingencies, a class of antecedent stimuli) that accounts for variance (i.e., changes in magnitude, duration, frequency) of a behavior problem. A causal relation is the form (e.g., linear, parabolic), strength, and direction (bidirectional or unidirectional) of the functional relation between a causal variable and the variable it affects (Haynes, 1992).[2]

Because of the importance of the clinician's causal model for a client, the behavioral assessment paradigm emphasizes identification of causal variables that are *important* (i.e., that account for a large amount of variance in a behavior problem), *contemporaneous* (rather than historical), and *modifiable* (i.e., are amenable to change). Some causal variables, such as chronic medical problems or traumatic life events, may be important causes of a client's problems but are less amenable to change. We refer to such variables as *original causal variables*.

Behavioral clinical case formulations may include specific cognitive, socio-environmental, setting, and contextual events as causal variables. The behavioral clinical case formulation emphasizes identification of contemporaneous causal variables for a client's behavior problem because these are most likely to directly and immediately affect the behavior problem. For example, peer pressure may have been an initial cause of the onset of alcohol use, but stress reduction and biological factors may more strongly affect its maintenance.

Causal relations can be complex. First, a behavior problem can be affected by multiple causal variables, each of which can influence a behavior problem through multiple causal paths. For example, the amount of alcohol consumed

---

[2]Because of epistemiological complexities associated with the idea of causation, behavioral assessors often emphasize functional rather than causal relationships (see discussion in Haynes & O'Brien, 1990; Haynes, 1992). However, inferences of causation underlie all behavioral interventions. Causal relationships are a subset of functional relationships. Two variables have a causal relationship when (a) they covary (i.e., when they have a functional relationship), (b) the causal variable reliably precedes the effect, (c) there is a logical mechanism for the causal relationship (i.e., a logical connection), and (d) alternative explanations for the observed covariance can be excluded (Haynes, 1992). Causal variables may trigger, moderate, mediate, or maintain a behavior problem. Furthermore, causal variables need not be necessary, sufficient, exclusive, important, or modifiable.

by a client might be affected by the number of life stressors he or she is experiencing, the social setting in which drinking occurs, the client's expectancies about the positive effects of alcohol, and the aversive physiological effects of abstinence.

Some types of causal variables and causal relations are more important and useful than others for selecting treatment targets. *Bidirectional causality* (i.e., *reciprocal determinism*), introduced in the preceding section, is an important form of causal relation. In reciprocal causal relations, a client's behavior problem affects the client's environment, which, in turn, affects the client's behavior. For example, life stressors can increase the chance that a client consumes alcohol, and alcohol consumption can also increase a client's life stressors (e.g., by impairing the client's functioning at work and with family members), which, in turn, can increase alcohol consumption.

Second, moderating and mediating variables often influence the effect of causal variables. Moderating variables influence the strength of a causal relation between two other variables. For example, the degree to which a client's stressful work experience leads to alcohol consumption might be moderated by the client's interactions with his or her spouse after work. Mediating variables "explain" a causal relation. For example, presleep worry might account for the disruptive effects of a stressful work experience on sleep.

Third, the variables affecting a clients' behavior problems can change over time. Causal relations are dynamic—sometimes new causal variables can appear, some variables disappear, and moderator variables can change. Also the form, strength, and direction of causal relations can change across time. As discussed earlier, social factors, such as peer influences, can be important initial causal factors for a clients' alcohol use. However, the relative importance of peer reinforcement can decrease and the importance of biological factors can increase as drinking continues.

Many behavioral treatments focus intervention efforts on introducing or strengthening moderating variables. For example, treatments that focus on strengthening social supports, increasing relaxation skills, and introducing self-statements are intended to affect moderating variables.

Fourth, we noted how the behavior problems of clients usually occur more often (or with greater intensity, or last longer) in some settings than in others (O'Donohue, 1998); we talked about this as the conditional nature of behavior problems. Differences in the occurrence of a behavior problem across settings and contexts can provide us with hints about what might be causing them. For example, differences in how a patient responds with different levels of anxiety to different coworkers or in different social contexts suggests that some aspect of the social interactions may be affecting the behavior problem.

Finally, what affects a behavior problem may not be the contemporaneous level of a causal variable (e.g., the amount of stress, the level of social support), but is perhaps the contrast between current and previous levels of the variables.

That is, causal relations may be a function of change in, rather than absolute level of, a causal variable. For example, alcohol consumption for a client may be associated more strongly with changes in his or her life stressors than with the absolute level of life stressors.

In sum, causal variables and causal relations are important components of a behavioral clinical case formulation because they are often the focus of treatment. Causal variables that have a strong relation to behavior problems, account for the maintenance or frequent onset of behavior problems, and are modifiable are often the most useful treatment targets. It is unsurprising, then, that response contingencies, setting variables and establishing operations, and antecedent stimuli (Martin & Pear, 1996) are often important components of behavioral clinical case formulations.

Strategies of Assessment

We noted that the validity of a behavioral clinical case formulation is affected by underlying assumptions about behavior problems and their causes. We also noted that the strategies used to understand a client's behavior problems affects the information we receive. In this section, we describe the strategies of behavioral assessment and their impact on clinical case formulation. We suggest that the validity of a behavioral clinical case formulation depends on the degree to which assessment strategies (a) provide valid measures of clinically important variables, (b) are sensitive to the dynamic nature of client behavior problems and causal variables, (c) are sensitive to the conditional nature of behavior, (d) provide measures of functional relations for behavior problems, (e) include multiple sources of data, and (f) emphasize observable behaviors relevant to the natural environment. Embedded in these strategies is the emphasis on a scholarly approach to clinical assessment. Behavioral assessment strategies are summarized in Table 3.1 and several are addressed as follows.

A Scholarly Approach to Clinical Assessment. Judgments about a client are most likely to be valid if the clinician takes a scholarly approach to clinical assessment. The purpose of this is to reduce measurement and clinical judgment errors. Clinical judgments based on assessment data are more likely to be valid if assessment strategies include precise and frequent measures of the client's behavior and potential causal variables. The clinician should obtain information about the client in different situations and focus on specific behaviors and thoughts rather than on abstract personality concepts or diagnoses. To achieve these goals, the clinician should use multiple validated assessment instruments and gather data from as many informants and in as many settings as is practical.

TABLE 3.1
Assessment Foci and Strategies of the Behavioral Assessment Paradigm

Focus of Behavioral Assessment Strategies	Definition/Explanation
Less inferential variables	Emphasis on the measurement of lower order, specific constructs versus higher order constructs
Observable behavior	Emphasis on behavior that is observable and therefore measurable versus hypothesized constructs such as intrapsychic events
Behavior in natural settings	Behaviors should be measured in their naturally occurring environment
Extended social systems	Measurement of the social systems (e.g., parents, coworkers) relevant for a client
Functional relations between variables	As opposed to merely descriptions of behavior and events
Strategies of Behavioral Assessment	
Idiographic assessment	Focus is on the client's specific goals and unique behavior problems, often in conjunction with nomothetic assessment instruments
Time-series measurement	Frequent measurement of independent and dependent variables
Hypothesis-testing approach	Ongoing testing of hypotheses to enhance and refine clinical judgments
Multiple sources of information	Use of multiple methods, multiple informants, multiple assessment instruments, and multiple assessment occasions
Use of validated measures	Use of instruments and methods that have been validated for the construct and context of interest

Use of Validated Instruments. Because clinical judgments depend on the information we obtain about a client, it is important that assessment instruments provide valid measures of the phenomena of interest. Invalid measures are likely to lead to invalid behavioral clinical case formulations and subsequent treatment decisions. However, validity of an assessment instrument (i.e., of the measures derived from an instrument) is conditional. Measures from an instrument should have been validated in conditions similar to those of the target assessment occasion (e.g., classroom setting vs. home setting), for samples relevant to the client (e.g., sex, ethnicity), and for the purposes for which the measures are to be used (e.g., treatment planning vs. screening).

Multiple Sources of Information. Clinical judgments based on many sources of information about a client are usually better than judgments based on a few sources. The behavioral assessment paradigm emphasizes use of multiple sources of information, each of which can capture unique aspects of behavior problems or provide information from unique perspectives. Multi-source assessment can also help reduce the effects of idiosyncratic and system-atic measurement error associated with any single source and can help iden-tify important causal variables and their functional interrelations. Multisource assessment involves use of multiple (a) informants (e.g., spouse, coworkers), (b) methods (e.g., self-report questionnaires, analog observations), (c) assess-ment instruments, and (d) assessment occasions (i.e., a time-series measure-ment strategy).

Different sources of information often provide information on unique as-pects of a client's behavior and causal variables. For example, interviews with different informants, such as health-care professionals and spouses, can pro-vide unique information about a client's paranoid behaviors. Alternatively, self-report questionnaires and client interviews can provide valuable informa-tion about what a client thinks or feels, which are often unobservable to oth-ers. Analog observation (e.g., observation in structured clinic settings; see the Special Section in *Psychological Assessment*, *13*, No. 1, 2001) of the same client can provide useful information such as the environmental triggers of his or her paranoid thoughts, which can be difficult for the client to identify.

The task of clinical assessment is further complicated because many behav-ior problems have *multiple modes* (e.g., cognitive, behavioral, physiological), each of which may best be assessed by different methods and instruments. Al-though different assessment instruments can use the same method and target the same variable, they can differ in the aspect or mode of the target construct being measured. For example, two analog observation instruments to evaluate marital communication can differ in the verbal behaviors that they measure and the degree to which they measure emotional and paralinguistic aspects of marital communication.

It is also useful to estimate functional relations for a client's behavior prob-lem from multiple sources of information. For example, observing a client role-play in a controlled clinic setting may help us understand the sequence of that client's verbally aggressive behavior toward his or her spouse. This in-formation can be augmented by asking clients to describe marital interactions during conflict or through questionnaires about how each spouse responds during such conflict.

Each source of information about a client introduces error, some proportion of variance in every measure fails to reflect "true" variance in the target variable. For example, information from spouses and family members can provide useful information about a client's aggressive behaviors, but the information also can reflect the informant's biases toward the client. Self-report questionnaires can reflect a client's need to present him- or herself positively.

In summary, errors in measurement and judgments about a client can often be reduced by using multiple sources of information when the sources pro-vide valid estimates of the variable. A behavioral clinical case formulation based on only one source is likely to reflect errors associated with that source. However, acquiring information about a client from multiple sources can also present problems for the clinician. Because they reflect the conditional nature of clients' behavior across situations and different sources of measurement error, data from multiple assessment sources can conflict. For example, information from analog observation, spouse reports, and self-reports could differ in the information they present about the characteristics and triggers for a client's panic episodes. Differences could reflect true differences in the phenomena measured by each source, or the differences could reflect biases and other errors associated with each assessment method. Integration of conflicting assessment data then presents additional challenges for the clinician (see discussion in Haynes & O'Brien, 2000).

Time-Series Measurement. Because the phenomena that we measure in clinical assessment can change rapidly, behavioral clinical case formulations should be based on frequent measurements of independent and dependent variables. Because of the dynamic nature of clinical phenomena, we should also expect that behavioral clinical case formulations of a client will change over time. Therefore, time-series measurement can be a powerful strategy for capturing the dynamic characteristics of behavior problems and causal variables. It is also a powerful tool for estimating functional relations relevant to a client's behavior problems.

Examples of time-series assessment strategies (many of which can be found in Franklin, Allison, Gorman, 1996; Kazdin, 1998; Kratochwill & Levin, 1992) include daily self-monitoring by a client of social contexts to identify social triggers of anger or verbal aggression. A depressed client with diabetes may complete a short self-report mood questionnaire and monitor blood glucose levels daily to identify the magnitude of covariance between these variables. The factors associated with onset and maintenance of panic attacks for a client might be identified with a time-series assessment design when those panic attacks and potentially relevant environmental and cognitive factors are measured concurrently.

Several attributes of time-series assessment strategies make them suitable for behavioral assessment and behavioral clinical case formulation: (a) They can capture the dynamic qualities of behavior and causal variables, (b) they are amenable to a focus of behavioral assessment on variables relevant to an individual client (an idiographic focus), and (c) they allow for the sensitive evaluation of an intervention (they are particularly useful for identifying failing interventions quickly).

When used with single-case experimental designs, time-series assessment strategies are particularly powerful methods of identifying functional and causal relations [i.e., interrupted time-series designs; ABAB withdrawal and reversal designs (Kazdin, 1998; Kratochwill & Levin, 1992; Repp & Horner,

2000)]. These designs involve the systematic manipulation of hypothesized controlling variables and the measurement of their effects on behavior problems.

Methods of Assessment

How we conceptualize a client's behavior problems and our decisions about the best ways to treat such a client depend on the information that we have about him or her and is, in turn, affected by our assessment methods. In this section, we briefly consider seven methods of assessment and summarize them in Table 3.2. We discuss their conceptual basis, sources of error, and utility for behavioral clinical case formulation. The methods differ in their assets, liabilities, applicability, and utility for behavioral clinical case formulation. However, all can be used to identify and specify behavior problems, acquire time-series data on dynamic variables, and examine functional relations relevant to a client's behavior problems.

The methods presented here are illustrated in the behavioral clinical case example in the latter part of this chapter. More extensive discussions of behavioral assessment methods and instruments can be found in books by Haynes and O'Brien (2000) and Bellack and Hersen (1998).

Several behavioral assessment methods are especially congruent with the assumption that understanding of a client's behavior problems is strongly facilitated by observing them. This leads to an emphasis on direct observation of a client, preferably in his or her natural environment. Direct observation allows the clinician to evaluate the situational specificity and conditional probability of behavior problems. It also helps address concerns with developing behavioral clinical case formulations solely on the basis of self-report interviews and questionnaires. Observation in the natural environment, participant observation and ratings, and self-monitoring allow the clinician to assess specifically defined behavioral and environmental events, acquire quantitative time-series data, and identify functional relations that are important for treatment planning. However, direct observation and other assessment methods differ in their applicability across behavior problems and settings, cost-efficiency, and sources of error.

Observation in the natural environment with external observers, such as observation of clients interacting with their family members during supper, is a powerful method of measuring clients' behavior and identifying important causal variables. However, it can be a difficult and expensive method of assessment, particularly with infrequently occurring or socially sensitive behaviors, such as partner aggression and substance use. Furthermore, data may reflect reactive effects of assessment in that the client may behave differently when observers are present. Data acquired by participant observers (e.g., spouses, psychiatric staff members) are less expensive and may be less influenced by

TABLE 3.2
Methods of Behavioral Assessment

Method	Examples	Data/Inferences Derived	Conceptual Basis
Observation in the natural environment	Observation of parent–child interactions in the home at supper time	Behavior rates, conditional probabilities, change across time	Data from natural environment, situation specificity, time samples, observation; highly specific
Analog observation	Observations of marital problem solving in a clinic setting	Behavior rates, conditional probabilities, change across time	Situation specificity, time-samples, observation; highly specific
Self-monitoring	Daily monitoring of mood, pain, and social interactions	Behavior rates, functional relations, ratings	Data from natural environment, situation specificity, time samples; highly specific
Participant ratings/monitoring	Psychiatric staff/teacher observations of patient's activity 4x/day	Behavior rates, functional relations, ratings	Data from natural environment, situation specificity, time samples; highly specific
Psychophysiological measurement	Ambulatory monitoring of blood pressure in stressful situations	Magnitude of response, latency of response, rate, response pattern	Multiple dimensions, time samples; highly specific
Interviews	Interview with person experiencing panic episodes; ratings to identify high-risk settings	All dimensions of measurement (e.g., rate, magnitude) and form of behavior; functional relations	Multiple dimensions, functional relations;
Questionnaires	Questionnaire about expected outcomes of drinking	All dimensions of measurement	Multiple dimensions, functional relations

reactive effects of the observation process. However, participant observers are often limited in the number of events they can monitor accurately and data may reflect their biases.

Self-monitoring, such as a client recording his or her level of discomfort in various social situations throughout the day, is perhaps the least costly of the observation methods and can be used to measure individual client behaviors and a wider range of modes. Although the utility and validity of self-monitored data can also be affected by the client's cognitive limitations, bias, and cooperation, these sources of error can often be minimized with instructions, practice, follow-up contacts, and carefully structured data acquisition procedures (see Special Section on self-monitoring in *Psychological Assessment, 11,* No. 4, 1999).

Analog observation, such as observing the interactions of a married couple as they try to discuss a problem in a clinic setting, is less costly than observation in the natural environment and can facilitate the idiographic observation of low-frequency events (see Special Section on analog observation in *Psychological Assessment, 13,* No.1, 2001). However, because it involves contrived settings, generalizability (ecological validity) is sometimes a concern and this method may be more susceptible to errors associated with assessment reactivity.

Psychophysiological assessment methods, such as ambulatory monitoring of cardiovascular reactivity to daily stressors, are often less susceptible to errors associated with self-report but can also be expensive to obtain (Cacioppo & Tassinary, 1990). However, when psychophysiological and other measurement methods, such as analog observation or self-monitoring, are used together, they can help the clinician identify settings and client states associated with psychophysiological responses.

Interviews and questionnaires can be easy to administer (although interviewers require training) and can be useful for examining functional relations involving all response modes. However, the resultant data can also reflect client biases, interviewer characteristics and skill, and degree of client cooperation. Their utility may also be affected by client cognitive impairments and errors in the development and scoring of the instruments.

BEHAVIORAL CLINICAL CASE FORMULATION

In the first sections of this chapter, we noted that behavioral clinical case formulations are guided by research-based assumptions about a client's behavior problems and their causes and by the information about the client derived from multiple sources and methods. In our efforts to understand a client, estimates of the importance of and functional relations among a client's multiple behavior problems and treatment goals, of the modifiability of causal variables, and of the strength and type of functional relations among causal variables are particularly important.

The purposes of a behavioral clinical case formulation strategy are to organize and communicate complex arrays of information and judgments about a client. The formulations are based on multiple measures of a client and on nomothetic research relevant to the client's behavior problems and treatment goals. The ultimate purpose is to design the best intervention program for the client. Behavioral clinical case formulation models inform the clinician about which variables are likely to be the most useful in treatment and help the clinician pick the best clinical assessment strategies. Behavioral clinical case formulation models also help reduce the biases and errors in clinical judgment.

Strategies and models for behavioral clinical case formulation have been proposed by Haynes and O'Brien (1990, 2000); Koerner and Linehan (1997);

Nezu, Nezu, Friedman, and Haynes (1997); Persons and Tompkins (1997); and Tanaka-Matsumi, Seiden, and Lam (1996). (See Eels, 1997, for a presentation of 14 behavioral and nonbehavioral clinical case formulation models.)

The five models we present differ in focus and components but are conceptually similar in several ways. All emphasize the importance of the identification and specification of a client's behavior problems and goals. Also, all emphasize individual differences in the characteristics of behavior problems, the importance of careful assessment before starting an intervention, the possibility that an individualized behavioral clinical case formulation can increase the effectiveness of treatment, and the clinical utility of a written or graphic presentation of a behavioral clinical case formulation.

In this section, we present an overview of models by Koerner and Linehan (1997), Nezu and coworkers (1997), Persons and Tompkins (1997), and Tanaka-Matsumi and coworkers (1996). In the subsequent section, we describe the functional analysis and functional analytic clinical case models of Haynes and O'Brien (1990, 2000).

A Problem-Solving Model

Nezu and coworkers (1997) described therapy as a problem-solving process in which the clinician solves the problem presented by the client. The problem-solving process includes several subproblems: problem analysis, target problem selection, treatment selection, treatment implementation, and treatment evaluation.

There are five components in the problem-solving process:

1. *Problem Orientation*: The clinician should think of the client's problem as multiply determined, with psychological, biological, and social influences.
2. *Problem Definition and Formulation*: The clinician conducts an idiographic assessment that includes information about response modes (i.e., behavioral, cognitive, affective, and physiological), the client's physical and social environments, historical and developmental information, and current information. Sources include subjective reports and less-biased sources such as standardized tests, behavioral observation, and psychophysiological measures.
3. *Generation of Alternatives*: The clinician uses brainstorming techniques to generate a large list of possible target variables and solutions or interventions.
4. *Decision Making*: The clinician evaluates the clinical utility of treatment alternatives, given the problem definition and formulation, and selects one that is likely to be the most effective.

5. *Solution Implementation and Verification*: The clinician implements the intervention/solution and monitors consequences of that implementation.

The Clinical Pathogenesis Map (CPM) is a flow diagram of the relations between stressful events, relevant stimuli, historical factors, and behavior problems. The CPM aids in the selection of the clinical goals and of the optimal treatment strategies (the authors also use a Goal Attainment Map for this purpose).

The clinician evaluates the match between predicted and actual effects of the intervention. Verification of the CPM proceeds throughout treatment, and the original conceptualization is reevaluated if predicted outcomes differ from actual outcomes.

Cognitive–Behavioral Case Formulation

Persons and Tompkins (1997) presented the Cognitive–Behavioral Case Formulation (CBCF) model, which emphasizes the causal role of cognitions (e.g., distorted thoughts) in client behavior problems. Similar to other models of behavioral case formulation, CBCF focuses on the form and causal mechanisms of behavior (structural assessment) and on the functions of behavior (functional assessment). Borrowing heavily from cognitive theories of depression and functional analysis, CBCF differs from other behavioral clinical case formulation models in that a central focus is the causal role of core beliefs (key distorted thoughts) for client behavior problems. Therefore, an important focus of assessment is the identification and specification of the client's core beliefs.

The Cognitive–Behavioral Case Formulation model has seven components:

1. *Behavior Problem List*: This is a comprehensive and specific list of all client behavior problems, regardless of their importance.
2. *Core Beliefs*: These are the client's specific beliefs about themselves, others, and the world. Early in the assessment process, the clinician begins forming hypotheses about the client's core beliefs and how they are operating as causal variables for the client's behavior problem.
3. *Precipitants and Activating Situations*: The clinician specifies environmental events and situations that trigger the client's core beliefs that lead to the behavior problem.
4. *Working Hypothesis*: The clinician links together the client's identified behavior problems and core beliefs and the triggering environmental events and situations. Together, these form a working hypothesis to guide assessment and treatment decisions.
5. *Origins*: The early learning history of the client is assessed with the intention of learning how his or her core beliefs were formed. Special

attention is given to significant experiences that involved parents or significant others.

6. *Treatment Plan*: Although not part of the behavioral clinical case formulation, Persons and Tompkins (1997) include "Treatment Plan" as part of the seven components to demonstrate how the Working Hypothesis is central to treatment planning.

7. *Predicted Obstacles to Treatment*: Using the information provided, predictions are made concerning problems that may arise during therapy, such as "power struggles" between client and therapist.

Dialectical Behavior Therapy Clinical Case Formulation

Koerner and Linehan's (1997) approach to case formulation, which predominantly focuses on work with individuals diagnosed with borderline personality disorder, is associated with Dialectical Behavior Therapy. This approach integrates a stage theory of treatment (prioritize therapeutic goals on the basis of threats to life and quality of life), a biosocial theory of etiology and maintenance of borderline personality disorder (equifinality for borderline personality disorder based on biological vulnerability and impact of the environment), learning principles (functional analysis and analysis of behavior chains), and a dialectical orientation to change (consideration of clients in their natural environments).

Dialectical Behavior Therapy Clinical Case Formulation emphasizes a three-stage approach to case formulation. The first stage involves gathering information on potential targets for therapeutic intervention. This includes identification of antecedents for important problems, such as parasuicidal behaviors, that can prevent successful therapy, and analysis of behavioral chains associated with behavioral problems. The second stage involves organization of information gained in the first stage to guide therapeutic interventions. This most commonly takes the form of a written narrative or a flowchart. The third stage calls for frequent revisions of the written case formulation as assessment and treatment continue. Because personality disorders are dynamic, frequent revisions may be necessary. These revisions may be minor adaptations of the original conceptualization or a sweeping reworking of the entire conceptualization, depending on the nature of new data.

Dialectical Behavior Therapy Clinical Case Formulation emphasizes both distal and proximal causal variables. Borderline personality disorders are assumed to result from emotional dysregulation caused by genetic predisposing conditions and invalidating historical environments (situations and settings that do not effectively teach goal-related behaviors to individuals). The maladaptive behaviors associated with borderline personality disorder (e.g., parasuicidal behavior) are assumed to result from difficulty regulating emotions. However, the causes for emotional dysregulation must be identified in order for effective treatment to occur. As a result, case formulations include current causal variables, such as behavior patterns, behavior chains, core beliefs, skills deficits, and current environmental reinforcement contingencies that lead to maladaptive behaviors.

Current causal variables are identified via interview, ongoing *in vivo* assessment, and traditional assessment instruments. The causal variables are assumed to vary across the contexts; Similar causal variables may result in different adaptive and maladaptive behavioral responses, depending on the setting. These contextual effects contributes to the dynamic nature of Dialectical Behavior Therapy Clinical Case Formulation.

Culturally Informed Functional Assessment Interview

The Culturally Informed Functional Assessment (CIFA) Interview, presented by Tanaka-Matsumi, Seiden, and Lam (1996), is a set of guidelines for developing behavioral clinical case formulation for clients whose cultural background differs from that of the clinician. As with other behavioral clinical case formulation models, the CIFA Interview seeks to identify and specify important controlling variables affecting a client's behavior problems. In addition, the CIFA Interview seeks to understand the specific cultural context in which a client's behavior problems occur. Thus, the CIFA Interview is congruent with and supplements the other models of behavioral clinical case formulation presented in this chapter.

Tanaka-Matsumi and colleagues outlined eight steps to a CIFA Interview. The steps relevant to assessment of a client's behavior problems are outlined as follows:

Step 1: Assessment of Cultural Identity and Acculturation. The clinician begins the assessment process by attempting to understand not only the client's cultural identity and level of acculturation but also the family's and that of their community (Dana, 1998; Suzuki, Meller, & Ponterotto, 1996). The clinician identifies discrepancies between the client's cultural identity and level of acculturation and that of his or her family and other primary support groups. The clinician then determines whether he or she is competent to work with the client, given the clinician's familiarity with the client's cultural background, or whether the client should be referred to another clinician. If the clinician continues with the assessment, he or she should consult the literature on relevant cultural issues and may choose to include a cultural consultant to insure that the assessment process is culturally sensitive.

Step 2: Specification of Presenting Problems. The clinician begins to identify and specify the client's behavior problems and their frequency, duration, and magnitude. The clinician also solicits the family's ideas about the client's problem and compares the client's problems with the norms of the client's cultural reference group via cultural informants or the family members themselves.

Step 3: Elicitation of the Client's Explanatory Model. The clinician solicits the client's causal explanatory model of his or her problem behaviors as well as the family's causal explanatory model of the client's behavior problems. Causal mechanisms leading to the client's problem behavior are explored collaboratively with the client and family. The client's causal explanatory model is compared with the norms of the client's cultural reference group to distinguish thought disorders or behavior problems from culturally normative explanatory models.

Step 4: Functional assessment. Important, modifiable causal variables, the client's motivation to change, and natural reinforcers are specified. Historical and contemporaneous factors related to the client's behavior problems are also specified. The consequences of the client's problems for family members as well as new problems that may result from treatment are explored. The client's reactions to particular stimuli (e.g., job-related stress) are compared with the typical reaction of his or her cultural reference group. Finally, a tentative clinical explanatory model is developed.

Step 5: Comparison and negotiation of Causal Explanatory Models. The clinician, client, and the client's family compare causal explanatory models. Discrepancies are collaboratively negotiated. In the case of clients with delusions and hallucinations, more emphasis is placed on the clinician's and the client's family's causal explanatory model.

Steps 6–8: Treatment. These are treatment related and beyond the focus of this chapter. These steps focus on the generation, comparison, and negotiation of treatment variables; data collection procedures; and the discussion of treatment duration, course, and expected outcomes. The clinician, the client, and the client's family negotiate treatment goals, target behaviors, agents of change, and methods of treatment. Treatment techniques from the client's cultural group are considered if proposed treatments are unacceptable to the client.

THE FUNCTIONAL ANALYSIS AND FUNCTIONAL, ANALYTIC CLINICAL CASE MODELS

The last model for behavioral clinical case formulation discussed is the functional analysis. *Functional analysis* is "The identification of important, controllable, causal and noncausal functional relations applicable to specified behaviors for an individual" (Haynes & O'Brien, 1990, p. 649). The functional analysis is similar to the four behavioral clinical case formulation models presented previously in that it is a clinician's working model of a client's problem behaviors and goals, the causal variables related to those problems and goals, and the functional relations among them. Functional Analytic Clinical Case Models (FACCMs) are vector diagrams of the functional analysis. The principal purposes of the functional analysis and FACCM are to help the clinician organize information and hypotheses from preintervention assessment and guide additional assessment decisions and the selection of intervention targets.

Components of the Functional Analysis

The functional analysis is composed of 11 clinical judgments that help the clinician decide on the best intervention targets. Decisions about intervention targets depend on judgments about the importance of and interrelationships among the client's behavior problems and the functional relations among behavior problems and causal variables. These judgments are outlined in Table 3.3.

All components of the functional analysis influence estimates of the relative magnitude of effect of focusing treatment on particular causal variables, which are the immediate targets of intervention. The functional analysis tries to answer the question, "What would be the relative effect on the client's behavior problems of focusing treatment on different causal variables?"

The overall purpose of the functional analysis is to organize the complex array of preintervention data and judgments about the multiple variables and functional relations for a client, integrate these data with data from nomothetic research, and communicate the results for the purpose of designing an individualized intervention program. The functional analysis helps the clinician estimate the degree to which each of the client's behavior problems (or intervention goals) is affected by each causal variable. The functional analysis helps the clinician estimate the relative magnitude of effect that would be expected if the treatment focused on the modification of each causal variable identified in the assessment process.

In FACCMs, estimates of the magnitude of treatment effects are aided by assigning each component of the functional analysis (e.g., strength of relations between variables, importance of the client problems) a numeric value. Thereby, expected magnitudes of effect can be estimated more easily with clients who have multiple behavior problems and multiple causal variables.

Characteristics of the Functional Analysis

The functional analysis has several characteristics. First, because its primary goal is to select the focus of treatment, the functional analysis emphasizes important, controllable, functional relations relevant to the client's behavior

TABLE 3.3
Components of the Functional Analysis

Component	Description
Client's behavior problems and intervention goals	Major behavior problems or intervention goals are identified in specific, measurable terms. Functional analysis may include different response modes (e.g., behavioral, cognitive) and dimensions (e.g., frequency, duration).
Relative importance of the client's behavior problems and goals	Most client's have multiple behavior problems that differ in importance (consider the relative importance for a client of minor tension headaches versus severe episodes of depression or drinking).
Functional relations among a client's behavior problems	A client's multiple behavior problems may have no functional relations, noncausal relations, and unidirectional or bidirectional causal (reciprocal) relations. Reciprocal causal relations are particularly important for intervention decisions because they can involve treatment effects that are magnified and sustained over time.
Effects of a client's behavior problems	Many behavior problems have important effects for the client. They may affect the client's or others' occupational, social, legal, medical, or family functioning and contribute to the estimated magnitude of effect of a particular intervention focus.
Causal variables that affect a client's behavior problems or treatment goals	Causal variables can include many classes of variables, such as genetic or learning experiences, but the functional analysis emphasizes contiguous antecedent environmental events and behavior, situational and setting factors, response contingencies, and cognitive variables.
Modifiability (treatment utility) of causal variables	Causal variables differ in the degree to which they are modifiable in an intervention program.
Type of functional relations between causal variables	The functional relations between a causal variable and behavior problems can be unidirectional or bidirectional.[a]
Strength of functional relations between causal variables and behavior problems	Causal variables can differ in their strength of impact or magnitude of their causal effect.
Relation among causal variables	Causal variables can interact with different types and strengths of functional relations.
Chains of causal variables	Behavior problems are often the result of chains of causal variables. Elements of the chain can point to several possible intervention points.
Mediating variables	Mediating variables explain "how" or "through what means" a causal variable affects a behavior problem (e.g., the effects of a life stressor on sleep may be mediated by presleep thoughts about the stressor). Mediating variables are particularly important intervention targets when unmodifiable variables (e.g., early life stressors or learning experiences) have important causal effects.
Moderating variables	Moderating variables affect the strength of relation between two other variables (e.g., social support might moderate the effect of a life stressor on mood).

[a] Causal relations can also assume different forms, such as parabolic, linear, or catastrophic (Haynes, 1992), but these are often beyond the measurement and inferential abilities of clinical assessment.

problems. *Importance* refers to the strength of the functional relation or the magnitude of impact of the causal variable. In a functional analysis, we are interested in those causal relations that account for the greatest proportion of variance in behavior problems: those variables that seem to most strongly affect the onset or duration of the behavior problem. Also, because of its focus on selecting the best treatments, the functional analysis emphasizes controllable causal variables. Many important causal variables (e.g., traumatic life events, genetic predisposition, head trauma) cannot easily be modified and are, therefore, less useful for the design of behavioral intervention programs. Consequently, the functional analysis often emphasizes response contingencies (e.g., how others respond to a client's behavior problems), settings (e.g., home vs. school, alone vs. with others), antecedent events (e.g., commands by a staff member, a critical comment by a friend), and cognitive events (e.g., a negative thought about oneself following a critical comment by another) as important causal variables for behavior problems.

Although they reflect clinical research findings, functional analyses are idiographic—they are likely to differ across clients with the same behavior problem. Nomothetic research on a behavior problem can point to possible causal relations for a client's behavior problem and guide initial assessment foci with that client. However, there are important between-person differences in the characteristics and causes of behavior problems, and the functional analyses of clients with the same behavior problem are likely to be substantively different (Haynes, 1992; Haynes & O'Brien, 2000).

The functional analysis can include many classes of variables and can be based on many methods of assessment. Physiological, cognitive, environmental, and behavioral variables can be important components of a functional analysis. Also, functional relations can be estimated through controlled manipulation of hypothesized causal variables, self-reports, observation in the client's natural environment, and multivariate time-series regression analyses.

A functional analysis is always hypothesized and tentative. It is an integration of the clinician's judgments at the time of its construction and reflects measurement and inferential errors. Consequently, it is also dynamic—the functional analysis of a client changes over time as new data are collected on the client, as conditions in the client's life change, and as treatment changes the causal variables and behavior problems.

More than one functional analysis can be valid for a client. For example, a functional analysis that emphasizes a strong functional relation between depressed mood and the loss of social reinforcement (e.g., through divorce or loss of a family member) does not preclude a strong functional relation between depressed mood and automatic negative thoughts.

A functional analysis can include extended social systems. Variables that affect others in the client's life can be important components of a functional analysis. Consequently, a client can be affected by variables far removed in time or place. For example, the spouse of a client may have work or family problems that affect his or her treatment of the client.

FUNCTIONAL ANALYSIS OF AN ADULT RECEIVING OUTPATIENT PSYCHOLOGICAL SERVICES

In this section, we describe the development of a functional analysis of a man referred to an outpatient mental health center following unsuccessful medical treatment of a painful work injury. The referring orthopedic surgeon suspected that psychological and environmental factors were affecting the maintenance of his persistent pain complaints. We discuss the methods and rationale of behavioral assessment across two sessions and how the functional analysis evolved as new information on the client was collected.

Referral and Initial Contact

Mr. Jordan, a 50-year-old married man of Asian–Caucasian descent, was referred to the pain management program of an outpatient mental health center by his orthopedic surgeon. The surgeon reported that, despite two surgeries, Mr. Jordan had experienced intractable pain for 6 months from neck and back injuries sustained at his job as a dock worker. The referring surgeon stated that the surgery, which occurred 2 weeks after the accident, was successful: the injuries had healed and several medical examinations revealed no organic etiology for his pain.

Mr. Jordan lived in a four-bedroom house with his wife of 25 years and two of their three children. The oldest child was in college. Mr. Jordan had been the sole provider in the household and was earning middle-class wages prior to the accident.

First Assessment Session

Mr. Jordan arrived for his first appointment at the clinic accompanied by Mrs. Jordan. The first 10 minutes were spent explaining the details of the assessment procedures and obtaining informed consent for assessment from both Mr. and Mrs. Jordan. At this point, Mrs. Jordan agreed to wait for Mr. Jordan in the waiting room while he was interviewed alone.

Based on information from the referring surgeon, Mr. Jordan completed a depression inventory [Beck Depression Inventory (BDI); Beck, Ward, Mendelson, Mock, & Erbaugh, 1961] and the Multidimensional Pain Inventory (MPI; Kerns, Turk, & Rudy, 1985) in the waiting room before his first assessment session. The pain inventory included questions about Mr. Jordan's pain and psychosocial factors that might affect pain expression.

In his initial session with Mr. Jordan, the assessor had several goals relevant to the development of a functional analysis: (a) to develop a supportive relationship with Mr. Jordan, (b) to survey for behavior problems related to Mr. Jordan's chronic pain, (c) to obtain specific qualitative and quantitative information about the pain and other behavior problems, (d) to identify Mr. Jordan's goals for therapy, and (e) to gather initial information on factors that might be maintaining Mr. Jordan's behavior problems. The information would be used to construct an initial FACCM and guide subsequent assessment strategies.

Unstructured Interview with Mr. Jordan. During the initial 15 minutes of the interview, Mr. Jordan reported that he had been experiencing severe neck and back pain and frequent nighttime awakenings since the accident, and that these problems had not been reduced by the surgery. He stated that he was unable to return to work and was concerned about meeting his financial obligations, such as his home mortgage payments, on the reduced income he was receiving from his worker's compensation. Mrs. Jordan had not worked outside the home since their marriage, and Mr. Jordan indicated that she was unwilling to initiate a job search. Mr. Jordan reported "some problems" in his marriage, but was reluctant to discuss these further. He identified his chronic pain and consequent inability to work at his previous job as his most important concerns.

Semistructured Interview with Mr. Jordan. The assessor then switched to a semistructured interview format to gather more specific information about Mr. Jordan's pain, sleep problems, and marital distress, and identify variables that may be functionally related to those problems.

Mr. Jordan reported that he had severe pain episodes 2 to 3 times a day, which usually lasted for 1 to 3 hours. He stated that his current pain level was about a 5 on a 10-point scale (1 = "no pain," 10 = "most pain imaginable"), but that the pain sometimes reached a level of 9, was not responsive to non-narcotic medication, and that the only thing that helped was to lie down and rest. The most severe pain episodes were in the evening when the children were home from school. During these episodes, he remained lying on the bed or couch.

Mr. Jordan shifted his position in his chair several times during the interview, winced, and commented that he could not sit comfortably for protracted periods of time. From his verbal tone, rate of speech, and self-reported mood, he appeared to be moderately depressed. He stated that he no longer engaged in any of the pleasurable activities that he once enjoyed, even those that were still physically possible for him (e.g., bowling, gardening). He stated that he could no longer lift anything heavy, such as a bag of groceries, or walk at even a moderate pace for more than 20 or 30 feet without experiencing "excruciating" pain.

In commenting on his marital relationship, he stated that his wife did not understand the depth of their financial problems or the uncertainty of their future and continued to spend money on unnecessary items for the house. He reported that they engaged in daily "fights" over money, usually in the evening, and that he just wanted her to leave him alone. He also stated that his wife did not understand the level of pain he was experiencing and expected him to help the children with their homework because he was just "lying around."

When questioned about his sleep patterns, Mr. Jordan stated that although he was able to fall asleep within an hour of going to bed, he was "never" able to sleep without waking 2 to 3 times per night due to pain. He stated that he was a "total wreck" during the day and that his "life was ruined" by the pain and sleeping problems.

When asked what his life would be like if his pain subsided, he stated that he felt he could go back to work part-time. He also stated that "at least we wouldn't be fighting so much." His primary goals for therapy included fewer and milder pain episodes and better sleep (more sustained sleep).

Self-Monitoring Homework. The frequent collection of data is an important aspect of behavioral assessment, particularly when assessing dynamic variables, such as pain, sleep, and mood (see Special Section on Self-Monitoring in *Psychological Assessment*, 1999, pp. 411–497). Consequently, the assessor and Mr. Jordan developed a plan to self-monitor pain episodes, mood over the course of the day, and sleep patterns. Each morning, Mr. Jordan was asked to estimate the previous night's latency to sleep-onset, number of times he awakened, the length of time spent awake, and presleep thoughts. Mr. Jordan also recorded the intensity and duration of his pain episodes, the setting in which each occurred, and the reactions of others. Mr. Jordan rated his mood on a 10-point scale (1 = "no depression," 10 = "most depressed ever") five times a day.

After meeting individually with Mr. Jordan, the assessor called Mrs. Jordan into the session to explain the purposes and procedures of the homework assignments. Mrs. Jordan also agreed to meet with the assessor individually during the second session. In addition, Mr. and Mrs. Jordan were asked to take home and complete the Dyadic Adjustment Scale (Spanier, 1976) to provide information on the extent of their marital problems.

Results of Assessment. Results from the BDI indicated that Mr. Jordan was moderately depressed (score = 20) and endorsed many somatic items (i.e., fatigue, sleep problems, and decreased sexual activity). Mr. Jordan's responses on the MPI indicated that pain was interfering with his work and social and family functioning, that he frequently received negative responses from his wife when he complained of pain, and that he participated minimally in daily activities.

Preliminary Functional Analysis. The FACCM in Figure 3.1 illustrates the clinician's functional analysis based on the information from the interviews,

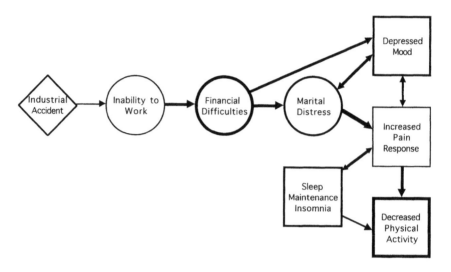

Estimated Relative Magnitude of Effect of Causal Variables

Financial Difficulties: 2.1
Marital Distress   1.9
Decreased Physical Activity   .5

FIG. 3.1. Preliminary functional analysis, illustrated by a Functional Analytic Clinical Case Model (FACCM), based on information from the first assessment session with Mr. Jordan. The functional analysis was based primarily on an interview with Mr. Jordan.

MPI, and BDI. The industrial accident was the original causal variable, but it is unmodifiable. The industrial accident resulted in Mr. Jordan's initial inability to work and consequent financial difficulties and marital distress (as indicated by the MPI and the interview). Several problems were initially identified: periodic increases in pain, sleep maintenance insomnia, decreased physical activity, and depressed mood. Mr. Jordan's pain appeared to increase during periods of marital distress and the pain has also led to a decrease in his physical activity. Mr. Jordan's pain was hypothesized to have a bidirectional causal relation with depressed mood and sleep maintenance insomnia. Decreased physical activity was exacerbated by Mr. Jordan's difficulty sleeping at night. The assessors surmised that Mr. Jordan's depressed mood was at least partially the function of his financial difficulties, but the mechanisms underlying that relation were unclear. Mr. Jordan's depressed mood and marital distress seemed to be related in a bidirectional manner. Figure 3.1 illustrates the hypothesized strength of these relationships and the estimated effect sizes associated with the causal variables.

Second Assessment Session

The purposes of the second assessment session, held 5 days after the first session, were to (a) further specify the variables and the functional relations depicted in the initial FACCM, (b) gather additional information on Mr. and Mrs. Jordan's marital distress, and (c) identify and specify other behavior problems, causal variables, and their functional relations.

Marital distress was a major focus of Session 2 because it was presumed to affect some of Mr. Jordan's other problems, especially the number of pain episodes he experienced. Homework assignments (i.e., self-monitoring and DAS) were scored and reviewed individually with Mr. and Mrs. Jordan. Mrs. Jordan was interviewed alone to gather sensitive information (i.e., sexual behaviors and other sources of marital distress) that might not be reported in the presence of her husband. Mr. Jordan was interviewed alone to review his self-monitoring data from the previous 5 days. Mr. and Mrs. Jordan were also interviewed jointly about their relationship and to provide the opportunity to observe their interactions in an analog behavior observation.

Marital Satisfaction Questionnaire.   Results of the DAS confirmed hypotheses regarding marital distress and further clarified specific concerns. With higher scores indicating a better relationship, Mr. and Mrs. Jordan scored 60 and 52, respectively, suggesting a low level of satisfaction with the relationship by both partners. The original standardization sample of normal, married people had a mean of 114.8 and a standard deviation of 17.8 (Spanier, 1976). An item analysis of Mr. Jordan's DAS revealed that he often disagrees with Mrs. Jordan on matters of recreation, making major decisions, and leisure time interests. He reported on the DAS that he and Mrs. Jordan rarely "think that things are going well" between the two of them. Mr. Jordan also reported infrequent positive verbal interactions as indicated by a low score on the affectional expressions subscale. Congruent with Mr. Jordan's DAS report, Mrs. Jordan also reported that they often disagree on matters of recreation, making major decisions, and leisure time interests. In addition, she reported that they often disagree on sex relations and the handling of family finances. Mrs. Jordan also reported that she rarely "feels things are going well" between the two of them and reported a low frequency of positive verbal interaction.

Semistructured Interview with Mr. Jordan.   Based on information provided in the initial interview and DAS information, a second semistructured interview focused on marital difficulties and further explored Mr. Jordan's views of himself. He stated, "I feel worthless after fighting with my wife. I don't remember my parents ever fighting about money or not being able to provide financially for the family." Follow-up questioning revealed that

Mr. Jordan holds strong, traditional beliefs regarding the roles of males in providing for the family. This belief may be consistent with traditional Arian ethnocultural beliefs.

Self-Monitoring of Pain and Sleep. The self-monitoring data on Mr. Jordan's pain and sleep over the previous week were reviewed with him and charted. The pain data were congruent with what Mr. Jordan had stated in the interview regarding the characteristics and associated settings: The self-monitoring data suggested that Mr. Jordan's pain was most intense (average of 7 on a 10-point pain scale) during and following conflicts with Mrs. Jordan. During other times, Mr. Jordan reported no to moderate levels of pain (rated 1 to 4). He experienced a total of 21 intense pain episodes (6 or greater) over the previous week. Twelve of the 21 pain episodes were preceded by verbal arguments with his wife, and seven were preceded by a verbal request from Mrs. Jordan to perform either a household chore or to help with the children. No antecedent events were reported for two of Mr. Jordan's intense pain episodes. Each intense pain episode would last at least an hour.

As part of the self-monitoring assignment, Mr. Jordan had rated his mood five times a day. Mr. Jordan reported feeling most depressed (8 or greater) during periods of intense pain (6 or greater). Levels of reported depression varied from 2 to 9, with a mean of 4.5.

In addition to the frequent awakenings throughout the evening (four to five times per night) almost every night (3 nights since the previous assessment session), Mr. Jordan also reported that he had developed difficulty falling asleep. Mr. Jordan's sleep latency was worse on evenings when Mr. and Mrs. Jordan had argued. Mr. Jordan reported that he often worried about their financial difficulties on nights that he had trouble falling asleep. It appeared from the self-monitoring data that arguments with his wife were associated with presleep worry and, in every instance, led to increased sleep maintenance difficulties at night. However, pain was evidently not a source for Mr. Jordan's sleep difficulties. Although he reported mild pain during the evening (average score of 1.5) , there were no obvious differences in reported pain levels between nights when he did and did not experience sleep difficulties. Mr. Jordan was asked to continue self-monitoring his pain and sleep so that the clinician could monitor response to treatment.

Semistructured Interview with Mrs. Jordan. Guided by the information from the DAS and the initial interviews with Mr. Jordan, a semi-structured interview was conducted with Mrs. Jordan. She was interviewed about areas of satisfaction and dissatisfaction with the marriage, events leading to conflict, goals for the relationship, and problem-solving strategies. Mrs. Jordan reported that the frequency and form of arguments over their financial situation were major sources of distress for her. According to Mrs. Jordan, arguments occurred at least once a day, every day, and they lasted for at least an hour. They often escalated to shouting and insults, but did not include physical aggression or intimidation. She also stated that, since Mr. Jordan's accident, he had withdrawn from family activities (e.g., he no longer sits at the dinner table and does not participate in weekend visits with other family members) and has refused to help with household chores or help the children with their schoolwork. She reported that whenever she asks Mr. Jordan to help around the home, he complains about his neck and back pain. Mrs. Jordan also reported a decrease in sexual activity from once a week to less than once a month. Finally, Mrs. Jordan indicated feeling angry toward her husband and that she is considering a divorce.

In addition to problems at home, Mrs. Jordan expressed concern about going to work outside of the home. She has never held a job and none of the women in her family have ever worked. She felt strongly that her primary responsibilities lay in areas of homemaking and caring for children. Furthermore, she felt strongly that her husband should fulfill his duty to provide a reasonable level of income.

Semistructured Marital Interview. A conjoint semistructured interview was conducted to further assess Mr. and Mrs. Jordan's marital relationship. The interview focused on each person's view of the positive qualities of the relationship, behaviors they would like to see increased as well as decreased, and ways each could improve the relationship. When asked about positive qualities of the relationship, Mr. Jordan indicated that his wife was very involved with the children's education (e.g., helps with homework) and extracurricular activities (e.g., school sports, boy scouts) and that she has done a "great job" at managing all household and parental responsibilities. However, Mr. Jordan reported that he would like for his wife to stop "nagging" him about the household chores and the children. Mr. Jordan stated that in order to fully recover from his injury, he needs to refrain from strenuous physical activity.

Mrs. Jordan was unable to identify any current positive qualities of the relationship, but noted several prior to her husband's injury. She stated that, before the injury, he communicated more, contributed to the managing of the household, and took an active role in the rearing of the children. Mrs. Jordan indicated that she wanted her husband to increase the number of household chores he performs and the amount of time he spends with the children (e.g., help them with homework more often). Finally, she stated that Mr. Jordan was using his injury as an excuse to avoid doing household chores and fulfilling his parental and financial responsibilities.

Analog Observation. A 15-minute analog observation was conducted toward the end of the interview with both spouses. The couple was asked to select a salient marital problem to discuss, and they chose "financial problems."

They were then asked to discuss their financial problems and try to reach a resolution. The clinician used a behavior checklist, idiographically constructed based on information learned from the interview, to quantify dimensions (i.e., frequency, duration, and intensity) of positive behaviors (e.g., compliments, agreements) and negative behaviors (e.g., insults, disagreements), compromise statements, and blaming statements. Qualitative impressions of the interaction were also recorded.

Initially, when discussing the problem, Mr. and Mrs. Jordan's voices were low in volume and conversational in tone with no interruptions. As the discussion advanced, their voices became louder and argumentative in tone, with an increase in the number of interruptions, blaming, and critical comments made by each spouse. During the observation session, Mr. Jordan was observed making 10 negative statements (e.g., "you're inconsiderate"), 4 positive statements (e.g., "you do help out a lot"), 7 interruptions, 2 negative attributions (e.g., "it's your fault I'm taking so long to heal"), and 2 compromise statements (e.g., "I can at least help with James' [son] homework"). In contrast, Mrs. Jordan was observed making 15 negative statements (e.g., "you're lazy," "good for nothing"), 2 positive statements (e.g., "I realize you are in pain"), 12 interruptions, 5 negative attributions (e.g., "it's because of you that our bills are getting paid late"), and no compromise statements.

Results of the analog observation suggested that Mr. and Mrs. Jordan each blamed the other for their financial circumstances. Their problem-solving strategies involved many negative and few positive interactions, and neither indicated that they were listening to the other. During debriefing, Mr. Jordan also noted that his back pain intensified during a period when the argument was particularly intense. This suggested that some of the muscle pain may have been related to muscle tensions.

Second Functional Analysis

Following the second assessment session, Mr. Jordan's functional analysis was modified to reflect the new assessment information (Figure 3.2). This FACCM included specification of marital distress (arguments over financial problems and wife's negative attributions) and the addition of thoughts of worthlessness and presleep worry. Additional behavior problems included decreased child-rearing involvement, decreased sexual activity, decreased physical activity, and sleep-onset insomnia.

Based on the additional data, it appeared that financial difficulties were leading to arguments between Mr. and Mrs. Jordan regarding financial problems, rather than leading directly to marital distress. The argument resulted in Mrs. Jordan making negative statements and attributions regarding her husband and also increased his presleep worry. In addition, his wife's negative comments increased Mr. Jordan's thoughts of worthlessness (which are viewed as a mediating variable between his wife's negative attributions and presleep worry),

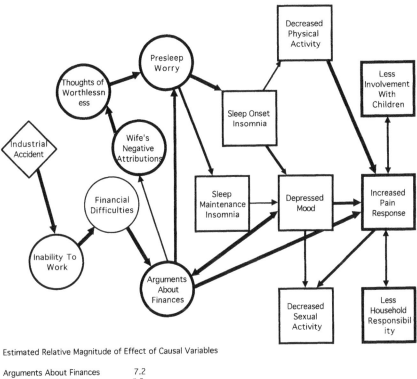

Estimated Relative Magnitude of Effect of Causal Variables

Arguments About Finances	7.2
Financial Difficulties	5.3
Presleep Worry	3.3
Thoughts of Worthlessness	2.6
Inability to Work	2.3
Wife's Negative Attirutions	1.7

FIG. 3.2. Functional analysis illustrated by an FACCM based on additional interviews with Mr. and Mrs. Jordan, self-monitoring data, self-report questionnaires, and analog behavioral observation of marital interaction.

which was also a source of his presleep worry. Mr. Jordan's presleep worry leads to both sleep-onset insomnia and sleep maintenance insomnia, sleeping difficulties that reduce his physical activity and increase his feelings of fatigue. Sleep maintenance insomnia also seemed to increase his depressed mood. Both depressed mood and increased pain response influenced marital interactions by decreasing the frequency of positive communication and sexual activity.

The addition of the new variables resulted in changes in the estimated effect sizes. The most important causal variable, from FACCM 1, was financial difficulties. However, the arguments over financial problems had a much larger estimated effect size (7.26) in the second FACCM. This FACCM suggested that a treatment focus on marital interactions with a specific emphasis on increasing positive interactions and decreasing arguments between Mr. and

Mrs. Jordan would be associated with the greatest treatment benefits for the client.

Clinical Case Conference

After designing the second functional analysis, the assessor organized a multidisciplinary case conference of pain program staff. The physiatrist, the occupational therapist, and the physical therapist attended the meeting. The physiatrist reviewed relevant medical data and confirmed that there was no known medical reason for Mr. Jordan's pain. However, Mr. Jordan had been using an increasing amount of pain medication, as indicated by increasing numbers of refills at the pharmacy.

The physical therapist reported no problems engaging Mr. Jordan in basic exercises. These exercises included weight lifting, stretching, and riding a stationary bicycle to increase endurance. These interventions were designed to counteract muscle atrophy that chronic pain patients often experience. Muscle atrophy can lead to a cycle wherein the pain patient stops physical activity and exercise due to pain; the muscles tend to atrophy from lack of use, which leads to reductions in strength and increased pain when the patient attempts to return to a normal level of activity.

The physical therapist reported that two problems emerged in spite of Mr. Jordan's initial cooperation. First, Mr. Jordan did not exercise at home. Second, if the physical therapist "pushed" Mr. Jordan to exercise more in the clinic (e.g., lift more weights), Mr. Jordan's pain complaints increased, his physical effort decreased, and he often asked for medication. However, when Mr. Jordan worked at his own pace, he completed all of the required exercises.

The occupational therapist reported that Mr. Jordan was showing acceptable progress in the occupational therapy program, which included training in new skills such as ways to move, lift, and carry items so that pain would be minimized. Similar to the physical therapists' report, the occupational therapist indicated that Mr. Jordan appeared unwilling to use newly obtained skills at home. For example, the client could carry up to 20 pounds at the clinic (usually in the form of groceries within a basket) without difficulty. However, Mr. Jordan reported an inability to carry a lightly loaded clothes basket at home; the occupational therapist reported that such baskets would usually weight between 15 and 20 pounds. This implied that Mr. Jordan was avoiding certain activities at home because such activities did not coincide with his view of a family provider.

FACCM 3

Team member reports led to changes in the function analysis (see Figure 3.3). Mr. Jordan's increased use of pain medications raised immediate concern—the team hypothesized that an increased reliance on pain medications was a way of

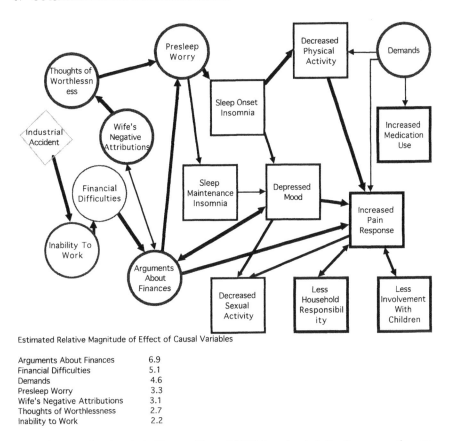

Estimated Relative Magnitude of Effect of Causal Variables

Arguments About Finances	6.9
Financial Difficulties	5.1
Demands	4.6
Presleep Worry	3.3
Wife's Negative Attributions	3.1
Thoughts of Worthlessness	2.7
Inability to Work	2.2

FIG. 3.3.   Functional analysis illustrated by an FACCM constructed after the case conference.

escaping from family and social demands. Support for this hypothesis comes from Mr. Jordan's responses to clinic staff when asked to work beyond his personal goals. This pattern seemed to parallel the pattern of interactions between Mr. and Mrs. Jordan. Thus, it appeared that social demands (Mrs. Jordan's demands for more spending money and help with the children) influenced Mr. Jordan's level of physical activity, response to pain, and use of medications.

In addition to reviewing information from individual providers, the psychologist presented FACCM 2 to the treatment team. The treatment team agreed with much of the model, but suggested that the relations between Mrs. Jordan's negative attributions exacerbated marital arguments over financial problems. Thus, this relationship was modified in FACCM 3 to represent a bidirectional relationship.

The four largest estimated treatment effect sizes were associated with marital arguments (6.9), financial difficulties (5.1), demands (4.6), and presleep worry (3.3). In addition to the previously mentioned intervention foci, the treatment team chose to focus on Mr. Jordan's responses to demands and advised marital therapy to decrease arguments and address Mrs. Jordan's negative attributions. (The team chose not to focus on financial difficulties because the team could not directly influence the family's financial situation).

Cognitive–behavioral family therapy included a focus on family goals in addition to Mr. Jordan's individual goals. The team recognized that both Mr. and Mrs. Jordan must learn to appraise the situation in a more positive light, develop better problem-solving strategies, and acquire new ways of communicating their needs and frustrations to each other. Mr. Jordan must learn methods of pain management and gain a higher level of functioning across a variety of situations. The team therefore chose to follow a model that addresses the effects of negative emotion in pain perception.

SUMMARY

The primary purpose of this chapter is to present behavioral approaches to clinical case formulation and the selection of treatment targets. We first present an overview of the concepts and methods of the behavioral assessment paradigm that affect case formulation. We note that treatment decisions are most likely to be useful and valid when assessment is based on data; involves multiple, validated assessment methods; gathers information from multiple sources; and focuses on identifying functional relations relevant to behavior problems. Assessment strategies should be sensitive to the dynamic nature of the client's behavior problems and causal variables, sensitive to the conditional nature of behavior, and emphasize observable behaviors relevant to the client's natural environment.

Behavioral assessment strategies and clinical case formulations on which treatment decisions are based are guided by assumptions about a client's behavior problems and their causes. Clients often have multiple behavior problems that can be the result of multiple interacting factors. Furthermore, the same behavior problem can occur in different forms and from different causes for different clients. Important causal factors often include a client's learning history, what the client thinks about his or her behavior problems and their causes, situational factors, and immediate social contingencies for the client's behavior. Multiple behavior problems can affect each other and a client's behavior problems can vary on multiple dimensions across settings and time. Causal variables can also vary across time, and those that are contemporaneous and modifiable are of most use in behavioral case formulation.

The strategies and methods of assessment guided by models of behavior disorders can strongly affect the validity of a behavioral clinical case formulation. The behavioral assessment paradigm emphasizes direct observation of a client in natural and analog settings and the identification of important functional relations relevant to the client's behavior problems. Self-monitoring and psychophysiological assessment is also emphasized, although self-report methods are important in behavioral assessment.

The complex array of assessment information on a client is organized and communicated through behavioral clinical case formulations. These formulations guide the clinician assessment efforts, reduce biases in clinical judgment, and help the clinician select the best treatment targets. Behavioral clinical case formulation models have been proposed by Haynes and O'Brien (1990, 2000), Koerner and Linehan (1997), Nezu and coworkers (1997), and Persons and Tompkins (1997).

The functional analysis emphasizes important, controllable, and functional relations relevant to the client's behavior problems. There is a particular emphasis on those causal relations that account for the greatest proportion of variance in behavior problems. The functional analysis often focuses on contemporaneous response contingencies, settings, antecedent events, and cognitive variables.

REFERENCES

Asher, X. X. (1976).

Beck, A. T., Ward, C. H., Mendelson, M., Mock, J., & Erbaugh, J. (1961). An inventory for measuring depression. *Archives of General Psychiatry, 4*, 561–571.

Bellack, A. S., & Hersen, M. (Eds.) (1998). *Behavioral assessment: A practical handbook* (4th ed.). Boston: Allyn & Bacon.

Cacioppo, J. T., & Tassinary, L. G. (Eds.) (1990). *Principles of psychophysiology: Physical, social and inferential elements.* New York: Cambridge University Press.

Dana, R. H. (1998). *Understanding cultural identity in intervention and assessment.* Thousand Oaks, CA: Sage Publications, Inc.

Eels, T. (1997). *Handbook of psychotherapy case formulation.* New York: Guilford Press.

Franklin, R. D., Allison, D. B., & Gorman, B. S. (Eds.) (1996). *Design and analysis of single-case research.* Mahwah, NJ: Lawrence Erlbaum Associates, Inc.

Garb, H. N. (1998). *Studying the clinician: Judgment research and psychological assessment.* Washington, DC: American Psychological Association.

Haynes, S. N. (1992). *Models of causality in psychopathology: Toward synthetic, dynamic and nonlinear models of causality in psychopathology.* Des Moines: Allyn & Bacon.

Haynes, S. N., Kaholokula, J., & Nelson, K. (1999). Idiographic applications of nomothetically derived treatment programs. *Clinical Psychology: Science and Practice, 6*, 456–461.

Haynes, S. N. & O'Brien, W. O. (1990). The functional analysis in behavior therapy. *Clinical Psychology Review, 10*, 649–668.

Haynes, S. N. & O'Brien, W. O. (2000). *Principles of behavioral assessment: A functional approach to psychological assessment.* New York: Plenum/Kluwer Press.

Huberty, X. X. (1996).

Kazdin, A. (1998). *Research design in clinical psychology.* Boston: Allyn & Bacon.

Kerns, R. D., Turk, K. C., & Rudy, T. E. (1985). The West Have-Yale Multidimensional Pain Inventory (WHYMPI). *Pain, 23*, 345–356.

Koerner, K., & Linehan, M. M. (1997). Case formulation in dialectical behavior therapy. In: T. D. Eells (Ed.), *Handbook of psychotherapy case formulation* (pp. 340–367). New York: The Guilford Press.

Kratochwill, T. R., & Levin, J. R. (Eds.) (1992). *Single-case research design and analysis: New directions for psychology and education*, Hillsdale, NJ: Lawrence Erlbaum Associates, Inc.

Martin, G., & Pear, J. (1996). *Behavior modification: What it is and how to do it* (5th ed.). Upper Sandle River, NJ: Prentice Hall, Inc.

Mash, E. J., & Terdal, L. G. (Eds.). (1997). *Assessment of childhood disorders*, 3rd edition. New York: The Guilford Press.

Nezu, A. M., & C. M. Nezu, C. M. (Eds.) (1989). *Clinical decision making in behavior therapy: A problem-solving perspective* (pp. 9–34). Champaign, IL: Research Press Co.

Nezu, A. M., Nezu, C. M., Friedman, S. H., & Haynes, S. N. (1997). Case formulation in behavior therapy: Problem-solving and functional analytic strategies. In: T. D. Eells (Ed.), *Handbook of psychotherapy case formulation* (pp. 368–401). New York: The Guilford Press.

O'Brien, W. H., & Haynes, S. N. (1993). Behavioral assessment in the psychiatric setting. In: A. S. Bellack & M. Hersen (Eds.). *Handbook of behavior therapy in the psychiatric setting* (pp. 39–71). New York: Plenum Press.

O'Donohue, W. (Ed.) (1998). *Learning and behavior therapy*. Needham Heights, MA: Allyn & Bacon.

Persons, J. B., & Tompkins, M. A. (1997). Cognitive–behavioral case formulation. In: T. D. Eells (Ed.), *Handbook of psychotherapy case formulation* (pp. 314–339). New York: The Guilford Press.

Repp, A. C., & Horner, R. H. (2000). *Functional analysis of problem behavior: From effective assessment to effective support*. Belmont, CA: Wadsworth Publishing Co.

Shapiro, E. S., & Kratochwill, T. R. (2000). *Behavioral assessment in schools*. New York: Guilford Press.

Spanier, G. B. (1976). Measuring dyadic adjustment: New scales for assessing the quality of marriage and similar dyads. *Journal of Marriage and the Family, 38*, 16–28.

Suzuki, L. A., Meller, P. J., & Ponterotto, J. G. (Eds.) (1996). *Handbook of multicultural assessment clinical, psychological, and educational applications* (pp. 319–347). San Francisco: Jossey-Bass Inc.

Tanaka-Matsumi, J., Seiden, D. Y., & Lam, K. N. (1996). The Culturally Informed Functional Assessment (CIFA) Interview: A strategy for cross-cultural behavioral practice. *Cognitive and Behavioral Practice, 3*, 215–233.

Part II

Specific Disorders

Major Depressive Disorder

Paula Truax
Pacific University

DESCRIPTION OF THE DISORDER

Depression is one of the most common reasons that people seek mental health care. It is also one of the most frequent and expensive mental health problems across the United States. From 5% to 9% of women and 2% to 3% of men meet criteria for Major Depressive Disorder (MDD) at any one time; from 10% to 15% of women and 5% to 12% of men will experience MDD at some point during their lives (American Psychiatric Association, 1994). Not only is depression experienced by a significant number of people, it may also have a chronic impact on those who experience it. Between 50% and 60% of those with one episode of depression will have a second episode; 70% of those with two episodes and 90% of those with three episodes will have another episode (APA, 1994).

According to the *Diagnostic and Statistical Manual of Mental Disorders, Fourth Edition* (*DSM–IV*; APA, 1994), MDD is characterized by a constellation of emotional, cognitive, behavioral, and physical symptoms (Table 4.1 for DSM–IV diagnostic criteria). There are four basic elements to a diagnosis of MDD. The first is presence of the hallmark emotional symptoms of MDD: sadness and anhedonia. At least one of these emotional symptoms must be present most of the day nearly every day for a minimum of 2 weeks. Although necessary for diagnosis, these mood symptoms are not sufficient to warrant a diagnosis of MDD. The second component is presence of behavioral and physical concomitants, such as sleep difficulties, appetite or weight

TABLE 4.1
DSM–IV Diagnostic Criteria for Major Depressive Disorder

A. Five (or more) of the following symptoms have been present during the same 2-week period and
   represent and change from previous functioning. At least one of the five is number 1 or number 2.

   1) Depressed mood *most of the day nearly every day*
   2) Markedly decreased interest or pleasure *most of the day nearly every day*
   3) Significant increase OR decrease in weight or appetite *nearly every day*
   4) Insomnia OR hypersomnia *nearly every day*
   5) Psychomotor agitation OR retardation *observable by others nearly every day*
   6) Fatigue OR loss of energy *nearly every day*
   7) Feelings of worthlessness OR excessive guilt *nearly every day*
   8) Difficulty concentrating OR making decisions *nearly every day*
   9) Recurrent thoughts of death or suicide
B. The symptoms do not meet criteria for a Mixed Episode (significant manic symptoms).
C. The symptoms cause clinically significant distress or impairment in important areas of
   functioning.
D. The symptoms are not due to a substance or general medical condition.
E. The symptoms are not better accounted for by Bereavement.

---

changes, psychomotor changes, and fatigue, as well as cognitive symptoms
of worthlessness or guilt, difficulty concentrating, and suicidal ideation. Note
that most of the symptom areas are multidimensional and may be coded as
present whether the symptom has significantly increased or decreased. Thus,
there can be great diversity among different people who meet the MDD diagnosis. The third necessary component is that symptoms must lead to clinically
significant distress. That is, clients must be experiencing notable difficulties
in their social, familial, occupational, or recreational life as a result of these
symptoms. Finally, it must be determined that symptoms are not better accounted by a diagnosis other than MDD. Common psychological conditions
that should be ruled out when determining whether a client meets criteria for
MDD are Bipolar Disorder, Dysthymic Disorder, Bereavement, Posttraumatic
Stress Disorder (PTSD), and Generalized Anxiety Disorder (GAD).

MDD and Bipolar Disorder differ in one important way: presence or absence
of manic symptoms. Any person meeting full criteria for MDD with a history
of even one diagnosable manic or hypomanic episode should be diagnosed
Bipolar Disorder I or II rather than MDD.

Dysthymic Disorder and MDD differ in two important ways: Dysthymic
Disorder is milder and longer lived than MDD. In contrast to MDD's "most
of the day, nearly every day" for 2 weeks requirement, Dysthymic Disorder
requires "more days than not" for 2 years. If a client meets full criteria for
current or past MDD, a Dysthymic Disorder diagnosis will not ordinarily
be made. One important exception is that when a full 2 years of Dysthymic
Disorder precedes the initial MDD episode, a comorbid diagnosis of MDD
superimposed on Dysthymic Disorder may be given.

MDD should also be differentiated from disorders that represent reactions to extreme events such as Bereavement and PTSD. Bereavement and MDD often appear similar and involve similar symptoms. The key difference is that bereft individuals have experienced the loss of a loved one to death within the preceding 2 months and their symptoms are directly related to the consequences of the loss. When symptoms do not begin abating 2 months postloss and/or they are more severe than would typically be seen with Bereavement (e.g., psychosis, extreme feelings of worthlessness or generalized guilt, significant suicidal ideation), a diagnosis of MDD should be considered. MDD also has a symptom profile similar to PTSD (e.g., loss of interest, sleep difficulties, difficulty concentrating), yet PTSD is unique from MDD in that it requires (a) the presence of a recent or past trauma (e.g., rape, natural disaster, childhood sexual abuse), (b) intrusive visual, emotional, or sensory memories of the trauma, and (c) active attempts to avoid thinking about the trauma. Therefore it is essential to assess significant life events and their role in the client's current symptoms for differential diagnosis in MDD.

The distinction between GAD and MDD is a subtle one. Some argue that they are two variants of the same construct (Burns & Eidelson, 1998). Still, there are some key differences in symptom profiles and prescribed treatments. Like MDD, GAD involves difficulty concentrating, fatigue, and difficulty sleeping. Unlike MDD, GAD's hallmark symptom is excessive and inappropriate worry about most issues in daily living. People with GAD find it difficult to stop worrying and relax. Because some evidence suggests that people who meet criteria for both MDD and GAD may be less amenable to standard treatments for depression (Bakish, 1999), it is important to evaluate the extent to which worry dominates the depressive symptoms.

Although the *DSM–IV*'s categorical distinctions are far from perfect, a growing body of literature on empirically supported interventions suggests that accurate diagnosis can enhance treatment, whereas inaccurate diagnosis hampers treatment. Cognitive–behavioral therapy, for example, is the most researched and the most supported therapy for MDD. In contrast, when the depression is severe or involves a manic component, psychotropic intervention should be part of the treatment plan. Similarly, when anxiety or avoidance dominates the client's presentation (e.g., PTSD, GAD), exposure interventions should be incorporated into treatment (see Nathan & Gorman, 1998, for a summary of treatments and empirically supported interventions).

METHODS TO DETERMINE DIAGNOSIS

Two commonly used methods for determining a diagnosis of MDD are the clinical interview and the Structured Clinical Interview for the *DSM–IV*–Clinician's Version (SCID–CV; First, Spitzer, Gibbon, & Wlliams, 1997). Unstructured clinical interviews are the most frequently used, but also the less reliable of the two (First et al., 1997). Essential factors in increasing the reliability of the typical clinical interview are the clinician's knowledge and systematic application of that knowledge during the diagnostic portion of the interview. Minimum knowledge areas include the following:

- Diagnosis of MDD: *DSM–IV* symptoms of MDD, time-frame (2 weeks), and severity (e.g., most of the day, nearly every day)
- Differential diagnosis: *DSM–IV* symptoms of other mood disorders and other diagnoses that may appear like MDD (e.g., GAD, PTSD, Bereavement, Adjustment Disorder with Depressed Mood)

Application of this knowledge requires the following:

- Asking specifically about each of the symptoms, time-frame, and severity
- Asking specifically about key symptoms from other diagnoses.

An example of how the diagnostic portion of the clinical interview may begin follows:

Therapist: Now I would like to ask you some fairly specific questions about how you have been feeling recently. I know you said that you have been feeling depressed and that it has been going on for about two months. Has there been a two-week period in the past month in which you felt depressed most of the day, nearly every day?

Client: Yes, I have felt depressed most of the day, nearly every day for the past two months.

Therapist: Okay. Can you tell me if the past two weeks have been characteristic of the past two months.

Client: If anything the most recent two weeks have been the worst. That is why I came to see you.

Therapist: OK then, let's focus on the most recent two weeks for the rest of these questions. [Establishing time frame] In the past two weeks, have you also lost interest or pleasure in things that you usually enjoyed? [Checking out specific symptoms]

Client: Yes.

Therapist: Has that been most of the day, nearly every day? [Severity]

Client: It has been constant. I can't get interested in anything.

Therapist: How about your weight and appetite? You mentioned earlier that you have gained twelve pounds in the past month because you are eating all the time due to depression. Did I get that right? [Time-frame, specific symptoms, severity]

Client: Yes; I understand some people lose weight when they feel depressed. I wish that were me.

Therapist: Depression is different for everyone. Weight gain is not uncommon. You also mentioned earlier that you have been having difficulty going to sleep; has that been nearly every day over the past two weeks? [Time-frame, specific symptoms, severity]

Client: It has been every day over the past two weeks. [Interviewes continues asking about all symptoms, time frame, and severity]

Once the therapist has asked about the symptoms of MDD and ruled out other diagnoses, a timeline may be drawn of the client's MDD history to assess the role of events and possible comorbidity with Dysthymic Disorder (p. 388, *DSM–IV*, APA, 1994). See Fig. 4.1 for MDD timeline of the case presented later.

The SCID–CV (First et al., 1997) is a semistructured interview for assessing the major *DSM–IV* Axis I diagnoses. The SCID–CV is a simplified version of the SCID Research Version designed to be more appropriate for the clinical environment. It is divided into modules (Mood Episodes, Psychotic Symptoms, Psychotic Disorders, Mood Disorders, Substance Use Disorders, Anxiety and Other Disorders) that can be used independently or as a comprehensive diagnostic interview. The Mood Episodes and Mood Disorders modules take about 20 minutes to administer. Administration time for the entire SCID–CV is approximately 90 minutes. The primary advantages of the SCID–CV over the less structured clinical interview are that it is more reliable and it prompts the interviewer to ask the appropriate diagnostic and differential diagnostic questions.

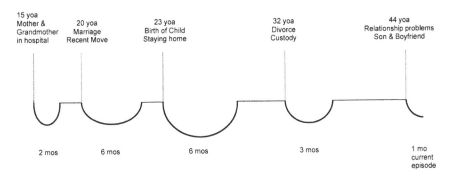

FIG. 4.1. Genevieve's Major Depressive Disorder (MDD) timeline (yoa, years of age; mos, months).

ADDITIONAL ASSESSMENTS REQUIRED

Medical Consultation

A thorough assessment of MDD should always involve a physical examination to determine potential physiological factors that may be causing or exacerbating the client's condition, such as thyroid problems, infections, toxic chemical levels, liver disease, cancer, or vitamin and mineral deficiencies. Such an evaluation is doubly important when a client is either taking or wishing to take psychotropic medication.

Self-Report Instruments

There are numerous self-report instruments for depression. Any measures selected should be practical, relevant, in common use, reliable, valid, and consistent with case conceptualization, treatment plan, and goals. Both symptomatic assessment and cognitive–behavioral assessment are presented in the following sections.

Symptom Measures

Depression Symptoms. The Beck Depression Inventory: Second Edition (BDI–II; Beck, Steer, & Brown, 1996) is one of the most commonly used self-report inventories for assessing depression severity. The BDI–II is a 21-item measure corresponding to the *DSM–IV* symptoms of depression. Each item is rated from 0 to 3, and completion time is approximately 5 minutes. Scoring and interpretation involves totaling the item scores and comparing the total score to the severity cutoffs in the BDI–II manual (0–13 = minimal; 14–19 = mild; 20–28 = moderate; 29–63 = severe). The BDI–II demonstrates good internal consistency with coefficient alphas of .93 and test–retest stability over 1 week ($r = .93$, $p < .001$). Discriminant and construct validity have been demonstrated with higher correlations between the BDI–II and depression measures than between the BDI–II and anxiety measures (see Beck et al., 1996, for a review of the psychometric properties of the BDI–II).

Other frequently used self-report measures of depression severity include the Hamilton Depression Inventory (HDI; Reynolds & Koback, 1995), the Center for Epidemiological Studies Depression Scale (CESD; Radloff, 1977), and the Minnesota Multiphasic Personality Inventory: Second Edition (MMPI–II) Depression Subscale (Graham, 1993).

Suicidal Ideation. Suicidal ideation is the most dangerous symptom of depression, and no self-report instrument can substitute for a careful interview assessment of suicidality. One instrument that can be used to augment the clinical assessment is the Beck Hopelessness Scale (BHS; Beck & Steer, 1993). The BHS is a 21-item true or false self-report inventory for measuring the extent of negative attitudes about the future. Completion time is about 5 minutes and its internal consistency (KR-20 = .82–.93) and test–retest reliability (r = .69, $p < .001$) are good. Although the BHS is highly correlated with the BDI ($r = .51–.64$, $p < .001$) for MDD patients, it is a better predictor of suicidal ideation and intent than depression measures. Scoring involves coding the items in the direction of hopelessness (true = 1, false = 0), reverse scoring items in the direction of hopefulness (true = 0, false = 1; items 1, 3, 5, 6, 8, 10, 13, 15, and 19), and summing the scores. Interpretation guidelines suggest that clients with scores exceeding 9 are at significant risk for suicidal ideation or intent.

Overall Psychiatric Symptoms. Because depression is often comorbid with other mental health problems, a standardized assessment of overall psychological distress enhances a comprehensive assessment of the client's psychological functioning. The Brief Symptom Inventory (BSI; Derogatis, 1993) is a frequently used 53-item instrument derived from the longer SCL–90, with items rated from 0 (not at all) to 4 (extremely). The BSI takes approximately 8 to 10 minutes to complete and yields nine subscale scores (Somatization, Obsessive–Compulsive, Interpersonal Sensitivity, Depression, Anxiety, Hostility, Phobic Anxiety, Paranoid Ideation, and Psychoticism) as well as summary scores such as the Global Severity Index (GSI). Scoring and interpretation involve computing averages for subscale items and comparing averages with appropriate t-test scores in the BSI Manual (Derogatis, 1993). Although reliability and validity analyses for the subscales are typically within acceptable ranges, the GSI is more stable (test–retest reliability, $r = .90$) and consistently discriminates between psychiatric and normal populations. These findings suggest the BSI may be a better measure of overall distress than of specific symptomatology.

Cognitive Behavioral Measures

According to Beck's (1979) widely supported cognitive–behavioral therapy (CBT) for depression, there are two primary components in the cause and maintenance of depressive symptoms: behavioral inactivity and dysfunctional cognitions. These dimensions are central to CBT conceptualization and treatment planning.

Behavioral Symptoms. The Mood-Related Pleasant Events Schedule (MRPES; MacPhillamy & Lewinsohn, 1982) is a 49-item instrument designed to evaluate the frequency (0 = not within past 30 days; 1 = one to six times in the past 30 days, and 2 = seven or more times in the past 30 days) and enjoyment

(0 = not pleasant; 1 = somewhat pleasant; 2 = very pleasant) of a list of mood-related activities such as "being in the country" or "having a lively talk." Completion time is approximately 10 minutes. Enjoyment and frequency averages are computed by summing and dividing by the number of items completed. Product scores are computed by multiplying each item's frequency score by its corresponding enjoyment score, summing the results, and dividing by the number of items endorsed. Scores may then be compared to normative scores of nondepressed subjects (Women: frequency $M = 1.37$, $SD = 0.25$; enjoyment $M = 1.54$, $SD = 0.26$, and product $M = 2.18$, $SD = 0.59$. Men: frequency $M = 1.31$, $SD = 0.27$; enjoyment $M = 1.47$, $SD = 0.29$, and product $M = 2.06$, $SD = 0.63$) or used to assess pre- to postchange in activity level.

Cognitive Symptoms. The Automatic Thought Questionnaire (ATQ; Hollon & Kendall, 1980) is designed to assess the frequency of depressogenic automatic thoughts. It is composed of 30 items such as "I can't finish anything" and "I can't stand this anymore" rated from 1 (not at all) to 5 (all the time). Scoring and interpretation involves summing the scores and comparing totals to scores for a depressed sample ($M = 79.64$, $SD = 22.29$) or a nondepressed sample ($M = 48.57$, $SD = 10.89$). Internal consistency is good, with an alpha coefficient of .97 and the ATQ significantly discriminates between depressed and nondepressed subjects.

CASE ILLUSTRATION: GENEVIEVE

Genevieve is a 44-year-old divorced, retired, master's-level computer programmer for a large company. Through a combination of fortuitous investments, generous company stock options, and frugal living, Genevieve has actualized a personal dream of early retirement at age 42. Her teenage son has recently moved out. Genevieve phoned the clinic for help with "a lifelong struggle with depression" when she read about the clinic services in the newspaper.

Presenting Complaints

During the intake interview, Genevieve presented with emotional, physical, behavioral, and cognitive concerns. She reported feeling very sad, empty, and apathetic for the previous 2 months. She noted that the sadness "comes and goes," but the feelings of interminable "emptiness" and ennui had been constant. She expressed "welcoming the sadness" because "at least I am feeling something."

Physically and behaviorally, Genevieve reported sleeping 12 hours a day, eating at least a third more than she usually did, gaining 12 pounds in the previous 2 months, and feeling "leaden." She described her sensation as "moving and talking through molasses." As a result, she had curtailed nearly all of her previously satisfying activities. Prior to this depressive episode, she had been active in theater, volunteer work, and training for a triathalon. She reported that over the previous 2 months she had gradually lost contact with all but one friend, was regularly canceling her volunteer work, and had not exercised once. She had neglected basic housework and yard maintenance, and reported more frequent arguments with family members.

Cognitively, her most troubling symptom was intermittent suicidal ideation. She reported that, over the previous 2 months, she had thought about suicide at least once weekly, although in the previous 2 weeks had been thinking about it daily. She denied having any plan or intent, but was very distressed that she was having these thoughts. Genevieve also reported anxiety and worry over the stability and adequacy of her relationships with her male partner and her son. When questioned, Genevieve either directly stated or implied that her beliefs about herself, others, and the world were negatively toned. Some of her most salient beliefs about herself were that she was unworthy of love and that she had to be perfect at all times to prevent the loss of affection from others. With regard to her closest relationships, she described believing that their love would dissipate as soon as her achievement diminished. She characterized the world as being unfair and unforgiving.

History of the Disorder

Genevieve described herself as a "cyclic depressive." Although she denied any manic episodes, she described four previous episodes of depression that coincided with difficult times in her life (see Fig. 4.1 for a timeline).

- *Episode 1, age 15*: Her first episode was at age 15, when her parents were considering divorce, her "soul-mate" had broken up with her, and both her mother and grandmother were hospitalized for suicidal depression. She said that after 2 months her mood and activities returned to her previous level, but her view of the world was never really "back to normal." She stated that her perfectionism solidified and that she continued to feel that she had to "earn the love of others."
- *Episode 2, age 20*: Genevieve's second episode began soon after her marriage to a man she was dating in college. She had just completed 2 years of college, and she and her husband moved to a small town to support his recent promotion. As a result, Genevieve transferred to a new college and lost many of the credits she had worked for. She was greatly distressed by the contrast between her husband's advancing success and her setback. She was bothered by thoughts that of an "unfair world," in which women

were expected to give up everything to follow their husbands. She also despaired about the emotional distance between her and her new husband. She described him as emotionally and sexually unresponsive. She had thoughts of suicide but no serious thoughts of attempting to kill herself. Through talking to a counselor in the college counseling center and increased involvement in classes and school activities, Genevieve gradually improved her mood over a period of 6 months

- *Episode 3, age 23*: It was 6 months after the birth of Genevieve's son that she lapsed into her third and most severe depressive episode. She had decided to take a year out of school to be with her new son and was now having mixed feelings about her choice. She feared that she was ineffectual as a parent and did not deserve to have this helpless infant dependent on her. Her husband continued to be absent much of the time as his prestige in his company grew. His success further accentuated her concerns that she was getting behind by taking time out of school. She reported that this was the first time she was convinced that she might be better off dead. She was so concerned about her suicidal thoughts that she self-referred for psychiatric hospitalization, in which she was treated with imipramine and released 3 weeks later. She stated that the imipramine was moderately helpful, although she experienced some side effects that eventually led her to terminate the medication 6 months later when her depression remitted. At that time, she returned to school and completed her undergraduate degree in mathematics. Although she did not have another full-blown depressive episode until her 30s, she reports that she continued to question her worth and competence.

- *Episode 4, age 32*: Genevieve's most recent previous depressive episode was during her divorce and custody battle, during which she vacillated between intense anger and morbid depression. She reported daily passive suicidal thoughts although no plan or actual intent. Her thoughts were dominated by emptiness, unworthiness, incompetence, and hopelessness. She began treatment with Prozac during this time and stated that the result was a "miracle." For the first time ever, she felt great. All of her depressive symptoms remitted within 3 months She continued on Prozac until 2 years ago, when she learned that her inability to have an orgasm was due to the medication. After discontinuing Prozac, she began Wellbutrin, which did not have the sexual side effects, but also did not have comparable antidepressant effects.

- *Current episode*: Genevieve's current episode was precipitated by relationship problems with her boyfriend and frequent arguments with her son about his current depression. The current episode had been ongoing for 1 month before she sought treatment. The primary problems with her boyfriend have been sexual. She said that all she wanted to do was have

TABLE 4.2
Genevieve's Self-Report Scores and Interpretations at Intake

Measure	Raw Score	Interpretation
BDI–II	34.0	Severe range
BSI GSI	2.9	t-score $= 70$, 98th percentile[a]
MRPES		
Frequency	0.9	1.9 SD below mean[b]
Enjoyment	1.1	1.7 SD below mean[b]
Product	1.0	2 SD below mean[b]
ATQ	83.0	Within 1 SD of the mean[c]

Note.
[a] For psychiatric outpatient women (Derogatis, 1993).
[b] For nondepressed women (MacPhillamy & Lewinsohn, 1982).
[c] For depressed subjects (Hollon & Kendall, 1980).

a "normal sexual relationship with someone!" Her ex-husband had no interest in sex, her previous boyfriend had been impotent, and her current boyfriend has had erectile dysfunction in their recent attempts at intercourse. She relayed these incidents with tearfulness and desperation. She expressed fear that her lack of a normal sex life reflected a fundamental flaw in her. These problems were exacerbated by a recent rift in her relationship with her son. She relayed a pivotal conversation in which the son had said he was going to stay away from her because of her "malignant influence." (See Table 4.2 for Genevieve's intake scores on the self-report instruments.)

Medical History

Genevieve's medical history was unremarkable. She reported that she had been in good health all her life. She denied significant illnesses or surgeries, stating that her only health concern was the recurrent depression and the side effects from the psychotropic medication. Her only current medication was Wellbutrin. She reported drinking 1 to 2 glasses of wine per week and taking over-the-counter vitamins.

Family History

Genevieve described her childhood as "happy, but pressured." She was the middle of three children and reported that both parents and siblings had advanced academic degrees and professional occupations in business and the arts. Although she remembered many happy times of family togetherness, she also noted that her father had a "dark side." She said that his temper was unpredictable and caustic. He would stay angry for several days and "everyone would walk on eggshells" to try to avoid his wrath. Although Genevieve and her mother rarely fought, they rarely talked either. Genevieve says that she grew up with a vague feeling that nothing she could do would be enough, and that she had nothing offer anyone.

Regarding her family's mental health history, Genevieve reported that both her mother and maternal grandmother had suffered from intermittent depression that often involved significant suicidal ideation. Genevieve's first MDD episode at age 15 was precipitated by the simultaneous psychiatric hospitalization of her mother and grandmother for suicidal depression. Genevieve's 19-year-old son had also experienced at least one episode of MDD. On her father's side of the family, an uncle and aunt had both died in their 50s of liver disease due to alcoholism.

Sexual History

Genevieve reported no history of sexual abuse or rape. She had her first sexual relationship with a boyfriend at age 16. She reported that this was the first and last relationship in which sexual experiences were consistently mutually satisfying. She described her husband as "asexual." According to her report, he had little interest in sex and she rarely had an orgasm when they had sex. She denied any extramarital affairs. In her relationships following her divorce, she also had difficulty in her sexual relationships. Her previous boyfriend had been unable to achieve or maintain an erection during their 5-year relationship, and her current boyfriend also had intermittent difficulties maintaining an erection for intercourse. These problems were exacerbated by Genevieve's own past difficulties in having an orgasm due to her Prozac side effects. Although Genevieve's orgasmic potential returned after discontinuing the Prozac, she continued to have beliefs that her failed sexual relationships were due to a fundamental flaw in her.

Mental Status Examination

Genevieve was well groomed, alert, and cooperative at intake. Her reported and observed mood was depressed (e.g., stooped shoulders, frequent tearfulness, down-turned mouth); her affect was restricted (i.e., limited to sadness and depression), and her speech and physical movements were markedly slow. Although she reported subjective difficulties with concentration and memory, no objective deficits were noted in the intake session. Genevieve was oriented to person, place, and time, and conducted serial 7s (i.e., subtracting 7 from 100 and resultant sums five times) without error. Her memory for recent and remote events appeared to be intact as she recounted her depression history in detail. No hallucinations or delusions were observed or reported. Although Genevieve reported some extreme beliefs about herself (e.g., I am empty and worthless), others (e.g., Others will not come through for me), and the world (e.g., The world is unfair and unforgiving), she was amenable to the possibility that they may be false. Her thought processes were goal-directed and detail oriented. Genevieve was aware of her depression and demonstrated good insight into solutions. According to her report, it was more difficult for her to make good judgments about social and familial relationships when depressed.

Prior Treatment

Genevieve had participated in both counseling and pharmacotherapy for her MDD. She reported being significantly helped by supportive counseling during her second episode of depression. In her third episode of depression, the primary intervention was imipramine. She reported that although it was helpful in alleviating her depressive symptoms, the side effects were too troubling to continue the medication over the long term. Pharmacologically, she reported the most benefit from Prozac during her fourth episode of depression, although the sexual side effects were prohibitive for maintenance on this medication. Her most recent intervention was Wellbutrin. She stated that it was about "half" as helpful as the Prozac for her depressed mood and sleep and energy disturbance, but because she did not have the sexual side effects she felt it was a better pharmacological solution for her depression than the Prozac.

DIAGNOSTIC ASSESSMENT

DSM–IV Diagnosis

Axis I:	296.32	Major Depressive Disorder, recurrent, moderate
	V61.20	Parent–Child Relational Problem
	V61.1	Partner Relational Problem
Axis II:	V71.09	No Diagnosis
Axis III:		Client is in good health with no significant medical conditions
Axis IV:		Problems with primary support group (son and boyfriend) and social environment (lack of social contact)
Axis V:		GAF = 50 (at intake)

Justification and Differential Diagnosis

Genevieve has experienced the following symptoms most of the day nearly every day for the previous month: depressed mood, reduced interest in previously enjoyed activities, hypersomnia, increased appetite and weight gain, fatigue, feelings of worthlessness, difficulty concentrating, psychomotor retardation, and daily thoughts of suicide. She reported four previous episodes also meeting full MDD criteria with full interepisode recovery. None of her depressive episodes had been precipitated by substance use or medical problems. Dysthymic Disorder and Bipolar Disorder were ruled out because her depressive symptoms had never lasted 2 years and she had no history of manic or hypomanic episodes. Although her depressive episodes were typically preceded by difficult situations, they did not involve the death of a loved one or traumatic events, ruling out Bereavement and PTSD. Because her symptoms and impairment were limited to the depressive episodes, GAD and Axis II disorders were also ruled out.

BEHAVIORAL ASSESSMENT

A central purpose of behavioral assessment is to increase understanding of the contextual factors that are maintaining the client's concerns. According to behavioral theory, the events that immediately precede and follow the target behaviors may be instrumental in their maintenance. The method of assessing a behavior's environmental context is known as functional analysis. The basic goals of a functional analysis are to gather information about overt, covert, and external events that increase and decrease the probability that an individual's behaviors will occur. For depressive behaviors, a functional analysis aims to assess antecedents that are likely to set the stage for a depressive reaction and the consequences that either strengthen or weaken the depressive response.

Functional Analytic Interview

Behavioral Targets

The first step in a functional analysis (FA) is to identify the covert (emotional, cognitive, physical) and overt (behavioral) targets for change. For Genevieve, her most disturbing covert experiences were feelings of emptiness (emotional) and thoughts of suicide (cognitive). She identified her most salient overt behavioral targets as inactivity and arguments with her son. She pointed to reducing her thoughts of suicide as the most pressing initial goal; therefore, the target in the following example is suicidal thoughts. (See Fig. 4.2 for Genevieve's functional analysis of her depressive behaviors.)

Antecedents

The second step in an FA is to identify the covert, overt, and environmental events that tend precede the targets. Information about antecedents may be

Genevieve's Functional Analysis

Behavioral Target	Antecedents	Exacerbating Factors (Reinforcers)	Consequences	
			Mitigating Factors (Punishers)	
Thoughts of suicide (covert)	**Covert** • emotional: despair, anger • cognitive: *I will never be normal. Things will never improve.* • physical: psychomotor retardation **Overt** • Sitting alone in darkened room **External** • Argument with son • Failed sexual encounter with boyfriend	**Covert** • cognitive: *I am bad for having these thoughts. This means I am going to end up in another downward spiral. I am just so worthless!* **Overt** • Sitting alone **External** • When people do not call to check on her	**Covert** • cognitive: I have done some worthwhile things in my life, even if I am not perfect. **Overt** • Calling for help, going for a walk* **External** • When people call to apologize or attempt to make amends	
Feelings of emptiness above an "8" on a scale of (0-10) (covert)	**Covert** • emotional: unable to feel any pleasure (anhedonia) • cognitive: *There is something fundamentally wrong with me. I would be better off dead* **Overt** • Being alone **External** • Argument with anyone • Lying in bed after partner had gone to sleep • Friends canceling social dates	**Covert** • cognitive: *I am truly flawed! I should be able to feel emotions like a normal person. I am unworthy of love.* **Overt** • Inactivity	**Covert** • cognitive: "It is normal for people to feel depressed once in a while". "I don't have to be perfectly responsive at all times" **Overt** • Calling a friend* • Getting out of the house* • Writing in journal* **External** • Friend calls to set up time to get together	
Inactivity (overt)	**Covert** • emotional: depressed mood over a "6" • cognitive: *I am just too tired to do anything. I would not enjoy or be successful at anything I did anyway* • physical: low energy **Overt** • Stay in bed, hit the snooze alarm • Unscheduled days • Staying in pajamas • Turning on the TV before breakfast	**Covert** • cognitive: *I haven't accomplished anything today, there is no use in trying at this point. This is just one more sign that I am getting more depressed* **Overt** • Going back to bed after breakfast • Keeping the TV on, channel surfing	**Covert** • cognitive: *OK! Get up do something! You know you will feel better.* **Overt** • Turning off the TV* • Staying out of bed* • Making plans for the day* • Getting dressed before breakfast* **External** • People calling to make plans with me	
Arguments with son (overt)	**Covert** • emotional: anger, guilt • cognitive: *I am an inadequate mother. He should appreciate all my efforts. He should not blame me for his mistakes. He should be nicer to me.* • physical: agitation **Overt** • Talking to son about his future **External** • Son making negative statements about her mothering*	**Covert** • cognitive: *I have failed! I am truly inadequate. All my son's problems are my fault.* **Overt** • Raising voice, trying to convince son I am good enough **External** • Son continues to put her down	**Covert** • cognitive: *I have done the best I can. No parent is perfect. He is going to have to take some responsibility for his happiness* **Overt** • Ending the conversation • Calling a friend to talk about it. **External** • When son calls to apologize	

* Factors identified by client as pivotal in preceding or following the target behavior

FIG. 4.2. Genevieve's functional analysis of depressive behaviors form.

collected on either (a) depressive behaviors as they usually occur or (b) a recent, specific depressive behavior. The former is likely to provide information about the client's theories about causes for their depression; the latter may provide more concrete information about a specific episode. Both are important in developing hypotheses about treatment and both should be assessed. For Genevieve, the assessment of antecedents proceeded as follows:

Therapist: Now Genevieve, I would like to get a better understanding of what is going on inside of you and outside of you when you get to feeling more depressed, and in particular when you have thoughts of suicide. This will be very helpful in helping you and I decide on a treatment direction.

Client: Okay. [Tentatively]

Therapist: First, I would like to ask you about what usually happens when you get so depressed that you have suicidal thoughts. Can you tell me how you are usually feeling before you begin to have suicidal thoughts?

Client: Absolute despair. I feel utterly hopeless that my life will ever improve! [Crying]

Therapist: So having suicidal thoughts is really the bottom of the barrel for you? [Client: Um, uh.] I really appreciate your willingness to answer some of these questions. I believe that through this work we are doing right now, we will get information that may help us figure out ways to reduce these thoughts.

Client: [Wiping eyes and nodding] Yes, I do believe this will be helpful, it is just difficult to think about this.

Therapist: Okay, so what kinds of thoughts tend to be going through your mind right before you think about killing yourself?

Client: It is just that I will never ever be normal and that nothing is ever going to work out for me.

Therapist: How about inside your body, how are you generally feeling before you begin to feel so depressed that you think about killing yourself?

Client: I am not sure, I just feel absolutely leaden. Like any movement would just be an impossible effort.

Therapist: What are you usually doing when you generally begin to think of suicide?

Client: I am usually sitting at home alone on the couch.

Therapist: Are there any types of events or situations that often precede your thoughts of killing yourself?

Client:	That is difficult; the situations all seem so different. Sometimes it is an argument with my son; sometimes it is a failed sexual encounter with my boyfriend; sometimes it is just me being alone, thinking I will always be alone.
Therapist:	Even though these events are different, do you have any thoughts about themes that might tie them together?
Client:	Well, I guess the theme that contributes to much of my feeling depressed is feeling that I have fundamentally failed and that no amount of anything I can do will make it right again.
Therapist:	Okay! This is very helpful for me in thinking about how we might choose to proceed. Now, let's talk about a specific time recently in which you were having suicidal thoughts and felt very depressed. What was the most recent time you had suicidal thoughts?
Client:	(deep breath) Well, I was thinking that my whole family might be better off without me yesterday.
Therapist:	Would you be okay with us using that as an example to get a better understanding of your depressed moods?
Client:	Yes, that would be fine. At least I can remember more about it since it was just yesterday.

Genevieve goes on to report that the primary covert events preceding her most recent suicidal thoughts were despair, anger, thoughts of hopelessness and failure, and feelings of restlessness. The primary overt event was pacing alone in the darkened living room after an external event of having a tearful conversation with her son in which he told her that she was the reason he was "so screwed up."

Consequences

The third step in an FA is to evaluate what internal and external events follow the target that either increase or decrease the probability that the depressive behavior will occur again. In traditional behavioral language, consequences that increase the target are called *reinforcers* and consequences that reduce the target are called *punishers*. It should be noted, however, that reinforcers are not always positive and punishers are not always negative. For example, a spanking may reinforce a child's acting-out behavior because if provides attention, even if it is not positive. Instead, the key issue is whether the consequence increases or decreases the probability that the behavior will occur again. In this chapter to avoid confusion between colloquial and technical definitions of reinforcement and punishment, the term *exacerbating consequences* is used in place of reinforcement and the term *mitigating consequences* is used in place of punishment.

For Genevieve, both exacerbating and mitigating consequences were assessed. See the following transcript:

Therapist: So, now that we have a good idea of what situations tend to come before you start having suicidal thoughts, let's take a look at what tends to happen after you start thinking this way.

Client: I think it is going to be difficult to separate out before and after, because everything just seems to run together.

Therapist: Many people describe just that sensation, that everything is a big blob. I think if we can get a bit more specific about just a few things, we can get a better understanding of what makes your depression better and worse.

Client: Okay, I'm willing to try.

Therapist: Let's start by looking your suicidal thoughts in general. Can you tell me about what you think or do that seems to make them worse?

Client: Wow! They always seem to get worse when they start. I guess I usually focus on how hopeless everything is and bad it is that I am having these thoughts again.

Therapist: And what are you usually doing that makes the thoughts worse?

Client: I guess I just sit there and let the thoughts take over. I don't do anything.

Therapist: What about other people; is there anything that anyone else does that makes the thoughts worse?

Client: Not really. I guess the only thing is that when no one calls to see how I am, I just assume I am right that I would be better off dead.

Therapist: Now, I know you said that the thoughts always get worse when they start; has there ever been a time that you have been able to stop the thoughts before they spiraled down? Is there anything that you can do to make the thoughts less severe or frequent?

Client: There have been a few times that I have not gotten to feeling a lot worse. Last night is at least a partial example. After I had sat for an hour or two, I just decided that I had to do something or I would end up in the hospital again. That was the ultimate humiliation. I never want to end up there again. So, I called you and set up an appointment. Then I went for a walk. I was able to think of a few reasons to live. When I got back, my son also apologized for what he said to me. That helped too.

> *Therapist:* So calling someone to talk to, getting yourself out of the house, and thinking about reasons to live rather than reasons to die seemed to make a positive difference for you?
>
> *Client:* Yes, this time it did. There have been a few other times that I have been able to pull myself out of feeling really low by just telling myself to "buck up" or getting myself moving.

The third type of consequences that should be assessed in an FA interview involves what negative consequences the client is able to avoid by the target behaviors. In this case, what is traditionally defined as *negative reinforcement* is termed *secondary gain*. Assessing how a client benefits from being in utter despair can be quite tricky, and the therapist should always be aware that clients are doing the best they can with the knowledge and skills they have. Typically, the best you can do early on in your relationship with your client is to develop some hypotheses through asking some of the following questions:

- How does your depression affect others around you?
- Is there anything you used to do before you were depressed that you have been unable to do since becoming depressed?
- How do people around you begin to act differently when you start to feeling less depressed?

It should be noted that the FA interview is based primarily on the client's perceptions of what precedes and follows their behavior. It has been well established that retrospective perceptions tend to have little relationship to objective observations. Although this discrepancy may be partly due to the fact that the client has exclusive access to internal information not visible to the outside observer, it is also likely that the time that elapses between target events and the interview further blurs the recall of the functional components. Because objective behavioral observation with outpatient adults is cumbersome and invasive, it is rarely used in the assessment of adult MDD. Instead, self-monitoring is typically used as an alternative.

Self-Monitoring

Self-monitoring refers to the client's daily recording of covert and overt experiences of depression as well as the events that precede and follow these experiences. This "in-time" monitoring circumvents some of the problems inherent in retrospective reports and affords the client–therapist team a number of advantages, such as (a) providing tentative tests to the hypotheses developed in the functional analyses; (b) increasing client awareness of mood variation, antecedents, and consequences; (c) increasing client mastery over mood and monitoring; and (d) providing an indirect measure of client compliance that may help to assess readiness to change.

Behavioral Targets

Target behaviors are commonly self-monitored along three dimensions: frequency, intensity, and duration. Behaviors that have a distinct beginning and end may be measured in terms of frequency (e.g., times walked around the block). Behaviors that vary in valence across occurrences and have no clear beginning and end (e.g., depressed mood) should be assessed in terms of intensity. Behaviors that vary in duration (e.g., arguments) should also be monitored along this dimension.

Beginning at intake, Genevieve self-monitored the following behaviors: overall depressed mood (average daily intensity from $0 =$ no depression whatsoever to $10 =$ the most depressed she can imagine feeling); feelings of emptiness (average daily intensity); suicidal thoughts (frequency, intensity, and duration); arguments with family (frequency, intensity, and duration). See Figs. 4.3 and 4.4 for Genevieve's monitoring forms.

Antecedents and Consequences

To test the hypotheses developed in the initial interview as well as increase the client's awareness of triggers and environmental variables, antecedents and consequences may also be self-monitored. The key issue is to identify a discrete behavior that cues the client to focus on what preceded and followed that behavior. Intermittent behaviors can be identified by their occurrence, whereas continuous behaviors can be identified by crossing a relevant threshold. For example, Genevieve's suicidal thoughts are intermittent. Thus, each time a suicidal thought occurred, she would write down (a) emotional, cognitive, physical, behavioral, and environmental events that immediately preceded it; (b) events that immediately followed the thought; and (c) her rating of the role of each of the antecedents and consequences in the suicidal thoughts. For her feelings of emptiness, she could track the antecedents and consequences when the feelings cross a threshold of 8 (on a scale of $0 =$ no feelings of emptiness to $10 =$ feeling utterly and completely empty).

CASE CONCEPTUALIZATION

The case conceptualization consolidates the information gained in the interview and assessment phase into cohesive hypotheses about cause, maintenance, and intervention. The premise here is that the most important information for

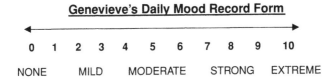

Genevieve's Daily Mood Record Form

0	1	2	3	4	5	6	7	8	9	10

NONE   MILD   MODERATE   STRONG   EXTREME

1. Using the scale above, rate your general level of DEPRESSION (D) and EMPTINESS (E) at the end of each day.

2. This rating is based on how you felt on average over the course of each day.

3. If you didn't feel a bit DEPRESSED or EMPTY mark 0.

4. If you felt really DEPRESSED or EMPTY (the worst you have ever felt or can imagine yourself feeling), mark 10.

5. If it was "so-so" mark 5.

	Mon		Tues		Wed		Thurs		Fri		Sat		Sun		Average	
Date																
Depressed (D) Empty (E)	D	E	D	E	D	E	D	E	D	E	D	E	D	E	D	E
Week 1																
Week 2																
Week 3																
Week 4																
Week 5																
Week 6																
Week 7																
Week 8																
Week 9																
Week 10																
Week 11																
Week 12																
Week 13																
Week 14																

FIG. 4.3. Genevieve's daily mood record form.

designing interventions is a thorough understanding of the remote and recent context of the depressive behaviors.

The concept of what actually causes a problem is elusive. It can never be truly known or tested. Nevertheless, developing hypotheses about how the past or a remote context may influence the current behavior may be pivotal for choosing interventions and therapy foci. All aspects of the biopsychosocial assessment are relevant for understanding this historical context. The following six areas are addressed for Genevieve: learning and modeling, significant life events, genetic factors, physical factors, substances, and sociocultural factors.

Genevieve's Frequency, Intensity & Duration Form

Please indicate the intensity and duration of YOUR ARGUMENTS WITH SON and SUICIDAL THOUGHTS each time they happens over the next WEEK.

ARGUMENTS WITH SON

	Example										Summary
Date	8/23/99										Total Frequency
Time	10:00										
Intensity (0–10)	7										Average Intensity
Duration (Min)	10 min										Average Duration

SUICIDAL THOUGHTS

	Example										Summary
Date	8/23/99										Total Frequency
Time	10:00										
Intensity (0–10)	7										Average Intensity
Duration (Min)	10 min										Average Duration

FIG. 4.4.   Genevieve's frequency, intensity, and duration form.

Modeling and Learning

Genevieve may have learned some of her depressive behaviors through operant conditioning and modeling. Although Genevieve reported that most of her social interactions were impaired while depressed, she also noted that some of her most satisfying human contact came from her friends and family expressing their concern and support. Thus, she may have been intermittently reinforced for feeling depressed. She may have also have been punished by her father for directly expressing her anger and directed it inward instead. His unpredictable outrage and her mother's unavailability may have initiated some of her fears that she is flawed. Finally, she may have modeled the depressive behaviors demonstrated by her mother and grandmother.

Significant Life Events

Genevieve has had several life events that may have influenced her beliefs that she is unworthy, unlovable, and flawed. Her mother and grandmother's simultaneous hospitalization that precipitated her first depression may have increased her fears of abandonment and being doomed to a flawed life. Her unhappy marriage and later divorce may have reinforced some of her beliefs that she is unworthy and unlovable. Likewise, her recent sexual problems and conflict with her son have further exacerbated her beliefs that she is flawed.

Genetics and Temperament

Genevieve's mother, grandmother, and son have all experienced MDD. This suggests that a genetic factor is at least a partial cause, although it is difficult to discern the extent to which her genetic and environmental heritage have interacted over time.

Physical Conditions

According to Genevieve and her physician's report, Genevieve has no current or past significant physical problems. Thus, these are an unlikely cause for her depression.

Drugs

Genevieve's only current prescription medication is Wellbutrin. Although she believes this medication has a positive effect on her depression, she notes her past Prozac use caused positive (depression relief) and negative effects (inability to have an orgasm). She states that although her ability to have an orgasm returned, her alarming thinking about her sexuality has persisted.

Genevieve drinks 1–2 glasses of wine a week and denies any other use of over-the-counter, prescription, or illegal drugs.

Socioeconomic and Cultural Factors

Genevieve is a white, educated, middle-income, middle-age woman. She grew up in a time when values about women's roles conflicted. Although she was educated and had earning power similar to her husband, societal pressures to stay in the home with her young child precipitated at least one of her depressive episodes. Similarly, the competition that colored her relationship with her husband may also have been rooted in conflicts about appropriate roles for women.

It appears that a number of factors may have been involved in the development of the beliefs and behaviors that characterize Genevieve's current depression.

The most researched and supported interventions for depression, such as CBT, are based in the assumption that the search for a cause is less important than knowledge of the factors that are maintaining the depressed mood. CBT theorists argue that even though the depression may have deep roots in past experiences, the most effective way to resolve the depression is through the current manifestations of past experiences in the form of beliefs and behaviors. Within CBT theory, dysfunctional beliefs and a reduction in satisfying pleasurable and mastery activities are common maintenance factors for depression. The functional analysis is vital in developing hypotheses about conditions that are keeping the depression going.

Genevieve has identified both behavioral and cognitive antecedents and consequences that are important in the maintenance of her depressed mood (see Fig. 4.3). In particular, she notes that her thoughts of being flawed, unworthy, or a failure tend to precede feeling depressed and worsen any depression she might already be feeling. In contrast, more moderate cognitions and increased activity appear to be instrumental in alleviating the depressed mood. Although these suppositions are based in the client's perceptions of the contingencies surrounding her depressed mood, they help to begin generating hypotheses about how to proceed with treatment.

Prioritization of Targets for Treatment

Prioritization of treatment targets should be a collaborative process between client and therapist that addresses client preferences, urgency, and the functional analysis. Genevieve's primary overall goal was to reduce her depressed mood. Subgoals within the overall goal were to reduce her suicidal ideation, feelings of emptiness, and inactivity. Her secondary concerns were to improve her relationships with her son and boyfriend. Her primary goal of depression reduction was targeted because it met all three criteria: the client preferred it, the suicidal ideation and discomfort made it urgent, and the functional analysis suggested that the depression was fueling if not causing the secondary concerns.

Selection of Treatment Strategies

Selection of treatment strategies should flow naturally from the case conceptualization about cause and maintenance while taking into account the following issues: empirical evidence, fit with client problems, client preferences, and therapist competence.

Empirically Supported Treatments for MDD. There are two primary psychosocial treatments for MDD that meet the APA Guidelines for empirically supported treatments (Nathan & Gorman, 1998): Cognitive–Behavioral Therapy (CBT) and Interpersonal Therapy (IPT). Beck, Rush, Shaw, and Emery (1979) developed CBT, the most extensively researched psychosocial treatment for depression. It is based in the idea that dysfunctional beliefs about self, others, and the world cause and maintain depressed mood. Treatment is designed to last 14–20 sessions and it involves three basic components: symptom reduction through increasing pleasurable and mastery activities (sessions 1–3), identifying and challenging logical errors in automatic thoughts (sessions 4–10), and identifying and rewriting core schema (sessions 9–16). Sessions are structured with collaborative agenda setting, didactic education, Socratic questioning, and weekly homework assignments.

The more recent development of IPT (Klerman, Weissman, Rounsaville, & Chevron, 1995), a 14–16 session individual therapy with somewhat different goals than CBT, focuses on the identification and resolution of the client's difficulties in interpersonal functioning related to the current MDD. Targets for intervention include unresolved grief, interpersonal disputes, role transitions, and social skills training.

Efficacy research suggests that CBT and IPT are largely comparable in overall outcome. Both lead to recovery in 53% to 83% of clients with MDD (Nathan & Gorman, 1998). Although little research has addressed the question of how to choose between the two, one study found that MDD clients with lower levels of depressogenic cognitions actually responded preferentially to CBT, whereas those with lower levels of social dysfunction responded better to IPT (Sotsky et al., 1991). These findings point to a "capitalization hypothesis," which poses that building on strengths is more effective than targeting weaknesses.

There is some controversy about the additive benefits of combining psychosocial interventions with psychopharmacological interventions. Comparisons between combined and monotherapies are inconsistent. Some researchers found that medication adds nothing to CBT; other research shows that medication deters long-term outcome for CBT; and still other researchers found that medication adds to CBT, especially for severely depressed patients (see Thase et al., 1997, for a review). Although clearly more research is needed to address this question, the trend across all these studies is that clients who are severely depressed tend to benefit more from combined therapies.

Client Preferences. In a discussion of treatment options, Genevieve expressed a preference for a CBT approach in combination with her ongoing Wellbutrin. As noted previously, she conceptualized her depression as having been maintained more by dysfunctional cognitions than relationship events. Although she admitted that relationship problems could be triggers for depressed mood, she believed that her beliefs played a more important role. Her pretherapy awareness of her beliefs and their role in her functioning also suggested that she might already have some mastery in this area on which one might build.

Therapist Competence. Therapists should have adequate competence in conducting any treatment they implement. Minimal competency requirements for any treatment modality include formal training and supervised experience. Therapists who do not meet these requirements should either get training and supervised experience or refer the client to a therapist who is competent to conduct the treatment.

Priority of Treatment Strategies

The following issues should be considered in prioritizing treatment strategies: the prioritization of target problems, the functional assessment, client preferences, and feasibility.

Together with her therapist, Genevieve developed the treatment plan with prioritized goals, assessments and interventions (Fig. 4.5). Genevieve's highest priority was to reduce her depression and the associated suicidal thoughts. Because the FA pointed to cognition as being more strongly related to these thoughts than activity level, she opted for beginning with work on automatic thoughts rather than increasing activities. Therefore, the therapeutic interventions were planned to begin with identifying and challenging automatic thoughts (sessions 1–4; see Table 4.3), followed by increasing activity level and monitoring automatic thoughts (sessions 5–10; see Table 4.4 and Fig. 4.6). In the final sessions her core beliefs would be addressed (sessions 11–13; see Table 4.5) followed by relapse prevention (Session 14; see Table 4.6).

Feasibility is a significant concern with managed care limitations on mental health care benefits. When a client's sessions are limited, potent

Genevieve's Treatment Plan

Client Name:	Date:
Genevieve Anyname (pseudonym)	5/5/99

Primary Concern:
Depressed mood, feelings of emptiness, lack of interest in pleasurable or mastery activities, suicidal ideation, sleeping 12+ hrs/night, eating 1/3 more than usual with a 12 lb. weight gain, difficulty concentrating on leisure or volunteer work.

Secondary Concerns:
1. Increased arguments with 19 year-old son, especially regarding his depression.
2. Increased arguments with boyfriend, especially regarding their sexual relationship.

Prioritized Goals:
1. Reduce depressed mood from the severe range (BDI-II = 34) to the minimal range (BDI-II < 13).
   a. Reduce suicidal ideation from an intake baseline of 7/week to 0/week.
   b. Reduce feelings of emptiness from an intake daily average subjective rating of 8 (0 = none, 10 = the most imaginable) to a 3.
   c. Increase pleasurable activities from an intake baseline of 3/week to 14/week.
   d. Increase mastery activities from an intake baseline of 3/week to 14/week
2. Reduce frequency of arguments with son from 3/week to 1/week
3. Increase frequency of positive interactions with boyfriend regarding sex from 0/week to 1/week.

Interventions (corresponding goals in parentheses)
1. Identify and challenge alarming automatic thoughts regarding self, others & the world (1, 1a, 2 & 3)
2. Increase activity level through goal-setting and reward (1, 1c & 1d)
3. Identify and challenge core beliefs regarding emptiness (1, 1b, 2, 3)

Referrals (medication, physical, assessment, other counseling provider, etc.)
1. Referral to primary care physician for a physical examination to rule-out organic causes
2. Collaborate with psychiatrist regarding continued Wellbutrin use.

Measurement of Each Goal	Schedule
1. BDI-II	Weekly
BSI GSI	Monthly
a. self-monitoring of frequency of suicidal ideation	Daily
b. self-monitoring of intensity of emptiness (0 = none, 10 = the most imaginable)	Daily
c. self-monitoring of frequency of pleasurable activities	Daily
d. self-monitoring of frequency of mastery activities	Daily
2. Self-monitoring of frequency of arguments with son	Daily
3. Self-monitoring of frequency of positive interactions with boyfriend	Daily

Client Strengths and Obstacles
Strengths: Client is intelligent, aware of connections between mood, behavior & thought, motivated for change and has had previous success in improving her mood.

Obstacles: Client is concerned that her core beliefs have been so long standing that they will not be changeable

Prioritized Summary and Time Frame
Total estimated treatment duration: 14 sessions (Sessions 1-5 Automatic Thoughts; Sessions 6-10 Behavioral Activation; Sessions 11-13 Core Beliefs; Session 14 Relapse Prevention)

Client Signature	Date	Therapist Signature	Date

FIG. 4.5. Genevieve's treatment plan.

interventions for symptom relief should be conducted first and the proposed treatment should fit within the sessions allotted. Because Genevieve's health insurance covered 20 mental health sessions a year, the proposed treatment plan targeted both early symptom relief and a step-by-step plan designed to be complete in 14 sessions.

TABLE 4.3
Objectives and Strategies for Automatic Thought (AT) Interventions

AT Objectives	AT Strategies	Session

Increase awareness of environmental triggers for depressed mood.	1. Therapist introduces the Automatic Thought Record (ATR; see Fig. 4.6)
	2. Therapist describes Activating Events (i.e., anything that triggers depressed mood)
	3. Therapist describes Consequences
	  a. Physical
	  b. Emotional (rated 0–10)
	  c. Behavioral
	4. Therapist models completion of the ATR columns Activating Events (A) and Consequences (C)
	5. Client practices columns A and C in session on situation in which they "got themselves more depressed than they wanted to be"
	6. Client practices columns A and C three times at home
		1

Increase awareness of the role of thinking in depressed mood.	1. Therapist introduces Beliefs (B) column
	  a. Predictions—what you expect to happen
	  b. Labels—one word generalizations for self, others, and the world
	  c. Standards—musts, have to's, shoulds, needs for self, others, and the world
	2. Therapist models completion of columns A, B, and C for previous example
	3. Therapist draws connection between extreme beliefs and extreme consequences
	4. Client practices columns A, B, and C on situation in which they "got themselves more depressed than they wanted to be"
	5. Client practices A, B, and C at home three times
		2–3

Identify alarming thoughts related to depressed mood.	1. Therapist identifies, circles, and labels beliefs from own example that represent the alarming beliefs (e.g., all-or-nothing thinking, extreme words, catastrophizing, mind-reading, overgeneralization, rigid standards) 2. Client identifies, circles, and labels beliefs from own example that represent the alarming beliefs	2–3

Learn to challenge alarming thoughts with more moderate, realistic helpful beliefs.	1. Therapist introduces the Disputation (D) and Effects (E) columns
	  a. Goal is to develop more moderate, realistic, and helpful alternative beliefs
	  b. Goal is to have additional perspectives to choose from.
	2. Therapist challenges beliefs in own example
	3. Client challenges beliefs in own example
	4. Client completes columns A, B, C, D, and E at home three times
		4–5

TABLE 4.4

Objectives and Strategies for Behavioral Activation (BA) Interventions

BA Objectives	BA Strategies	Session

Identify pleasurable and mastery activities	1. Therapist introduces BA rationale and downward spiral
	2. Client generates a list of 25 potentially pleasurable activities
	3. Client generates a list of 10 potential mastery activities that would be completed if not depressed
	4. Activities in either category should cover a variety of areas
	  a. Relationships (family, social, intimate)
	  b. Education/employment/career
	  c. Hobbies/recreation
	  d. Volunteer work/charity/political activities
	  e. Physical health issues (diet, sleep, exercise, etc.)
	  f. Spirituality
	  g. Psychological issues (issues other than depression you would like to explore or improve)
	5. Client assesses baseline pleasurable and mastery activity level by assessing daily frequency of items on list
		6

Set goals for increasing pleasurable activity	1. Therapist introduces rationale and procedures for SMART goal setting
	  a. Specific
	  b. Measurable
	  c. Attainable
	  d. Realistic
	  e. Time to check-in
	2. Client sets three SMART pleasurable goals
	3. Client implements pleasurable goals
	4. Client continues to monitor frequency of pleasurable and mastery activities
		7–10

Plan rewards for goal accomplishment	1. Therapist introduces rationale for rewarding goal accomplishment
	2. Client generates a list of rewards that are
	  a. Simple
	  b. Possible
	  c. Pleasurable
	  d. Repeatable
	  e. Non-sabotaging (e.g., spending $300 on dinner when money and weight management are a problem)
		8

Set goals for increasing mastery activities	1. Therapist reviews rationale and procedures for goal setting 2. Client sets three SMART mastery goals 3. Client sets a reward for accomplishment of each goal 4. Client implements mastery goals and rewards self 5. Client continues to monitor frequency of pleasurable and mastery activities	8–10

HOW DO WE GET OURSELVES DEPRESSED??

Directions: When you notice your mood changing, ask **What's going through my mind right now?** and quickly jot down any thought or image in the Belief Column.

Date/Time	Activating Event — Describe events or thoughts that happened right before you started to feel more depressed.	Beliefs or Automatic Thoughts — 1. Write automatic thoughts that precede emotions.	Consequences — What was your response to the activating event?	Disputation / Alternative Response — Write response to automatic thoughts, using the questions at the bottom of this form.	Effects — Re-rate your consequences after alternative thoughts
		2. Predictions (What are you predicting for the future?)	Physical (What was going on in your body?)	Predictions	Physical (What was going on in your body?)
		Labels (What words are you using to summarize yourself, others and the situation?)	Emotional (How did you feel? Rate from 0-10)	Labels	Emotional (How did you feel? Rate from 0-10)
		Standards (What shoulds, musts, have-tos are you applying?)	Behavioral (what did you do?)	Standards	Behavioral (what did you do?)

Questions to help compose an alternative response: (1) What is the evidence that the automatic thought is true? Not true? (2) Is there an alternative explanation? (3) What's the worst that could happen? Could I live through it? What's the best that could happen? What's the most realistic outcome? (4) What's the effect of my believing the automatic thought? What could be the effect of changing my thinking? (5) What would I like to do about it? (6) If _____ (friend's name) was in this situation and had this thought, what would I tell him/her? (7) What's a more reasonable and helpful way to view this situation?

FIG. 4.6. Automatic thought record form.

TABLE 4.5
Objectives and Strategies for Core Belief (CB) Interventions

CB Objectives	CB Strategies	Session
Education about role of core beliefs in mood	1. Therapist introduces rationale for role of core beliefs in mood and automatic thought 2. Therapist introduces rationale for identifying and modifying core beliefs in preventing relapse	11

Identify core beliefs	1. Therapist introduces two methods for identifying core beliefs
	  a. Examining automatic thoughts for themes
	  b. Downward arrow
	2. Client identifies core beliefs by examining automatic thoughts for themes (Beck et al., 1979)
	  a. In order to be happy, I have to be successful in whatever I undertake
	  b. To be happy, I must be accepted by all people at all times
	  c. If I make a mistake, it means that I am inept or incompetent
	  d. I can't live without you (a particular person)
	  e. If somebody disagrees with me, it means that person doesn't like me
	  f. My value as a person depends on what other people think of me
	3. Client identifies core beliefs through serial downward arrow questioning of automatic thoughts
	  a. Why would this be so upsetting for you?
	  b. What is the meaning of this for you?
		11–12

Challenge core beliefs	1. Client uses challenging beliefs worksheet to challenge core beliefs
	2. Client evaluates pros and cons of holding the core belief and answers the following questions:
	  a. How is this belief affecting how you feel?
	  b. How is feeling this way affecting your life?
	  c. Are you gaining anything from holding this belief?
	  d. Are you losing anything from holding this belief?
	  e. Are you losing more than you are gaining?
	3. Client conducts behavioral experiments to challenge beliefs
	  a. Behaving opposite to belief and assessing outcome
	  b. Collects evidence to challenge belief
		12–13

Dealing with Complicating Factors

Although any variety of factors can complicate the treatment of MDD, three common complications include difficulty with treatment compliance, managing suicidal ideation, and prioritizing treatments with comorbid diagnoses.

Homework Compliance. MDD is characterized by its low interest, low energy, hopelessness, and general pessimism. Thus, the very symptoms that are treatment targets may interfere with homework completion. Therapists should anticipate and plan for some of these difficulties. First, the homework rationale should be thorough and well integrated into the other therapy material with an

TABLE 4.6
Objectives and Strategies for Relapse Prevention (RP) Interventions

RP Objectives	RP Strategies	Session
Education about relapse vs. lapse	1. Therapist introduces rationale for relapse prevention 　a. The less prepared, the more likely that relapse will occur 　b. People with more than three episodes of depression have a 90% chance than depression will recur 2. Therapist introduces relapse as a process, not a discrete event 　a. A lapse is a "slip-up"—feeling depressed for a few days 　b. A relapse is giving in to the slip-up and accepting depression as inevitable 　c. A lapse or a relapse is a learning experience rather than a failure	14
Identify high-risk triggers for depression	1. Client identifies potential triggers for depressed mood in the future through the following: 　a. Identifying past precipitants for depression 　b. Noting present triggers for feeling more depressed 　c. Predicting known and anticipated future events that may precipitate depressed mood 2. Client lists the anticipated triggers and the elements that would be pivotal 3. Client lists early warning signs that they are getting more depressed	
Increase coping skill with high-risk situations	1. Client lists coping skills for each element of the anticipated triggers considering behavioral and cognitive skills 2. Therapist and client practice coping with triggers through the following: 　a. Role-play 　b. Guided imagery	
Reduce harm of relapse	1. Client develops a list of "lessons learned" from past and current episodes 2. Client develops a list of beliefs that facilitate learning from a future lapse 3. Client develops a plan for how future lapses will be handled	

emphasis on the potential benefits of homework completion. Clients who understand that completing a daily mood record may increase their awareness of depression triggers and may even inadvertently improve their mood are more likely to complete the assignment than the client who is simply handed the daily mood record and asked to complete it. Second, the homework assignments should be realistic and specific. It is important to begin with something that the client is almost certain to have success with before increasing the quantity of homework. Third, behavior that is reinforced is likely to occur again; behavior that is punished is likely to be extinguished. The therapist should take time at the beginning of the session to review clients' homework and reinforce their efforts. Errors should be taken as opportunities for learning rather than occasion for punishment, however subtle. When a client does not complete the homework, the therapist can take session time for the client to complete that assignment. Fourth, helping the client to schedule a time each day for homework may also enhance participation. Fifth, a client's investment in completing work outside the session may be increased through designing assignments collaboratively with the client. If a client does not believe that an assignment is going to be helpful, the therapist may invite client revisions that would increase its helpfulness. Finally, treating skepticism as a hypothesis to be tested may help the client be willing to take the risk and engage in the assignment.

Suicidal Ideation. Suicidal ideation is frequently part of a client's symptom profile. Both client safety and modification of suicidal beliefs should be given treatment priority. Ensuring client safety involves initial and ongoing assessment as well as a safety contract. If a client has experienced current or past suicidal ideation while depressed, a verbal check-in should be made weekly. Because all clients with MDD are at risk for developing suicidal ideation, weekly screening instruments such as item 9 on the BDI–II (0 = I don't have any thoughts of killing myself; 1 = I have thoughts of killing myself, but I would not carry them out; 2 = I would like to kill myself; 3 = I would kill myself if I had the chance) should be reviewed. A written safety contract should also be established with any client who is having more than passive thoughts of dying. Contents of the safety contract would typically include the following:

- a promise to not hurt self
- a promise to follow the steps in the safety contract (e.g., calling a friend, engaging in a distracting activity, calling the therapist, calling the crisis hotline, taking themselves to the hospital)
- signatures by client and therapist

Suicidal beliefs should also be addressed as a goal for change and a topic for therapy. Genevieve's suicidal beliefs were addressed directly by targeting them as activating events for depressive feelings and depressive beliefs. Depressive beliefs elicited by suicidal ideation included: "I will never be normal"; "I am headed for another downward spiral"; and " I am just so worthless, I should be dead." Alternative beliefs were developed in much the same manner as for other alarming thoughts. Alternatives were: "I am in the habit of feeling depressed and having suicidal thoughts"; "Habits can be changed"; and "I have had successes and failures like most people, this does not mean that I deserve death."

Comorbid Diagnoses. MDD commonly co-occurs with other present-ing problems such as dementia, panic disorder, phobias, GAD, PTSD, eating disorders, and relationship problems. Such comorbidity can pose significant challenges for treatment planning. Prioritization of treatment goals and strate-gies may be facilitated through examination of the FA, the client's preferences, and the interaction of the symptoms across disorders. If, for example, a client meets criteria for both Panic Disorder and MDD and the FA points to thoughts of worthlessness being the primary trigger for panic attacks, MDD may be a priority for treatment. If, however, the client has restricted most pleasurable and mastery activities due to a fear of panic attacks, reducing the panic at-tacks would be the priority. Second, any successful intervention requires client "buy-in." Therefore, the client's conceptualization of their concerns is impor-tant to treatment choices with comorbid conditions. If the client believes that the depression is responsible for the panic attacks, the therapist should con-sider trying depression interventions first. Third, treatment decisions should take into account how the symptoms of one condition affect the treatment of the other condition. A client with both panic and depression who is unable to engage in depression treatment (e.g., pleasurable or mastery activities) be-cause of panic attacks, may benefit from a reduction in panic before depression interventions are implemented.

Role of Pharmacotherapy in the Case

Depression treatment often involves the concomitant use of antidepressant medication and psychotherapy. Although the data are conflicting on its additive benefit, the trends do appear to support combined therapy, especially for more severe MDD (cf. Nathan & Gorman, 1998).

Decision making regarding referrals for antidepressant medication should take into account the following factors: client preferences, previous success with medication, severity, and lack of success with psychotherapy alone. First and foremost, the client's preferences should be assessed and considered in treatment planning. If a client desires a medication referral and it is not con-traindicated, it should be considered. Likewise, if a client is adamantly opposed to medication, nonpharmacotherapeutic options should be explored. Similarly, if a client has had previous success with medication and wishes to take med-ication again, a referral would be in order. Finally, depression severity and response to psychotherapy should be considered. A client who is severely depressed or has significant suicidal ideation should always be considered for a medication adjunct to psychotherapy for two basic reasons. First, there is some evidence to support that medication may enhance therapy outcome for severely depressed clients (cf. Nathan & Gorman, 1998). Second, because some clients respond better to medication and other patients respond better to psychotherapy, the severely impaired client should be given the best possible chance of experiencing an effective therapy as soon as possible. Also, a client who is not responding to psychotherapy alone should be coached on the potential benefits of adding a psychotropic intervention to treatment.

Therapists who work with clients taking psychotropic medications can increase the probability that the client will benefit from the combined therapy by collaborating regularly with the prescribing physician, helping the client be an educated consumer, and addressing the client's attributions about the source of therapeutic gain. Collaboration with a client's physician can be helpful for learning when to refer for medication, how to aid in enhancing medication compliance, and how to facilitate tapering off of psychotropic medication. Therapists can also help their clients get more information about the effects and side effects of their medications and encourage and support clients in taking the initiative to discuss their concerns with their physicians. In addition, therapists can be aware of and probe for information about the client's change attributions. A client who attributes all of their gains to medication has a higher risk of relapse than a client who takes some responsibility for the therapeutic gain (Kavanaugh & Wilson, 1989). The therapist may work with the client to reframe and challenge these external attributions and beliefs of helplessness.

Managed Care Considerations

Providing compassionate and effective care for MDD within a managed care environment necessitates special attention to the client's needs as well as attention to the managed care requirements.

Working with Clients in Managed Care. A client often has had a combination of bad experiences and alarming beliefs about managed care that can impede treatment. It is important that the therapist minimize any hardship to the client while openly addressing any beliefs that may interfere with therapy.

To minimize any negative impact, the therapist must be knowledgeable about a client's managed care parameters, understand the limits of confidentiality, collaboratively design a treatment plan within these parameters, and ensure the client understands how managed care limitations will be addressed. Therapists can increase their knowledge of a client's managed care issues through education by the client and direct contact with the managed care organization. Any limits to sessions, benefits, or confidentiality must be discussed promptly and clearly so that the client can make informed decisions about their mental health care. Therapists must also be aware of and abide by any documentation requirements and ensure that treatment planning take any insurance limitations into account. Because insurance coverage for sessions is often limited, it is vital the client's most pressing concerns are addressed first. Finally, therapists have a responsibility to inform the client of their policies regarding session limits, advocacy, pro bono work, and fees for their services.

Above all, therapists should never abandon clients during a crisis, regardless of reimbursement limits.

Clients' previous managed care experiences combined with a depressogenic thinking style may lead to beliefs about managed care with themes of helplessness (e.g., "I have no control over my health care"; "I am trapped in a system that doesn't care about me") and hopelessness (e.g., "No one will be able to help me"; "I will never get enough sessions to really help me"). The therapist can address these beliefs in much the same was as any alarming belief in therapy through direct challenges, experiments, and behavioral changes. Therapists' awareness of their own beliefs about managed care are also important. Therapists who communicate (however subtly) that managed care is an abysmal arrangement reinforce these beliefs in clients. Instead, therapists should convey positive expectancies and optimism. Consider the potential results of the following therapist responses to learning about an eight-session limit for insurance coverage.

Therapist A: Eight sessions? Well, Okay. We'll do what we can in that time. It's not ideal. We may be able to begin addressing your first goal, but I don't think we are going to be able to get at the stuff that's really keeping this depression going.

Therapist B: Excellent! We can do some very good work in eight sessions! This will challenge us to work hard and stay focused. Let's set some specific goals for each of our sessions so that we can map out our work together.

Therapist C: Eight sessions? Wow! It seems like the limits just keep getting shorter and shorter. I would really like to have more time to work with you, but I think we are kind of stuck with what your insurance company says.

Therapists A and C have inadvertently reinforced the client's hopelessness and helplessness beliefs, respectively, whereas Therapist B has potentially set the stage for one of the most salient features in therapy effectiveness—the client's positive expectancies.

Working with Managed Care Organizations. Managed care organizations are charged with providing the best possible care to the greatest number of people for the least cost. Within mental health care, this has lead to some basic assumptions

- The primary problem is the symptom
- Symptom relief is the goal
- Selected treatments should target symptoms and have empirical support

- Client progress should be closely monitored
- Step-care models provide the most ethical and cost-effective treatment planning

Therapists working with MDD clients in managed care situations should target the observable and/or measurable symptoms of depression in their treatment goals (e.g., inactivity, sleep changes, weight changes) as well as the observable results of depression symptoms (e.g., decreased work performance due to difficulty concentrating, increased arguments with spouse due to feelings of hopelessness, reduced social contact due to anhedonia). Treatment should then be related directly to the goals and have research to support its effectiveness. Two good choices for depression are cognitive–behavioral therapy (CBT) and interpersonal therapy. Both have significant research support and both target symptom relief. The client's progress must then be monitored regularly with reliable, valid, relevant, and commonly used weekly measures of depression (e.g., BDI–II), and monthly overall measures of psychiatric symptomatology (e.g., BSI).

Perhaps the greatest challenge for contemporary therapists is creativity. Weekly sessions with an individual therapist may not be the best fit for all clients. Some clients may do the best with more frequent shorter sessions or less frequent longer sessions. Other clients may generalize the new information most effectively when they attend two or three weekly sessions followed by a month hiatus to apply the new skills. Still other clients may benefit from other interventions with comparable outcomes to individual therapy, such as group therapy (McRoberts, Burlingame, & Hoag, 1998) or bibliotherapy (Cuijpers, 1997). One service delivery model that is consistent with both managed care and client needs is the step-care model. The basic tenets are as follows:

- Treatment involves time, cost, and risk to the client
- Ethical treatment minimizes time, cost, and risk
- Services should be available at various intensities
- The least intrusive intervention likely to have significant benefit should be tried first
- Treatment intensity is increased when lower level treatment is ineffective

SUMMARY

Major Depressive Disorder is a common and debilitating psychological concern. Accurate diagnosis, biopsychosocial assessment, and a functional analysis of depressive behaviors are central to developing a case conceptualization that involves hypotheses about the cause, maintenance, and interventions. The treatment plan should then flow from these hypotheses and include specific goals, assessments, and interventions. The primary factors in prioritizing goals and interventions are the client's safety, the client's preferences, empirical literature, and feasibility issues. These form the trunk and branches of the decision tree. Therapists have a professional and ethical responsibility to help clients address the goals they are seeking help for as well as to provide therapy that is efficacious and feasible. Within a managed care environment, feasibility often equals brevity. Therefore, therapists should be prepared to help clients prioritize their concerns effectively and then provide brief empirically supported interventions. Additional research on tailoring manualized treatments to individual clients and the role of medication in psychotherapy will also augment treatment planning.

REFERENCES

American Psychiatric Association. (1994). *Diagnostic and statistical manual of mental disorders—4th Ed.* Washington, DC: Author.

Bakish, D. (1999). The patient with comorbid depression and anxiety: The unmet need. *Journal of Clinical Psychiatry, 60(Suppl 6)*, 20–24.

Beck, A. T., Rush, A. J., Shaw, B. F., & Emery, G. (1979). *Cognitive therapy of depression.* New York: Guilford Press.

Beck, A. T., & Steer, R. A. (1993). *Manual for the Beck Hopelessness Scale.* San Antonio: The Psychological Corporation.

Beck, A. T., Steer, R. A., & Brown, G. K. (1996). *Manual for the Beck Depression Inventory: 2nd Edition.* San Antonio: The Psychological Corporation.

Burns, D. D., & Eidelson, R. J. (1998). Why are depression and anxiety correlated? A test of the tripartite model. *Journal of Consulting & Clinical Psychology, 66*, 461–473.

Cuijpers, P. (1997). Bibliotherapy in unipolar depression: A meta-analysis. *Journal of Behavior Therapy & Experimental Psychiatry, 28*, 139–147.

Derogatis, L. R. (1993). *Administration, scoring and procedures manual for the Brief Symptom Inventory.* Minneapolis: National Computer Systems.

First, M. B., Spitzer, R. L., Gibbon, M., & Williams, J. B. W. (1997). *User's guide for the Structured Clinical Interview for DSM–IV Axis I Disorders–Clinician Version (SCID–CV).* Washington, DC: American Psychiatric Press.

Graham, J. R. (1993). *MMPI–2: Assessing personality and psychopathology: Second Edition.* New York: Oxford University Press.

Kavanagh, D. L., & Wilson, P. H. (1989). Prediction of outcome with group cognitive therapy for depression. *Behaviour Research and Therapy, 27*, 333–343.

Klerman, G. L., Weissman, M. M., Rounsaville, B., & Chevron, E. S. (1995). Interpersonal psychotherapy for depression. *Journal of Psychotherapy Practice & Research, 4*, 342–351.

Hollon, S. D., & Kendall, P. C. (1980). Cognitive self-statements in depression: Development of an automatic thoughts questionnaire. *Cognitive Therapy & Research, 4*, 383–395.

MacPhillamy, D. J., & Lewinsohn, P. M. (1982). The Pleasant Events Schedule: Studies on reliability and validity and scale intercorrelation. *Journal of Consulting and Clinical Psychology, 50*, 363–380.

McRoberts, C., Burlingame, G. M., & Hoag, M. J. (1998). Comparative efficacy of individual and group psychotherapy: A meta-analytic perspective. *Group Dynamics, 2*, 101–117.

Nathan, P. E., & Gorman, J. M. (Eds.) (1998). *A guide to treatments that work.* New York: Oxford University Press.

Radloff, L. S. (1977). The CES-D Scale: A self-report depression scale for research in the general population. *Applied Psychological Measurement, 1*, 385–401.

Reynolds, W. M., & Kobak, K. A. (1995). Reliability and validity of the Hamilton Depression Inventory: A paper-and-pencil version of the Hamilton Depression Rating Scale Clinical Interview. *Psychological Assessment, 7*, 472–483.

Sotsky, S. M., Glass, D. R., Shea, M. T., Pilkonis, P. A., Collins, J. F., & Elkin, I. (1991). Patient predictors of response to psychotherapy and pharmacotherapy: Findings in the NIMH Treatment of Depression Collaborative Research Program. *American Journal of Psychiatry, 148*, 997–1008.

Thase, M. E., Greenhouse, J. B., Frank, E., Reynolds, C. F. III, Pilkonis, P. A., & Hurley, P. A. (1997). Treatment of major depression with psychotherapy or psychotherapy–pharmacotherapy combinations. *Archives of General Psychiatry, 54*, 1009–1015.

5

Panic and Agoraphobia

Andrew J. Baillie
and Ronald M. Rapee
Macquarie University

DESCRIPTION OF THE DISORDER

Panic Disorder and Agoraphobia are characterized by a fear of anxiety and its consequences. These disorders share four elements that are present to varying degrees in all cases:

- *Panic attacks* are sudden attacks or spells of fear, anxiety, or uneasiness accompanied by strong physical sensations and a fear of death, losing control, and/or going crazy. Physical sensations include a racing or pounding heart, shortness of breath, choking, trembling, shaking, a dry mouth, depersonalization, derealization, dizziness, light-headedness, sweating, tightness or pain in the chest, nausea or discomfort in the stomach, numbness or tingling sensations, and hot flushes or chills. Attacks can be completely unexpected, more likely in feared situations, or occur only in the presence of feared stimuli. Attacks that are completely unexpected are the essential feature of Panic Disorder. Panic-like peaks of anxiety involving less than four of the symptoms listed previously are called *limited symptom attacks.*
- *Situational fears or phobias* involve fear and avoidance of situations from which escape may be difficult or help cannot easily be reached in the event of anxiety and are a feature of Agoraphobia. Feared situations typically include crowds; standing in a line; being away from home alone; crossing bridges; travelling by car, bus, or train; and shopping centers.

Agoraphobia without Panic Disorder is the diagnosis given when the typical Agoraphobic pattern of avoidance occurs in a person who has never experienced a full panic attack. Instead, people with this condition typically experience peaks of anxiety that are not technically panic attacks, but may be limited symptom attacks.

In addition, more subtle behaviors intended to reduce the perceived danger may also develop: for example, carrying a mobile phone to call for help in the event of a panic attack or carrying a bottle of water to prevent choking from a dry mouth.

- *Fear and avoidance of sensations* that are similar to those experienced in anxiety or panic attacks is also common. For example, physical exercise may be avoided because it produces a pounding heart and sweating; getting into a car that has been parked in the hot sun may be avoided because it may produce sensations similar to a hot flush and difficulty breathing. Drinking alcohol may be avoided because alcohol may produce sensations that are interpreted as being out of control.

- *Anticipatory anxiety.* Anxiety in anticipation of a future event is a common feature. Persistent worries about when the next attack might occur or worries that an attack might lead to something catastrophic are required for a diagnosis of Panic Disorder. When situational fears and phobias are present, these are often anticipated fearfully.

Epidemiology

It is estimated that 15% of the adult U.S. population will experience a panic attack at some time in their lives, 3.5% will experience Panic Disorder during their life, and 1.5% will currently meet criteria for this disorder (Eaton, Kessler, Wittchen, & Magee, 1994). Agoraphobia effects 6.7% of the adult U.S. population at some time in their life, and 2.3% currently have this disorder (Magee, Eaton, Wittchen, McGonagle, & Kessler, 1996).

Panic Disorder can occur in children and adolescents, but is usually much less frequent than in adults. This is a slightly controversial issue, and several papers have been devoted to the question of whether Panic Disorder can be diagnosed at all in prepubescent children. However, there is little doubt that Panic Disorder is relatively infrequent in children prior to puberty and increases in frequency after that. Even in adolescents it is a relatively low frequency disorder, and high levels of Panic Disorder really do not appear until late adolescence to early adulthood. When Panic Disorder presents in younger people, it is very similar in form to that found in adults. The main difference is usually a stronger focus on the somatic symptoms, with less-focused and clearly verbalized fears, especially in younger adolescents. For example, fears of death and heart disease typically found in adults with Panic Disorder (see later) are often not as clearly articulated in younger people, and these fears are more likely to be reported as vague feelings of impending doom.

Sex, employment, income, and education are associated with different rates of Panic Disorder and Agoraphobia. Panic Disorder and Agoraphobia are more common in women. Panic Attacks can begin at a number of points in the lifespan from the late teens to the 40s. Students and those who work in the home are more likely to suffer Panic Disorder and Agoraphobia. Eaton et al. (1994) report that those with lower educational levels but not lower income are more likely to suffer Panic Disorder. Both lower educational level and lower income are related to higher rates of Agoraphobia (Eaton et al., 1994; Magee et al., 1996).

The disturbing physical sensations experienced in panic attacks bring sufferers into contact with health services at a greater rate than other mental disorders. The challenge for health services is to diagnose panic attacks correctly rather than wasting health resources on unnecessary investigations.

Panic Disorder and Agoraphobia are not trivial conditions; they often cause substantial disruptions to the lives of sufferers and their families. The World Health Organization (WHO) and the World Bank have recently estimated that Panic Disorder is the 32nd most burdensome of all health problems in the developed world, contributing 0.6% of disability and years of life lost due to all health problems.

Typical Cognitive–Behavioral Therapy Formulations

Why do people who experience Panic Disorder continue to believe they are in danger during an attack when the consequences they fear do not occur? Despite their fears, people do not die, go crazy, or lose control of themselves in panic attacks. A cognitive theory of Panic Disorder, such as that developed by David M. Clark (1999), proposes that catastrophic misinterpretations, attentional biases, and safety behaviors are the maintaining factors in Panic Disorder.

People with Panic Disorder misinterpret symptoms of anxiety as an indication that their fear is about to happen. A pounding heart is interpreted as a sign of imminent heart attack and death. When an attack does not eventuate, the sufferer is more likely to make an attribution that maintains their fear: "I was lucky that time, but the next time it will happen."

Attentional biases may mean that sensations related to feared outcomes (e.g., feeling light-headed is related to fainting) are more readily noticed and misinterpreted as signs of impending catastrophe. Anecdotally, people with Panic Disorder often report scanning their bodies for any possible sign of an impending attack.

Many people with Panic Disorder take precautions that they believe reduce the likelihood of their feared outcomes. These precautions or safety behaviors may lead to a short-term reduction in anxiety because of such belief. However, the person may also come to believe that the feared outcome would have occurred had they not carried out the safety behavior despite the fact that these feared outcomes seldom occur. In this way, safety behaviors make a feared outcome seem more likely.

The role of safety behaviors in the maintenance of Panic Disorder is clear in the following example. Sally fears vomiting in public place and carries a plastic bag with her. She says the plastic bag would reduce the embarrassment of vomiting in public. However, as Sally has never vomited in public, carrying the bag around may only be serving to convince her that vomiting is a possibility, when it probably is not.

Typical cognitive–behavioral therapy (CBT) formulations of Panic Disorder link continued panic attacks to catastrophic beliefs about the consequences of panic and to actions such as avoidance and other safety behaviors that serve to prevent the disconfirmation of catastrophic beliefs.

For a comprehensive review of theories of Panic Disorder, see McNally (1994).

METHODS TO DETERMINE DIAGNOSIS

A clinical interview is the main tool in the diagnosis of Panic Disorder and/or Agoraphobia. Typically, information gathered in a clinical interview is used for diagnosis and functional analysis or formulation of the client's problems. In this section, we focus on information required for diagnosis and leave formulation to the following section.

The task in a diagnostic interview is to find the diagnosis that best fits the client's problems and rule out alternative explanations. For a diagnosis of Panic Disorder, the clinician is looking for evidence of panic attacks and for fear of these attacks as a maintaining factor. Information about avoidance and fear of specific situations is needed for a diagnosis of Agoraphobia. The clinician is also looking for information that may rule in or out other causes for panic attacks, such as general medical conditions, other anxiety disorders, and other mental disorders.

People suffering with Panic Disorder usually focus on their experiences of panic attacks. General opening questions such as, "What has brought you here today?" usually elicit a description of episodic physical sensations. Establishing whether these experiences meet the criteria for a panic attack is the first step. A panic attack begins suddenly, reaches a peak in no more than 10 minutes, and involves 4 or more of the list of 13 symptoms given in the *DSM–IV*.

A slow build-up of anxiety that reaches a peak over more than 10 minutes is not technically a panic attack and is often anticipation of a feared situation or event. While a sudden experience of anxiety that involves less than four of the *DSM–IV* symptoms is called a *limited symptom episode*, not a panic attack.

The next step is to inquire about the context of these attacks. Are the attacks completely unexpected? Are they out of proportion to their context? Are the attacks more likely in particular situations?

Establish that the anxiety experienced in the attack is unreasonable or out of proportion to the situation. For example, panic attacks for fear of being assaulted may be in proportion to the actual danger in cases of domestic violence. Fear of particular physical sensations and their consequences may be reasonable in some general medical conditions. For example, fearing loss of bowel control when this actually occurs in those suffering Crohn's disease, or fearing loss of balance when this occurs in Ménière syndrome. Of course, anxiety may play a role in amplifying these disorders, and if this is suspected, a more detailed assessment is required.

A diagnosis of Panic Disorder requires recurrent unexpected panic attacks at some point in the history of the disorder. Many who suffer with Panic Disorder and Agoraphobia no longer have unexpected panic attacks but did so at some time in the past.

Attacks that are expected because they follow a period of worrying about having an attack or worry about the mental or physical consequences of an attack are entirely consistent with a diagnosis of Panic Disorder. A significant change in behavior following an attack may also be evidence of fear of panic attacks.

Expected panic attacks may be part of Agoraphobia, a Specific Phobia, Social Phobia, or Post Traumatic Stress Disorder. If attacks are restricted to particular places, events, or stimuli then these diagnoses should be considered. Panic attacks that are limited to social situations where the client is the center of attention may provide evidence for a diagnosis of Social Phobia. If attacks occur only in response to memories of traumatic experiences, or are triggered by situations related to trauma, then a diagnosis of Post-Traumatic Stress Disorder (PTSD) should be considered.

If attacks occur in situations in which the client fears that he or she would not be able to escape or help could not easily be obtained, then Agoraphobia may be diagnosed. These situations typically include being outside the home alone, traveling by car or public transport, crossing a bridge, or being in a crowd or queue.

Asking about the worst outcome of a panic attack may assist in differentiating Panic Disorder from other anxiety and mood disorders. To make the distinction between Panic Disorder and/or Agoraphobia and Social Phobia, the clinician must consider whether the worst outcome is of embarrassment or humiliation (the social consequences of anxiety) or of the personal physical or mental consequences. For example, Steve fears choking and is concerned about the fuss that would be made if he were to choke during a panic attack

TABLE 5.1
General Medical Conditions That May Cause Panic-like Reactions

Hyperthyroidism
Hypothyroidism
Pheochromocytoma
Fasting hypoglycemia
Hypercortisolism
Mitral valve prolapse
Caffeine, cocaine, amphetamine, or other stimulant intoxication
Alcohol, sedative, or hypnotic withdrawal

in a public place. However, he has little fear of choking and little anxiety when he is alone at home. Emma seeks the company of others during anxious times so someone is able to resuscitate her or call for help if she were to choke. Steve may be more likely to suffer from Social Phobia, whereas Emma fears the physical or mental consequences of anxiety, reflecting Panic Disorder.

Panic attacks can occur in the context of Major Depressive Disorder (MDD) without meeting criteria for a diagnosis of Panic Disorder. For example, a depressed person may experience a peak of anxiety when faced with a difficult decision or when reminded of the hopelessness of the future. The key is the focus of the panic. For a diagnosis of Panic Disorder, the fear must be focused on the actual attack and more commonly on feared bodily sensations.

Persons suffering psychotic disorders can experience peaks of anxiety and panic attacks. Again, the key to differential diagnosis is the client's beliefs and fears. Are these beliefs delusional in nature? Is the anxiety in response to a hallucination?

Panic attacks and other peaks of anxiety can occur in the context of general medical conditions (Table 5.1). Most clients have had many medical assessments before consulting a mental health practitioner about panic attacks. However, if there is insufficient evidence for fear as a maintaining factor, it may be useful to consult a medical practitioner to rule these conditions out.

ADDITIONAL ASSESSMENTS REQUIRED

After reaching a diagnosis of Panic Disorder and/or Agoraphobia, the clinician can apply a standard package of cognitive–behavior therapy (such as Barlow & Craske, 1999). However, a more detailed assessment and functional analysis allows the clinician to tailor treatment to the individual by providing a formulation of factors that maintain the client's problems.

Interview

Information gained in a diagnostic interview is a starting point for a formulation. However, more detailed information about antecedents of anxiety; the physical, cognitive, emotional, and behavioral aspects of anxiety; and the consequences of anxiety is required.

Antecedents of Panic Attacks. Although unexpected panic attacks are the hallmark of Panic Disorder, it is usually possible to identity triggers for panic attacks. Situations in which attacks previously occurred, thoughts related to attacks, and sensations similar to those experienced in attacks can trigger attacks. It can be useful to ask the client, "What was the first thing you noticed?" Clients often do not recognize these events as triggers because they are seen as out of proportion to the intensity of the attack.

Physical Aspects of Panic Attacks. In addition to the list of physical sensations required to reach a diagnosis, it is useful to ask the client which sensations they fear the most. Which sensations as the most distressing? These questions may help identify catastrophic fears. For example, Emma is most distressed by butterflies in her stomach and tightness in her throat. These sensations match her fear of death by choking on her own vomit.

Information about the clients' perception of, and response to, these sensations in other contexts such as sports and excitement is useful. Do they fear or avoid activities that might normally be expected to bring on similar sensations? Are they scanning or monitoring their bodies for these sensations?

Behavioral Aspects of Panic Attacks. How do clients act in an attack? Are they able to remain in the situation or continue the activity they were involved in when the attack began? What do they do to handle the attack? What makes attacks easier—"Having a friend or relative come with you?" In the search for safety or rescue behaviors it is useful to ask, "What makes it easier to be in that situation?" or "What do you do to help yourself cope in that situation?"

Actions taken during panic attacks, such as avoidance and escape, must be assessed because they may prevent the client from getting feedback that would disconfirm their catastrophic beliefs. The client who avoids catching elevators because of fears of suffocation in a panic attack is prevented from finding out that he does not suffocate by this action.

When looking for safety behaviors, remember that the actions taken may be relatively common and benign but the intention may be to protect the client from an impossible or unlikely outcome. Many people carry a cell phone; however, feeling compelled to carry a cell phone in case of being disabled by panic is a safety behavior. A discussion of safety behaviors may lead to questions about anxiety management through the use or abuse drugs and alcohol.

Emotional Aspects of Panic Attacks.   Fear or terror is the predominant emotion described in panic attacks. How distressing and unbearable is an attack? Is the distress in proportion to the catastrophic thoughts identified? If not more careful assessment of beliefs and interpretations is warranted.

Cognitive Aspects of Panic Attacks.   Beliefs, thoughts, and cognitions in panic attacks reflect an inflated probability of anxiety and an inflated cost of anxiety. So those suffering Panic Disorder and/or Agoraphobia believe that panic attacks are more likely to occur and that the attacks have more severe consequences.

Most clients are quickly able to report their catastrophic fears so detailed questioning is seldom needed. Typically, thoughts involve catastrophic events such as death, losing control, or going crazy. There is usually both an inflated probability of anxiety and its feared consequences and an inflated cost to anxiety.

There is usually a consistency among the sensations feared most in an attack, the actions taken to cope with an attack, and the client's catastrophic fears. For example, those nominating tightness in the throat as their most feared sensation are often fearful of choking. Those fearful of going crazy or of having a stroke or brain tumor often nominate depersonalization or derealization. The client who prefers to be a passenger in a car may fear losing control of the car if they were the driver; however, the client who prefers to be the driver may fear being unable to flee from the situation if that were necessary. If clients are unable to report their catastrophic fears, a hypothesis may be generated from information already gained and questions framed to confirm or deny the hypothesis. Sam was fearful of travelling by underground train but found it difficult to describe why. For many years he had spent considerable effort avoiding travelling in closed-in, air-conditioned trains and avoid travelling without a companion to engage in conversation. It is likely that he was also employing cognitive avoidance techniques that worked so well that he was not of aware of any beliefs or thoughts behind his fear. It is likely that Sam's catastrophic thoughts were about not being able to escape or not being able to breathe given his pattern of avoidance. Often catastrophic thoughts become clearer when clients expose themselves to feared situations without distracting themselves.

Catastrophic thoughts are often supported or maintained by other cognitions. The clinician must be on the lookout for thoughts that protect a catastrophic thought from disconfirmation by experience. For example, Emma fears that she would choke and die if she were to vomit in a panic attack. When she experiences anxiety and does not choke (as would be expected), she believes she was simply lucky. In this way experiences that might disconfirm her catastrophic fears are discounted.

Consequences of Panic Attacks. What are the consequences of an attack? Do any voluntary actions after an attack maintain the attacks? For example, retreating to bed after an attack may reflect tiredness from the physical exertion of an attack, but may also reinforce inflated beliefs about the severity of attacks.

Clients often interpret the experience of another panic attack in a negative and self-defeating fashion. These thoughts may lead to low mood and actions that help maintain the cycle of panic. Emma told herself that she was stupid for having another attack, and this reinforced her belief that she was powerless to control attacks. These beliefs made it more likely that she would avoid feared situations.

Additional Information to be Gathered in the Clinical Interview. In addition to assessing the dimensions of anxiety, it is also important to assess the effects of anxiety problems on work, family, and social life; the client's expectations for outcome; previous treatment experiences; and the client's view of what causes his or her problem among other issues that are part of a standard cognitive behavioral assessment.

Self-Report Questionnaires

Self-report questionnaires can be used as another source to support information gathered in the clinical interview and as a yardstick to measure the success of treatment. Bouchard, Pelletier, Gauthier, Cote, and Laberge (1997) give an excellent review of self-report measures.

It is useful to include measures of the key aspects of Panic Disorder and Agoraphobia:

1. Physical symptoms of a panic attack (e.g., Beck Anxiety Inventory, Panic Attack Questionnaire, Bodily Sensations Questionnaire)
2. Fear experienced in and avoidance of situations (e.g., Fear Questionnaire, Mobility Inventory for Agoraphobia, Albany Panic and Phobias Questionnaire)
3. Beliefs about physical sensations, panic attacks, and their consequences (e.g., Agoraphobic Cognitions Questionnaire, Anxiety Sensitivity Index)
4. Vulnerabilities and personality (e.g., Neuroticism via Eysenck Personality Questionnaire, NEO-PI)
5. Disability (e.g., Medical Outcomes Study Short Form-36, or Short Form-12, Sheehan Disability Questionnaire)

Self-report questionnaires can also assess depression, drug and alcohol use, and other comorbid concerns.

CASE ILLUSTRATION

In the remainder of this chapter, we take you through the assessment, formulation, and treatment of Claudia,[1] who suffered from Panic Disorder and Agoraphobia.

Presenting Complaints

Claudia (age 37) was referred by her family physician for attacks of unreality and dizziness that came without warning. Along with these symptoms came a pounding heart, lightheadedness, tingling, numbness, and a fear that she would die. Claudia was convinced that she was experiencing a stroke. She was unable to drive more than a few blocks from her home for fear she would have a stroke, lose consciousness, or crash the car and injure other drivers or her passengers, particularly her children. Family resources were stretched transporting Claudia and her husband Stan's children, Emily (age 8) and John (age 3).

Claudia nominated the problems shown in Table 5.2 as her priorities for treatment.

History of the Disorder

Spells of dizziness and unreality began after the birth of her second child at age 34. Claudia went to her family physician, believing she was having a stroke. All tests were negative and Claudia was told that she "was just stressed" and should get some help to look after her children. Despite this reassurance, Claudia experienced panic attacks between one and six times a month over the next few years.

About 18 months before she was referred for treatment, Claudia's attacks worsened after she read an article in a magazine about "silent strokes." The article included a recommendation to seek urgent medical attention in the event of any unusual symptoms. At this time, her avoidance of driving alone and being away from home increased. In the year before her referral, Claudia had felt increasingly frustrated and hopeless about her continuing problems and the lack of effective help she received.

---

[1]This is not the description of an actual person, but an amalgamation of a number of people who have consulted us over the years. We have done this to protect the confidentiality of our clients.

TABLE 5.2
Claudia's Problem List and Goals for Treatment

Problem	Priority	Goal
Having unexpected panic attacks	1	To stop having panic attacks
Driving alone with the children	2	To be able drive to the local mall and do the weekly shopping
Being unable to take a vacation	4	To drive with the family for a vacation next summer
Feeling low	3	To spend more time with my friends
		To do more things I enjoy

Family History

Claudia said that her family had always described her maternal aunt as "suffering with nerves." She recounted family stories that her maternal grandfather rarely left his farm. Claudia was unaware if either had sought formal treatment.

Mental Status Examination

Claudia was neatly dressed and was oriented to time, person and place. At the beginning of the interview, she had difficulty sitting still and appeared agitated. Later in the interview, she was teary when discussing the effects of her anxiety on her family. The affect displayed in the interview was consistent with the material being discussed. No signs of formal thought disorder were present. Memory and concentration were somewhat reduced.

Prior Treatment

Since her attack began, Claudia had taken a variety of vitamin preparations, including B_{12}, magnesium, and zinc, which were recommended to her for stress. Claudia's family physician started her on fluoxetine 5 months before referral after diagnosing depression. However, she resisted taking medication for 6 months, preferring to rely on her vitamins. The initial effect of fluoxetine was to reduce the intensity of the panic attacks and depression. Claudia reported no further benefits and was skeptical that the medication had done anything. She was sure the initial effects were due to a change in vitamins.

CASE CONCEPTUALIZATION

Modeling and Learning

Claudia reported that her parents had often allowed her to stay home from school if she was sick, whereas "other kids had much meaner parents who would make them go to school." Her mother frequently took Claudia and her brother, Frank, to visit the family doctor "just to be sure" in response to their frequent stomach pains and nausea. It is possible that these experiences influenced Claudia to be wary of unexpected bodily sensations.

Life Events

Claudia gave up work as a teacher before the birth of her first child, Emily, 8 years before referral. This change in Claudia's lifestyle removed most of her social support and left her feeling increasingly lonely and isolated. Panic attacks began after the birth of her second child (John), possibly in response to increased stress and hormonal and physiological changes.

Genetics and Temperament

From the brief information about Claudia's mother's family it seems likely that her maternal grandfather and aunt suffered some kind of anxiety disorder. On the one hand, Claudia described herself as a confident, outgoing, though frequently stressed child; on the other hand, she reports many visits to her doctor for minor stomach complaints. At initial assessment, Claudia scored 20 on the Neuroticism Scale of Eysenck's Personality Questionnaire, suggesting a high level of trait anxiety. Taken together, this information would suggest an anxious temperament.

Socioeconomic and Cultural Factors

Claudia's family was placed under financial pressure when she stopped working before the birth of her first child. Her husband, Stan, compensated by working longer hours to earn more money, but this only increased Claudia's isolation.

Overall Conceptualization

The following formulation or model was developed in collaboration with Claudia (see Figure 5.1).

Problem Development. Claudia was probably vulnerable to some form of anxiety and depression because of her family history and temperament. As a child, she frequently experienced stomach pains and her mother's response to these pains reinforced their seriousness.

Changes in lifestyle following the birth of her children provided Claudia with increased stress and reduced the social support that may have helped her deal with that stress. The hormonal changes associated with the birth of her second child may have lead to an increase in somatic sensations. This, coupled

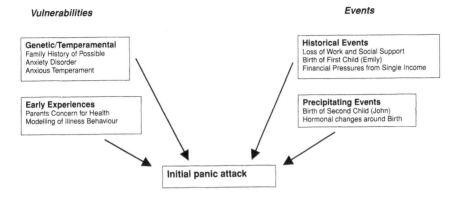

FIG. 5.1.   A formulation of the development of Claudia's problems.

with her psychological vulnerability, may have caused her to interpret these sensations as signs of a stroke and to experience her first panic attack.

Problem Maintenance.   After her first attack, Claudia quickly fell into a pattern of regular panic attacks maintained by (a) her belief that she was experiencing a stroke and would lose control of herself causing injury to others, (b) vigilance for sensations of dizziness, (c) generally heightened arousal, and (d) safety behaviors, such as seeking medical reassurance and avoiding driving.

As her avoidance of driving increased, Claudia's social isolation increased and her panic attacks continued. She became increasingly hopeless about her ability to cope and overcome her problems.

A formulation of the maintenance of Claudia's problems is shown in Fig. 5.2.

Diagnostic Assessment

Axis I	300.21	Panic Disorder with Agoraphobia
	296.21	Major Depressive Disorder, single episode, mild
Axis II	V71.09	No diagnosis or condition on Axis II
Axis III		None
Axis IV		Lack of social support
Axis V	GAF = 42	(Current)
	GAF = 55	(Highest level in previous year)

Behavioral Assessment

A detailed discussion of recent panic attacks and situations that Claudia avoided gave evidence for the formulation described previously. Claudia completed a diary for the week between her first and second sessions. An extract is shown in Table 5.3.

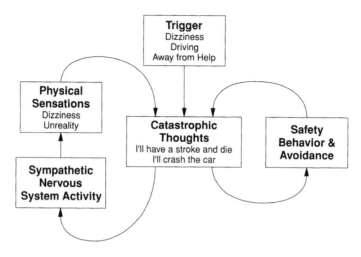

FIG. 5.2.   A formulation of the maintenance of Claudia's problems.

Information from interviews with Claudia and from her diary can be sum-marized as followings. Sensations of dizziness or blurred vision sometimes from changes in posture were triggers for attacks. During these attacks, she believed that she was having a stroke and would die. In response to this fear, her safety behaviors were staying close to her husband (Stan), carrying a cell phone and a list of local doctors' phone numbers in the event of an attack, and driving very slowly. She avoided being alone or away from her family, driving on two-lane roads, driving alone, and stopping at traffic lights. Claudia

TABLE 5.3
An Example of Claudia's Diary From the First Week

Situation	Thoughts (% belief)	Emotion (0–100)	Actions
Friday evening—After relaxing in the bath, I stood up and felt dizzy and my vision was blurry.	I'm relaxed—this can't be a panic attack; it must be a stroke (85%). Lucky Stan is home.	Anxiety 80	Grabbed towel rail to steady myself. Called Stan to help me into bed.
Monday afternoon—Spent all day trying to hype myself up to drive to pick up Emily from school. In the street outside my house I was dizzy.	I'm going to crash the car. I can't control it (70%). I can't make it to the school (89%).	Anxiety 60 Hopeless 80	Pulled over to curb. Sat for 5 minutes. Edged the car back into the garage. Rang the school and Stan's mom (who lives 30 miles away) to ask her to pick Emily up.

described some relief after she fled a feared situation, but this was followed by strong guilt.

Prioritization of Targets for Treatment

From her problem list, Claudia nominated the goals for treatment shown in Table 5.2. The most pressing concerns were reducing her panic attacks and fear of driving. We anticipated that some success toward these goals would lift her mood and, through greater ability to travel, reduce her feelings of isolation and loneliness.

Is it better to focus on panic attacks and then work on phobias? Where the same core fear motivates both panic attacks and phobias, we prefer to tackle both at the same time. Confronting feared situations provides an ideal opportunity to practice dealing with peaks of anxiety and this practice can increase confidence to better handle unexpected attacks.

Selection of Treatment Strategies

The core components of a cognitive–behavioral treatment for Panic Disorder and Agoraphobia are psychoeducation, cognitive restructuring, exposure to feared situations, and exposure to feared sensations. Relaxation and breathing techniques are sometimes used for anxiety reduction. For a review of the effectiveness of these treatment strategies, see Gould et al. (1995).

Priority of Treatment Strategies

The first priority is to develop a formulation of the problem with the client, give a thorough rationale for treatment, and provide educational material about anxiety. Exposure is the most important component, but is more easily targeted to disconfirm the client's core fears if cognitive restructuring is conducted concurrently.

Treatment for Claudia proceeded as follows. In the second appointment, the formulation shown in Figs. 5.1 and 5.2 was developed collaboratively and psychoeducation about the nature of anxiety was begun. Claudia was asked to keep a diary and read material about anxiety (cf. Rapee, Craske, & Barlow, 1996).

The third session began with a review of Claudia's understanding of the formulation, the psychoeducational materials, and her diary. Basic cognitive restructuring was introduced, and Claudia was asked to challenge unhelpful thoughts on paper (Table 5.4) during the next week.

After checking her understanding of the formulation and reviewing her diary, exposure was introduced in the fourth session. An exposure hierarchy was developed (Table 5.5) and Claudia agreed to work on the first steps in the next

TABLE 5.4

An Example of Claudia's Thought Diary From the Third Week of Treatment

Event Situation	Thoughts (% belief)	Emotion (0–100)	Challenges (% belief)	Actions
Thursday—During my exposure task to drive to the local convenience store, I was stopped at traffic lights and experienced dizziness.	I'm having a stroke (40%). I'll go unconscious and my foot will slip onto the gas (50%) and I'll cause an accident (20%). My kids will be killed (10%).	Anxiety 50	I felt like this many times before and have never had a stroke, so I'm unlikely to this time (50%). In the past when I've panicked I've always been able to get myself home in the car without causing an accident, so I probably will get home this time (30%).	I slowed down or sped up so I didn't have to stop at the traffic lights.
Saturday—At home watching TV I stood up to get a drink and became dizzy all of a sudden	I'm not stressed (90%), so this must be a stroke (80%). Who will look after Emily and John (40%)?	Anxiety 80	I've often had attacks out of the blue and they haven't turned out to be a stroke or anything else dangerous (60%). It's more likely that this is a panic attack (40%). I always get through panic attacks, so there is no need to worry about John and Emily (50%).	I rang my Doctor but he wasn't in. I rang Mom to call an ambulance and she tried to talk me down. I took more vitamins.
Afterwards when I had calmed down	I'm never going to get better (90%); this treatment is not working (80%).	Hopeless 90	Its true!	I stayed in bed until late the next day and didn't bother with exposure task.

TABLE 5.5
Claudia's Graded Exposure to Driving Hierarchy

Goal	To drive on my own across town, over the river, to the Mega Mall with the kids in the car at a busy time of day	
	Steps	*Anticipated Anxiety (0–100)*
1	Drive on single-lane road with traffic lights at a quiet time with the kids in the car	35
2	Drive to local convenience store (about 2 miles) on a two-lane connecting road at a quiet time with kids in the car	50
3	Drive to local convenience store on a two-lane connecting road at a busy time with kids in the car	60
4	Drive to local mall (about 5 miles) on two-lane connecting road at a busy time with kids	75
5	Drive on freeway (about 10 miles) and take last off-ramp before bridge over river	80

week. Key situational details that relate to Claudia's fears are described in the goal and at each step. Each step was constructed with the aim of disconfirming Claudia's core fear as directly as possible. Claudia began exposure from the first step with her children in the car so that she could quickly disconfirm her fear that they will come to harm if she has a panic attack. She had no access to childcare, so this was the only practical way to begin exposure. Our own practice is to begin exposure by discarding as many safety behaviors as possible at the beginning. In this way, each step in exposure is more likely to disconfirm the client's core fears, and exposure proceeds faster.

The fifth session began as usual with a check on Claudia's view of the formulation, a review of her overall progress, and a review of her diary. At this point, Claudia expressed doubts about continuing with treatment—How could she have a panic attack when she relaxed? She believed that the clinician was telling her that "stress causes panic attacks" despite agreeing with the formulation shown in Figs. 5.1 and 5.2. This was discussed in more detail, and it became obvious that Claudia had not fully understood the formulation. She was taken back through the unexpected attack she recorded in her diary step by step, looking for evidence consistent with the formulation. Claudia was able to recognize that she was fearful of dizziness because she believed it indicated a stroke, and realized that standing up quickly from watching TV might cause some mild dizziness. This discussion led to the rationale for interoceptive exposure.

Cognitive restructuring techniques provide more information with which to target exposure. Table 5.4 gives an extract from Claudia's thought diary. The entry for Thursday shows Claudia using a new safety behavior, slowing down

TABLE 5.6
Claudia's Interoceptive Exposure Worksheet

Exercise	Anticipated Anxiety	Actual Sensations	Actual Anxiety	Physical Similarity
Hyperventilating for 1 minute	50	Dizzy, lightheaded, unreal, dry mouth	35	60
Shaking head from side to side for 30 seconds	30	Dizzy, tense in neck, headache	30	20
Standing up suddenly after sitting with head down between knees for 30 seconds	25	Dizzy, lightheaded	35	40
Spinning around for 30 seconds	60	Dizzy, out of control, sweaty, nauseated	70	50

or speeding up to avoid stopping at traffic lights. Pointing this out and asking Claudia to deliberately try to stop at traffic lights in the following exposure tasks is more likely to target these tasks at her fear of causing an accident.

The main topic covered in the fifth session was interoceptive exposure. Exposure to feared sensations (interoceptive exposure) is associated with better outcome in Gould et al.'s (1995) meta-analysis of treatment outcome research. Standing up suddenly may produce some mild dizziness (see Table 5.4), which Claudia misinterpreted as the sign of a stroke. Exposure to these sensations through exercises like those described in Barlow and Craske (1999) or shown in Table 5.6 has the aim of reducing these misinterpretations. In the session, Claudia was asked to read a description of each exercise and rate how much anxiety she anticipated that she would experience if she were to carry the exercise out as written. Spinning and hyperventilating were the two exercises she rated as the highest anticipatory anxiety. Claudia carried out these exercises in the session with her therapist, and made ratings of the anxiety she experienced and how similar the experience was to her panic attacks. Claudia was asked to test the other exercises shown in Table 5.6 for homework and to repeat those exercises that gave her similar sensations to her panic attacks.

Conducting these exercises in the session provides an opportunity for the clinician to observe how the client responds to anxiety and to encourage the client to tolerate sensations until they pass without using safety behavior.

The sixth session focused on reviewing progress with exposure and cognitive restructuring, discussing any difficulties that emerged, and making specific plans to continue exposure.

A specific plan to deal with relapse was developed in the seventh session. Claudia planned to make a weekly check on her level of avoidance. She identified future obstacles and planned methods to avoid them, planned steps to carry out in case of an unexpected panic attack in the future, and listed resources she could use in case of relapse.

Dealing with Complicating Factors

In Claudia's diary (see Table 5.4), you can see how an unexpected panic attack led to feelings of hopelessness and thoughts that CBT was not working. She then gave up on her next exposure task. In our experience, this type of setback is relatively common. Taking Claudia through the experience step by step uncovered the following sequence of thoughts:

1. Seeing a psychologist means they think my dizzy attacks are caused by stress.
2. If I'm not stressed before I get dizzy, then it can't be a panic attack, so it must be a stroke.
3. Doing all this therapy stuff is not going to help a stroke, and it will stop me from getting help, making it more likely that I'll die. Who will be left to care for my kids?

Despite carefully discussing the formulation and rationale with Claudia, she retained the model that stress caused dizziness. Helping her to see that unexpected panic attacks were understandable and consistent with the broader formulation led to a better understanding of the rationale for treatment and greater motivation to continue.

Role of Pharmacotherapy in the Case

It appeared that fluoxetine improved Claudia's mood and reduced the intensity of her panic attacks. She continued this medication, but was increasingly skeptical about its benefits.

Our usual practice is to encourage clients who have not previously had treatment to choose either antidepressant medication or a program of CBT. We encourage people who continue to take antidepressants to wait until they have stabilized before we begin a program of CBT. Clients are then more able to attribute any gains made in therapy to their own hard work. This attribution improves motivation and assists in dealing with inevitable setbacks (Sanderson & Wetzler, 1993).

Managed Care Considerations

Cognitive–behavioral therapy for Panic Disorder and Agoraphobia can be effective in a small number of sessions. Detailed self-help workbooks (cf. Barlow & Craske, 1999), treatment in groups, and treatment by telephone are some of the effective ways to maximize the effectiveness of a smaller number of face-to-face contacts. Some clients need more therapist contact and others less. Although there is little evidence to use as a guide, clients whose problems are more focused, who are more prepared to work and tolerate anxiety, and who agree with the clinician on the formulation are more likely to benefit from a smaller number of sessions.

SUMMARY

Panic Disorder and Agoraphobia are characterized by a persistent fear of catastrophic consequences of anxiety. Thought processes (e.g., "I was lucky"; "It won't last") and actions (safety behavior and avoidance) that prevent the sufferer from disconfirming their catastrophic beliefs maintain this fear. Cognitive–behavioral treatment targets these maintaining factors through psychoeducation, cognitive restructuring, and exposure.

ACKNOWLEDGMENT

Andrew J. Baillie is supported by a National Health and Medical Research Council Public Health Postgraduate Research Scholarship.

REFERENCES

Barlow, D. H., & Craske, M. (1999). *Mastery of anxiety and panic–III*. San Antonio, TX: Psychological Corporation.

Bouchard, S., Pelletier, M. H., Gauthier, J. G., Cote, G., Laberge, B. (1997). The assessment of panic using self-report: A comprehensive survey of validated instruments. *Journal of Anxiety Disorders, 11*, 89–111.

Clark, D. M. (1999). Anxiety disorders: Why they persist and how to treat them. *Behaviour Research and Therapy, 37*, S5–S27.

Eaton, W. W., Kessler, R. C., Wittchen, H. U., & Magee, W. J. (1994). Panic and panic disorder in the United States. *American Journal of Psychiatry, 151*, 413–420.

Garssen, B., de Ruiter, C., & van Dyck, R. (1992). Breathing retraining: A rational placebo? *Clinical Psychology Review, 12*, 141–153.

Gould, R. A., Otto, M. W., & Pollack, M. H. (1995). A meta-analysis of treatment outcome for Panic Disorder. *Clinical Psychology Review, 15*, 819–855.

Magee, W. J., Eaton, W. W., Wittchen, H. U., McGonagle, K. A., & Kessler, R. C. (1996). Agoraphobia, simple phobia, and social phobia in the National Comorbidity Study. *Archives of General Psychiatry, 53*, 159–168.

McNally, R. J. (1994). *Panic Disorder: A Critical Analysis*. New York: Guilford Press.

Rapee, R. M., Craske, M., & Barlow, D. H. (1996). Psychoeducation. In: C. G. Lindemann (Ed.), *Handbook of the treatment of the anxiety disorders*, 2nd ed. (pp. 311–322). Northvale, NJ: Jason Aronson, Inc.

Sanderson, W. C., & Wetzler, S. (1993). Observations on the cognitive behavioral treatment of panic disorder: Impact of benzodiazepines. *Psychotherapy, 30*, 125–132.

6

Specific Phobia

Brad Donohue and James Johnston
University of Nevada, Las Vegas

DESCRIPTION OF THE DISORDER

Specific Phobia constitutes a marked and persistent fear that is excessive or unreasonable and that is cued by the presence or anticipation of a specific object or situation, such as heights, receiving an injection, or seeing blood (*DSM–IV*; American Psychiatric Association, 1994). Exposure to the phobic stimulus usually provokes an immediate anxiety response, which may result in a panic attack. Adults recognize that the fear is excessive or unreasonable, although this may not be the case in children. The phobic object or situation must be avoided or endured with intense discomfort, and there must be a significant impairment in functioning (e.g., occupational, academic, social activities, relationships, marked distress). Fears include animals, the natural environment (e.g., heights, storms, water), blood injection or injury; situations (e.g., airplanes, elevators, enclosed places), choking, vomiting, contracting an illness, loud sounds, and costumed characters. Oftentimes multiple fears are experienced concurrently.

Although most people experience fears, they rarely result in sufficient impairment or distress to warrant the diagnosis of Specific Phobia, as prevalence rates for this disorder are usually about 10%. Specific phobias typically develop in early childhood (e.g., 4 years for animal phobias) to early adolescence (e.g., 12 years for dental phobias). However, some phobias (e.g., heights, claustrophobia) have a much later onset.

Although the development of Specific Phobia is influenced by genetic predisposition, it is often a result of environmental factors, such as associative learning, modeling, and negative reinforcement. In respondent conditioning (associative learning), an aversive or traumatic stimulus (unconditioned stimulus, i.e., bite of a snake) is associated with a stimulus that did not previously bring about fear (neutral stimulus, i.e., the snake itself). If these stimuli are repeatedly associated or if the unconditioned stimulus is perceived to be especially aversive, presentation of the neutral stimulus by itself may subsequently elicit the fear response (the neutral stimulus would hence be referred to as a *conditioned stimulus*). The strength of this conditioning would depend on several factors, including similarity and temporal closeness of the neutral and unconditioned stimuli. In modeling, the phobic develops the phobia in response to watching others demonstrate fear reactions consequent to being exposed to the feared stimulus. For instance, if a child observes her mother screaming in response to seeing a spider, she may learn vicariously to fear spiders. Fear responses are often maintained by negative reinforcement. For instance, if an individual approached a spider, grew anxious, and consequently withdrew from the spider, anxiety would be attenuated. This reduction in anxiety would reinforce the individual to withdraw from spiders in the future, and therefore assist in the maintenance of the fear.

METHODS TO DETERMINE DIAGNOSIS

Methods that may be used in the assessment of Specific Phobia include clinical interviews, self-report measures, behavioral observation, and physiological/biological evaluation. As indicated in the following sections, each method yields unique insights. Therefore, Specific Phobia is best understood when multiple assessment approaches are used. The following sections provide a brief overview of effective assessment measures.

Clinical Interview

Typically categorized as structured, semistructured, or unstructured, the clinical interview yields qualitative and diagnostic information. In the unstructured clinical interview, the content of the interview is determined by the clinician, who is trained to ask questions that appear most appropriate. Unstructured interviews should always be used to some extent, as the unstructured format allows an assessment of factors that are unique to the client. Unstructured interviews are typically implemented during the first or second session and usually focus on establishing rapport and gaining an understanding of the condition. These interviews should include an exploration of fear responses, including the type and history of fears; consequences; precursors; concomitants of fear responses (e.g., feelings, behaviors, thoughts); reactions of significant others when the fear response occurs; family history of fears and anxieties; extent of caffeine intake; alcohol and drug use; medical history; problems in functioning due to the phobia; patient expectations of treatment; comorbid psychiatric diagnoses; and environmental stressors that exacerbate the fear response. It is beneficial to assess fear patterns in a chronologic order whenever possible, beginning with premorbid functioning. A chronologic assessment also provides an understanding of the functions of fear responses across various developmental stages and situations that change over time.

Structured interviews include standard (prescribed) questions and usually target specific content domains. The client's response is typically recorded following a forced-choice format (e.g., 1 = no history of panic attacks, 2 = history of panic attacks, 3 = history of panic attacks is questionable). Although structured interviews necessitate familiarity with the interview format, they are reliable and assist the interviewer in remaining unbiased. Therefore, structured interviews are often used in research, and are popular with relatively inexperienced clinicians who are trained in their use. The Anxiety Disorders Interview Schedule–Revised (ADIS–R; DiNardo et al., 1985) is a popular clinical interview in the assessment of specific phobia. This structured interview allows a broad assessment of the major anxiety disorders as well as reliable assessment of the nature of phobic symptoms. This instrument also assesses the extent of avoidance, presence and severity of associated physiological symptoms, and mode of onset. Other interviews yield useful information relevant to particular types of specific phobia. For instance, Kleinknecht and Lenz (1989) developed a semistructured interview to assess blood/injury phobia.

In the semistructured interview format, the clinician is typically provided standard questions that assess particular content areas. However, unlike the structured interview format, the clinician is free to choose the questions that appear most appropriate, given the client's unique circumstances.

Self-Report Measures

Self-report measures include questionnaires and behavioral self-monitoring procedures. Many questionnaires have long been established in the assessment of Specific Phobias. For example, questionnaires have been developed to assess fears relevant to snakes and spiders (Klorman et al., 1974) and dental anxiety (Corah, 1969). Other questionnaires have been developed to assess problematic thoughts that are contribute to specific phobia (e.g., the Rational Behavior Inventory; Whiteman & Shorkey, 1978). The most frequently used self-report measure in Specific Phobia is the subjective units of discomfort/distress scale (SUDS). In this procedure, patients use a Likert-type scale to indicate their level of fear/anxiety while in the presence of the feared object/situation (e.g., 0 = not at all anxious, 4 = extremely anxious). These subjective assessments of fear have been shown to correspond closely to physical symptoms of severity (e.g., heart rate) and are useful in treatment. For instance, in graduated exposure-based interventions (exposing the phobic to increasingly greater anxiety-provoking fear situations), phobics may use the SUDS to place fear scenarios in ascending order of anxiety. The SUDS may also be used as an ongoing assessment of the phobic's level of fear throughout exposure to feared stimuli during treatment, as well as an indicator of progress in therapy.

Behavioral Observation

Behavioral observation procedures involve observations of fear-relevant behavior during exposure to feared stimuli. In the Behavioral Avoidance Task (BAT), the clinician assists the phobic in constructing a hierarchy of situations that are increasingly anxiety-provoking, as mentioned above (e.g., standing next to a snake in a glass jar, touching the jar, putting hand in jar, touching snake). The phobic is encouraged to progressively expose him/herself to these situations, and observations of fear responses are performed. Behavioral checklists may be utilized to record the presence or absence of specified behavioral indicators of fear (e.g., trembling, facial tension, hesitation, withdrawal from the feared stimulus). Sometimes, Likert-scales are used as an attempt to quantify the overall severity of anxiety (e.g., 1 = no distress, 5 = extremely distressed).

Physiological Evaluations

Physiological evaluation procedures provide an objective assessment of specific phobia. Heart rate monitors are often utilized in this approach, as heart rate generally increases when phobics are initially exposed to fear provoking stimuli (note: heart rate decreases in the presence of blood for most phobics). Most heart rate monitors include disposable chest electrodes, which are connected to a small rubber casing with a battery and electronic transmitter. A wristwatch receiver records heart rate at a predetermined interval (e.g., every 15 seconds). These monitors are easily implemented during exposure based training programs, and complement subjective feelings of fear (i.e., SUDS ratings).

CASE ILLUSTRATION

Mary, a 27-year-old Hispanic woman, referred herself to an outpatient community mental health center shortly after she determined that her fear of elevators was interfering with her responsibilities as a maid in a high-rise hotel casino. She usually avoided elevator travel, and instead often used the stairs, which interfered with her job efficiency because it was very time consuming. Although

Mary reported that she had always been "a little" anxious in elevators, severity of this condition was intensified after an intoxicated member of a local fraternity attempted to pull the blouse off her body in one of the elevators at her work. Mary was able to exit the elevator prior to sexual contact. However, she reportedly grew increasingly fearful of elevators after this incident.

Mary reported no history of medical problems (including heart conditions) or use of prescription drugs. However, she did report consumption of up to four cups of caffeinated coffee prior to work each morning since the attempted rape in the elevator. She stated that her mother had an intense fear of heights and riding in airplanes. When asked if her mother was afraid of elevators, Mary abruptly responded: "She hates being in them because she worries that the elevator will fall." Other than the aforementioned assault in the elevator, Mary reported no history of sexual victimization. She was oriented to person, place, and time, and she did not evidence a formal thought disorder (e.g., delusions, hallucinations). Reporting no history of suicide, her affect was pleasant and her mood was cheerful. When asked if she had received previous psychological or psychiatric treatment, she responded: "I saw a shrink for nine sessions. He did nothing but ask me questions about my childhood; I decided to quit because he just wasn't helping me."

CASE CONCEPTUALIZATION

Modeling and Learning

Development of Mary's elevator phobia was greatly influenced by classical and operant conditioning. Along classical conditioning lines, the elevator (neutral stimulus) was associated with the assault (unconditioned stimulus), which resulted in fear (unconditioned response). After this incident, exposure to elevators without the assaultive behavior (conditioned stimulus) resulted in fear (conditioned response). Mary reported many occasions in which she would approach the elevator, become anxious, and withdraw from it. This withdrawal behavior, of course, resulted in immediate reductions in anxiety, and thus negatively reinforced her to withdraw from elevators in the future. In regard to modeling, Mary's mother modeled fear reactions in response to heights and being enclosed in elevators throughout Mary's childhood. Therefore, Mary learned vicariously to fear elevators and heights at a very young age.

Genetics and Temperament

The development of Mary's elevator phobia may have been influenced by genetics, as Mary's mother reportedly had a long-standing history of similar fears, and fears have been shown to be influenced by genetic endowment.

However, it is difficult to determine the relative extent genetics may have had in the development of Mary's phobia because environmental influences were also present (e.g., her mother modeled fear reactions).

Physical Conditions

Mary's thoughts interact with her symptoms of arousal to exacerbate the severity of her elevator phobia. Indeed, Mary reported that upon being exposed to elevators she gets nervous, her heart beats faster, she gets a lump in her throat, and she begins to perspire. As reported by Mary, "I set myself up to get scared. I'll tell myself I'm going to freak out, or that something bad is going to happen. After I do this, my heart starts to beat faster, which makes me even more nervous and upset. In fact, I sometimes think I'm going to have a heart attack, which leads me to believe I'm going to die. Then I start sweating like a pig."

Drugs

Mary reported daily use of caffeinated coffee. Caffeine is a central nervous system stimulant that increases physiological arousal; therefore, her use of caffeine is likely to have increased her arousal while traveling in the elevators at work and is likely to have exacerbated her subjective experience of anxiety during these times, as indicated previously.

Socioeconomic and Cultural Factors

Mary reported marital difficulties with her husband since the assault. Being raised in a traditional Hispanic and Roman Catholic background, Mary reported that she felt guilty about "not being home" to raise her teenage daughter, who had recently been arrested for possession of marijuana. Mary refused to quit her job because she believed her family needed her income. She reported that her husband thought she was "weak" for letting her fear of elevators interfere with her work productivity, and was also concerned that she would lose her job if she continued to avoid elevators.

Overall Conceptualization

The development of Mary's elevator phobia was multiply determined. Her presumed genetic background probably influenced her to develop fear reactions, as did her mother's modeling of fear reactions to elevators when Mary was a child. However, other environmental and biological influences appeared to be the primary determinants in the development of her fear of elevators. Indeed, the intensity of her phobia was reportedly exacerbated after associative learning occurred (i.e., the sexual assault), and was later maintained by negative reinforcement (withdrawal/avoidance behavior) and her use of central nervous system stimulants (i.e., coffee prior to work). Her husband's lack of support and guilt regarding her daughter's drug use probably contributed to stress, which usually exacerbates anxiety-based disorders.

Diagnostic Assessment

In determining Mary's *DSM–IV* diagnosis, the Anxiety Disorders Interview Schedule–Revised was administered during the initial assessment session after a brief unstructured interview. The results of the ADIS–R indicated that Mary clearly met criteria for Specific Phobia, as she persistently experienced marked anxiety in elevators, and her frequent avoidance of elevators interfered with her work productivity. She reported occasional panic attacks (i.e., sudden rapid heart beat, perspiration, dizziness), which often indicate Panic Disorder with or without Agoraphobia. However, this disorder was ruled out as it was determined that the panic attacks occurred exclusively in the presence of elevators. Caffeine-Induced Anxiety Disorder was ruled out during the unstructured interview when it was determined that Mary evinced many of the symptoms associated with Specific Phobia before the attempted rape. Thus, her daily use of caffeine may have exacerbated her fear of elevators, but caffeine could not have induced this fear.

Behavioral Assessment

Mary agreed that it would be important for the therapist to observe her reaction to elevators. Therefore, the therapist met Mary at her place of employment for the second assessment session. The therapist explained the SUDS rating scale (0 = no anxiety, 4 = extremely anxious), and informed her that she would be asked to provide SUDS ratings throughout her upcoming exposure to one of the hotel elevators. Mary then attached a heart rate monitor to her body so that an objective baseline measure of her heart rate could be determined. Her heart rate 5 minutes prior to being exposed to the elevator was 81 beats per minute. Her SUDS rating during this time was reportedly 0 and she demonstrated no physical signs of anxiety. She was then led to the elevator. Committed to going to the fifth floor with the therapist (10 floors total), Mary took several deep breaths, and spontaneously commented, "I hope this works out because my SUDS rating is already a 1" (heart rate = 90). As she entered the elevator, she reported that her SUDS rating had jumped to a 3. She started to tap her feet and appeared to tighten her facial muscles, particularly those muscles surrounding her jaw. Her rate of breathing increased, consistent with her heart rate (100 beats per minute). Immediately after pushing the button for the 5th floor, she shut her eyes and took another deep breath. As the elevator began to move, she reported that her SUDS rating was a 3.5 and that she was starting to feel dizzy. Her high rate of breathing continued, and she told the therapist that she was upset and wanted to get off the elevator (heart rate = 108 beats per min). Leaving the elevator on the 3rd floor, she exclaimed, "Thank God! I thought I was going to go crazy in that damn thing!" Immediately after she left the elevator, she reported that her SUDS rating was a 2. Within 3 minutes of leaving the elevator, her SUDS rating was reportedly a 0. Behavioral observations at the time she reported this last SUDS rating indicated that her rate was 82. Thus, behavioral assessment procedures indicated that Mary's subjective perceptions of anxiety severity (i.e., SUDS ratings) were consistent with objective therapist observations of behavior and physiological arousal (i.e., heart rate).

Prioritization of Targets for Treatment

It was decided mutually between Mary and her therapist that the primary goal of therapy would be for her to travel comfortably in elevators, particularly the elevator at her place of employment. Anchoring this goal to behavioral indices, she expressed a desire to ride the elevator at her work to the top floor (10th floor) with a SUDS rating of a 1 or 0 within four intervention sessions (two scheduled sessions per week). After the therapist informed Mary that her use of caffeinated coffee would probably interfere with her therapy goals, she agreed to eliminate caffeine from her diet immediately. She reported that she had been able to eliminate equivalent amounts of caffeine from her diet in the past, and therefore believed this goal was easily attainable.

Selection of Treatment Strategies

After several empirically derived treatment approach rationales were provided to Mary (e.g., flooding, graduated exposure in vivo, systematic desensitization, cognitive restructuring), she agreed to implement graduated exposure in vivo combined with cognitive restructuring procedures. These interventions were selected due to their demonstrated efficacy in controlled treatment outcome studies (see Sturges & Sturges, 1998).

Priority of Treatment Strategies

The basic treatment plan was to teach Mary cognitive–behavioral skills that could be used by her to decrease anxiety while traveling in elevators. It was explained to Mary during the second assessment session that the initial intervention session would occur in the therapy office. The purpose of this initial intervention session was twofold: (a) develop the format of her elevator exposure trials, and (b) teach her to perform cognitive–behavioral skills that would enable her to accomplish her goal of riding in elevators comfortably. She was told that the subsequent three sessions would occur at her place of employment so that she would have opportunities to practice her skills during her exposure trials in the elevator.

In the first intervention session (90 minutes), a hierarchy of fear severity was constructed that was relevant to riding one of the elevators at her work. This hierarchy advanced in fear severity and was consistent with two themes: fear of heights (1st floor to 2nd floor, 2nd floor to 3rd floor, etc.) and safety (e.g., travel with husband, travel alone, travel with stranger). A sketch of these trials is as follows:

1. Standing in front of the elevator door on first floor, pressing elevator button, husband present
2. Standing inside elevator on 1st floor with door open, pressing the button for the 2nd floor, husband present
3. Standing inside elevator on 2nd floor with door open, pressing the button for the 3rd floor, husband present
4. Standing inside elevator on 3rd floor with door open, pressing the button for the 7th floor, husband present
5. Standing inside elevator on 7th floor with door open, pressing the button for the 10th floor, husband present
6. Standing inside elevator on 1st floor with door open, pressing the button for the 2nd floor, alone in elevator
7. Standing inside elevator on 2nd floor with door open, pressing the button for the 3rd floor, alone in elevator
8. Standing inside elevator on 3rd floor with door open, pressing the button for the 7th floor, alone in elevator
9. Standing inside elevator on 7th floor with door open, pressing the button for the 10th floor, alone in elevator
10. Standing inside elevator on 1st floor, door open, press the button for the 2nd floor, alone, male stranger(s) walks in
11. Standing inside elevator on 2nd floor, door open, press the button for the 3rd floor, alone, male stranger(s) walks in
12. Standing inside elevator on 3rd floor, door open, press the button for the 7th floor, alone, male stranger(s) walks in
13. Standing inside elevator on 7th floor door open, press the button for the 10th floor, alone, male stranger(s) walks in

After the fear hierarchy was constructed, Mary was taught relaxation procedures (e.g., progressive muscle relaxation, imagining calm/peaceful situations) to be used during her exposure to the aforementioned trials. Briefly, she was taught to tense and relax each of the major muscles in her body. Once a state of relaxation was achieved, she learned to focus on a relaxation cue word (i.e., "calm"). She was assigned to practice these relaxation exercises at home each night (after the second intervention session, Mary was instructed to omit the tension component during her relaxation exercises).

Also during this initial treatment contact, Mary was taught to identify the dysfunctional self-statements that she made while traveling in elevators. She learned that statements such as, "I hope this works out," "I don't know if I can do this," and "I think I'm going to have a heart attack," are likely to lower her confidence and raise expectations of failure. Specifically, the therapist provided several generic examples of dysfunctional statements that were identified in the assessment phase to be consistent with Mary's thinking patterns. For each statement, Mary was asked to report why the statement was dysfunctional, if she could provide personal examples of having made similar statements, and she generated statements that were more positive and objective. For instance, she learned that an alternative statement to "I think I'm going to have a heart attack and die" is, "I feel my heart starting to beat faster, so I'm going to take a few deep breaths to slow my heart rate, and get calm." To conclude the session, Mary was asked to switch to decaffeinated coffee and monitor her daily intake of all major sources of caffeine (e.g., soda, coffee).

In the second session (90 minutes), Mary and her husband, John, met the therapist at the hotel. John was briefly informed of Mary's phobic condition, including her treatment plan. He was informed that his primary role would be to support Mary while she attempted to ride the elevator during her exposure trials, and that critical statements would be very deleterious to her treatment. The therapist modeled several supportive statements (e.g., "I know it's tough, just try to do your best, you're doing great"), and instructed John to practice similar statements. The heart rate monitor was not used because Mary's heart rate closely corresponded to her SUDS ratings throughout her behavioral observation assessment trials. However, Mary and John were each given a cell phone that allowed them to talk to the therapist during Mary's exposure trials (therapist remained on the first floor throughout all exposure trials). Mary and John were then instructed to perform the first trial (i.e., standing in front of the elevator door on the first floor and pressing the elevator button). Mary reported that her SUDS rating was 1 immediately after she pressed the elevator button. The therapist instructed her to remain standing in front of the elevator, and to practice her relaxation exercises and objective/positive self-statements. As she entered the elevator, she commented, "I feel a little nervous, but I'm going to do this." She reported that her SUDS rating was still a 1. The therapist consequently instructed John to complement Mary on her positive and objective thinking. John told her she was doing fine, and that he was proud of her effort. She then pressed the button for the 2nd floor. As the elevator was lifted to the 2nd floor, Mary commented that she did not think she would make it to the 10th floor with her husband that day. Mary was told, by the therapist, to concentrate on things that were associated with her second trial only. She quickly agreed, and said, "I need to take things one step at a time. I'm doing this, I just need to slow down my heart rate by taking long, deep breaths." Her husband spontaneously stated, "That's it, just keep trying, Mary. You're doing great." When the door opened at the second floor, Mary was instructed by the therapist to practice her relaxation exercises and to remain in the elevator with the door open until her anxiety dissipated. John rubbed her back. After 2 minutes, she reported that her SUDS rating was 0 and she pressed the button for the 3rd floor. Mary progressed through the next two trials in a similar manner.

In the sixth trial (standing in the elevator on 1st floor with door open, pressing the button for the 2nd floor, alone in elevator), John was instructed to stand next to the therapist, and Mary was asked to perform her first trial alone. When she pressed the button for the 2nd floor, an increase in her rate of breathing was observed and she stated that her anxiety level had risen to a 3. As the elevator started to move, she reported to the therapist that she was starting to get dizzy and that her SUDS rating had increased to a 3.5. Knowing that it would be important to end the trial without anxiety, the therapist instructed Mary to engage in her relaxation exercises, and concentrate on the cue word, "calm." As Mary reached the 2nd floor, her husband was instructed to tell her that she had accomplished a great deal in one day and that he was proud of her accomplishments. As the elevator door opened, she was instructed by the therapist to remain in the elevator and practice her relaxation exercises until her SUDS rating decreased to a 1 or 0. Approximately 30 seconds later she reported that her anxiety was 0, and she exited the elevator. John and the therapist met her on the second floor, and they all subsequently took the elevator to the first floor. Mary, John, and the therapist then went to a room in the hotel, where they discussed her accomplishments (e.g., reaching the 2nd floor by herself, efforts to relax herself on cue, use of objective/positive thoughts). John was praised for his support, and Mary was given a therapy assignment to practice her relaxation exercises at home (omitting the tension component). Mary was also instructed to practice riding the elevator with her husband at least once a day until the next session. As for her goal to abstain from caffeine, Mary reported that she was able to avoid all major sources of caffeine since the second assessment session, and that her abstinence from caffeine had influenced her to be "irritable" throughout the week. John replied that he understood what she was going through because he had a similar experience several years ago when he first quit smoking cigarettes. The session ended after the therapist urged John to continue assisting Mary in her avoidance of caffeine. He was also prompted to provide Mary with supportive statements during their practice exposure trials.

The third intervention session (90 minutes) was conducted at Mary's work-place. Mary was scheduled to begin her exposure training with Trial 5 to enhance the likelihood of starting the session on a successful trial. However, John was unable to attend the session, and Mary reported that she felt comfortable starting with Trial 6. She progressed through trials 6–9 with SUDS equal or less than 3.

As indicated previously, exposure trials 10–13 required a male stranger to walk into the elevator. Therefore, these trials were performed in an elevator that was located in a busy section of the hotel. For each step in the hierarchy (trial), Mary waited in the elevator with the door open. If a male entered, she proceeded with the exposure trial (i.e., pushed the appropriate elevator button). However, if a woman entered the elevator, she simply left the elevator, waited for the elevator to return, entered the elevator alone, and waited for a male to enter. Although time consuming, entering and leaving the elevator frequently with no anxiety appeared to assist in deconditioning her fears. Mary accomplished trials 10–13 uneventfully. In reviewing her efforts after the hierarchy steps were accomplished, Mary reported that she felt confident in her abilities to travel in the hotel elevators without anxiety. She reported no use of caffeine during the previous week. She was given a therapy assignment to continue her relaxation exercises at home on a daily basis. In addition, she was encouraged to practice positive and objective self-statements while traveling in at least three separate elevators each day prior to her next session.

The last session (fourth intervention session, 60 minutes) consisted of Mary traveling six times to the 10th floor in the busy hotel elevator. She reported no anxiety during these trips. During the last 25 minutes of the session, Mary was prompted to discuss her accomplishments, including the specific skills that she had acquired during intervention. She reported no use of caffeine, or irritability since the last session. Follow-up calls with Mary, conducted 1, 3, and 6 months after her last intervention session, indicated no anxiety while traveling in elevators.

Dealing with Complicating Factors

Prior to intervention, Mary's employer had threatened to terminate Mary's employment if she continued to do poorly in her work. To assist Mary in this problem, a release of information form was signed by Mary that permitted the therapist to discuss Mary's diagnosis and treatment plan. After a professional rationale for Specific Phobia was provided by the therapist, the employer made arrangements that allowed Mary to perform her practice trials during her scheduled hours of employment. He also agreed that he would not discuss her fear of elevators for the duration of her treatment, as Mary thought this would allow her to feel more relaxed.

Role of Pharmacotherapy in the Case

Psychopharmacological drugs have consistently been found to be ineffective in the treatment of Specific Phobia (see Lydiard, Roy-Byrne, & Ballenger,

1988). Moreover, ingestion of these agents during exposure trials may interfere with long-term reductions in anxiety (Marks, 1981). Indeed, substantial improvement may be noted initially; however, discontinuation of medication usually results in relapse. Drugs were not prescribed for Mary.

Managed Care Considerations

Mary's employment agency provided her with health insurance that paid 80% of her therapy expenses (i.e., $120 of the $150 fee per session). The therapist was asked by his employer to collect an additional $35 for each session that was conducted at Mary's workplace to compensate the community mental health center for travel expenses. Mary's insurance policy would not compensate Mary for this latter charge, which was a concern for her because she evidently was experiencing financial difficulties. Therefore, recognizing the necessity of conducting in vivo exposure training, the clinic director waived this additional charge.

SUMMARY

Specific Phobia constitutes a marked and persistent fear that is excessive or unreasonable, and that is cued by the presence or anticipation of a specific object or situation. Most people have experienced fears in the general population. However, the prevalence rate of Specific Phobia is estimated to be about 10% in the general population. Although specific phobia is influenced by genetic predisposition, its development is often significantly influenced by environmental factors, such as associative learning, modeling, intake of caffeine, and negative reinforcement. There are many methods that may be used in the assessment of Specific Phobia. Common instruments include clinical interviews, self-report measures, behavioral observation, and physiological/ biological evaluation. Treatments for Specific Phobia usually involve exposure of the individual to the feared stimulus. To expedite treatment effectiveness, exposure is usually graduated in severity of anxiety, and these individuals are often taught relaxation exercises and cognitive interventions, to be utilized during exposure training.

REFERENCES

American Psychiatric Association. (1987). *Diagnostic and statistical manual of mental health disorders*–3rd ed., Rev. Washington, DC: Author.

Corah, N. L. (1969). Development of a dental anxiety scale. *Journal of Dental Research, 48*, 596.

Dinardo, P. A., Barlow, D. H., Cerny, J., Vermilyea, B. B., Vermilyea, J. A., Himadi, W., & Waddell, M. (1985). *Anxiety Disorders Interview Schedule–Revised*. Albany, NY: Phobia and Anxiety Disorders Clinic, State University of New York at Albany.

Kleinknecht, R. A., & Lenz, J. (1989). Blood/injury fear, fainting and avoidance of medically-related situations: A family correspondence study. *Behaviour Research and Therapy, 27*, 537–547.

Klorman, R., Weerts, T. C., Hastings, J. E., Melamed, B. G., & Lang, P. J. (1974). Psychometric description of some specific-fear questionnaires. *Behaviour Research and Therapy, 5*, 401–409.

Lydiard, R. B., Roy-Byrne, P. P., & Ballenger, J. C. (1988). Recent advances in psychopharmacological treatment of anxiety disorders. *Hospital and Community Psychiatry, 39*, 1157–1165.

Sturges, J. W., & Sturges, L. V. (1998). In vivo systematic desensitization in a single-session treatment of an 11-year old girl's elevator phobia. *Child & Family Behavior Therapy, 20*, 103–115.

Whiteman, V. L., & Shorkey, C. T. (1978). Validation testing of the Rational Behavior Inventory. *Educational and Psychological Measurement, 38*, 1143–1149.

7

Social Anxiety Disorder

Brigette A. Erwin, Erin L. Scott,
and Richard G. Heimberg
Adult Anxiety Clinic of Temple University

DESCRIPTION OF THE DISORDER

Social anxiety disorder, also known as social phobia, is characterized by fear and frequently avoidance of social and/or performance situations in which embarrassment may occur (*DSM–IV*; American Psychiatric Association [APA], 1994). Almost everyone who has gone on a first date, interviewed for a job, or presented a formal speech has experienced concerns related to being under the close scrutiny of others. However, social anxiety disorder is distinguished by the severity and persistence of anxiety symptoms as well as the degree to which anxiety interferes with the adaptive functioning of the individual.

Individuals with social anxiety disorder typically fear that others will judge them to be inadequate on the basis of their behavior (e.g., not knowing the right thing to say to a new acquaintance) or that their anxiety symptoms will be visible to others (e.g., shaking while giving a speech) and lead to negative social consequences. For example, whereas individuals without social anxiety disorder may become nervous about an upcoming formal speaking engagement, the anxiety usually dissipates shortly after the speech begins and they will likely judge their performance to have been adequate, although not necessarily perfect. Individuals with social anxiety disorder, however, may find it impossible to think of anything else for days before the event, making persistent negative predictions about their upcoming performance. Although the anxiety may decrease somewhat during the speech, socially anxious individuals regard their performance as inept and may conclude that the audience could "see" their anxiety (e.g., sweating or shaking) and was put off by it.

For individuals with social anxiety disorder, attempts to engage in feared social situations or even anticipation of such attempts almost invariably produce distress. In some individuals, this fear may take the form of a surge of physiological arousal (e.g., trembling, blushing, sweating) or a situational panic attack. To the socially anxious individual, the experience of somatic symptoms may serve as additional evidence of one's inability to handle the situation and serve to further increase anxious arousal. In addition, the presence of symptoms that may be visible to others, such as blushing or sweating, may increase the individual's fears of negative evaluation by others.

A wide range of social situations may become the focus of one's social anxiety, including interacting with unfamiliar people, dating, giving a prepared speech, talking to persons in authority, participating in classes or meetings, eating or drinking in public, or using public restrooms. On the basis of the range of feared situations, individuals with social anxiety disorder can be further characterized as having either generalized or nongeneralized forms of the disorder. As defined by *DSM–IV*, generalized social anxiety disorder is marked by fear of most social situations; in contrast, those who experience distress in fewer situations are often referred to as having the nongeneralized type of social anxiety disorder. Generalized social anxiety disorder begins earlier in life and aggregates in families more than nongeneralized social anxiety disorder. Persons with generalized social anxiety disorder are more likely to experience severe impairment in educational, work, and social domains. Research has yet to determine whether specific interventions are differentially effective for each subtype, although treatment for generalized social anxiety disorder is likely to be more protracted.

Given the aversiveness of the experience of severe social anxiety, it is not surprising that individuals with social anxiety disorder frequently attempt to avoid or escape from social interaction and performance situations. For some, avoidance may take the form of overt behavior, such as persistent refusal to attend parties or not taking classes that include public speaking. However, avoidance behavior can be much more subtle, as in the case of a socially anxious person who attends parties but talks only to the one person he or she already knows, or the student who sits in the back of the classroom so as not to be called on to participate. Other individuals may not avoid situations as frequently, but instead endure them with extreme distress. For individuals who fear many situations, it is common to find some situations avoided completely whereas others are endured, depending on the degree to which the individual believes that he or she can "get away with" avoiding the situation. For example, socially anxious lawyers may not avoid depositions and discussions with opposing counsel because they feel that they "must" do these things in order to keep their jobs;

nonetheless, these same individuals may totally avoid dating situations and interactions with potential dating partners. Although the desire for interaction with potential partners may be very important, momentary loneliness may not motivate as strongly as the fear of losing one's job. Nevertheless, in more severe cases of social anxiety disorder, nearly all situations may be avoided.

Although only recently recognized as a distinct disorder, social anxiety disorder appears to be highly prevalent in the general population. The most recent large-scale psychiatric epidemiologic study conducted in the United States, the National Comorbidity Study (NCS), estimated the lifetime prevalence of social anxiety disorder to be approximately 13%, making it the third most common psychiatric disorder of those assessed (Magee, Eaton, Wittchen, McGonagle, & Kessler, 1996). This rate is considerably higher than the lifetime prevalence rate of 2.4% reported in the National Institute of Mental Health Epidemiological Catchment Area (ECA) study (Schneier, Johnson, Hornig, Liebowitz, & Weissman, 1992). The rate increase may be due, in part, to methodologic differences and the use of different sets of diagnostic criteria in the two studies. Whereas the ECA study based its diagnosis of social anxiety disorder on the presence of fear of and interference in one of three specific social situations (eating in front of others, public speaking, and speaking to strangers or meeting new people), the NCS examined three additional situations (using public restrooms, writing while being watched, and sounding foolish in front of others). Given that both studies allowed for a diagnosis of social anxiety disorder if the individual indicated significant interference in a single situation, the likelihood of receiving a diagnosis of social anxiety disorder in the NCS should have been much greater. However, it also appears that the prevalence of social anxiety disorder is increasing over time. Data from the NCS study reveal a cohort effect, such that social anxiety disorder is more prevalent in individuals age 15–24 than in those 25 and older. This is despite the fact that one might expect older individuals, having lived through a longer period of risk, to show higher lifetime prevalence rates.

Social anxiety disorder tends to occur more frequently in women and in people who are less well educated, single, and of lower socioeconomic status (Magee et al., 1996; Schneier et al., 1992). Despite the greater rate of social anxiety disorder among women in the general population, however, men and women present in approximately equal numbers to treatment settings. This may be at least partially explained by societal expectations for the behavior of men and women. For example, shy and reserved behavior may be accepted among women and viewed in a positive vein as "feminine." It is unlikely that the same behaviors would be judged as positively among men because they are in conflict with many notions of masculinity.

Individuals with social anxiety disorder often report additional concerns, including but not limited to other anxiety problems, depression, and substance abuse or dependence. In fact, the majority of individuals with social anxiety disorder meet criteria for at least one other psychiatric disorder during their lifetime. In the ECA study (Schneier et al., 1992), 69% of individuals with social anxiety disorder had at least one comorbid disorder. In the NCS study (Magee et al., 1996), the rate of comorbidity was 81%. In most cases, the onset of social anxiety disorder was earlier than that of the comorbid disorder, suggesting that social anxiety disorder may be a risk factor for the development of other psychiatric disorders (Magee et al., 1996; Schneier et al., 1992).

In the NCS, 56.7% of persons with social anxiety disorder met criteria for another anxiety disorder and 41.4% met criteria for any affective disorder (37.2% major depressive disorder). Social anxiety disorder is also associated with an increase in thoughts of suicide, and the rate of suicide attempts is increased in individuals with social anxiety disorder and a comorbid psychiatric disorder (Schneier et al., 1992). Substance use disorders are also relatively common among individuals with social anxiety disorder. In the NCS, nearly 40% of individuals with social anxiety disorder met the criteria for one of the substance-related disorders, 30% of individuals with social anxiety disorder were diagnosed with alcohol abuse or dependence, and 20% of individuals were diagnosed with drug abuse or dependence (Magee et al., 1996).

Although not assessed in the major epidemiologic studies, the comorbidity of social anxiety disorder and avoidant personality disorder (APD) is of significant interest. The essential feature of APD, as defined by *DSM–IV*, is the presence of "a pervasive pattern of social inhibition, feelings of inadequacy, and hypersensitivity to negative evaluation that begins by early adulthood and is present in a variety of contexts" (APA, 1994, p. 662). After reviewing the diagnostic criteria for APD, it is not surprising that various studies have found extremely high overlap between social anxiety disorder and APD. In fact, Heimberg (1996) questioned the utility of separating the two disorders onto separate axes. The combination of social anxiety disorder and APD may simply represent a more severe form of social anxiety disorder. In fact, individuals with social anxiety disorder with or without APD appear to respond equally well to cognitive–behavioral and pharmacological treatments.

Social anxiety disorder can be extremely debilitating and is frequently associated with significant impairment in educational, occupational, and social functioning (Schneier et al., 1992). Individuals with social anxiety disorder often find it difficult to initiate and maintain friendships and romantic relationships. They may refuse to participate in classes or make presentations for fear of being evaluated negatively. They may drop out of school or not seek higher education, thereby limiting their ability to succeed in the workplace. Once out of school, individuals with social anxiety disorder may choose jobs that will not trigger their social fears but that may be far below their educational level and ability. Not surprisingly, individuals with social anxiety disorder are more likely to require financial assistance through welfare or disability payments. Despite these difficulties, however, those with uncomplicated social anxiety disorder (i.e., without a comorbid diagnosis) are no more likely to seek treatment for emotional problems than those without a psychiatric diagnosis. This suggests that, despite significant impairment, individuals with social anxiety disorder may be unlikely to seek treatment, perhaps because of lack of awareness of the disorder, uncertainty over where to go for help, or fears of scrutiny by others.

METHODS TO DETERMINE DIAGNOSIS

The most common method of clinical assessment in research settings is the semistructured diagnostic interview. Semistructured interviews guide the clinician through the systematic assessment of diagnostic criteria while allowing the clinician flexibility to follow up on patients' areas of primary concern. One of the most frequently used semistructured interviews for the diagnosis of social anxiety disorder is the Structured Clinical Interview for *DSM–IV* Axis I Disorders–Patient Edition (SCID–I/P; First, Spitzer, Gibbon, & Williams, 1996). The SCID is a relatively time-efficient, broad-ranging interview that covers all Axis I disorders, allowing for ease in making differential diagnoses. The SCID uses multiple screening questions that allow the clinician to "skip out" at many points throughout the interview if specific diagnostic criteria are not met. Although this method provides for faster administration and more efficient collection of diagnosis-relevant information, the information collected may lack the depth necessary for treatment planning.

The Anxiety Disorder Interview Schedule for *DSM–IV*–Lifetime Version (ADIS–IV–L; DiNardo, Brown, & Barlow, 1994) is a semistructured interview designed to examine current and lifetime anxiety disorders. In addition, the interview contains modules for other disorders that commonly co-occur or overlap with anxiety disorders, including mood disorders, substance use disorders, and somatoform disorders, as well as screening questions for other major disorders (e.g., psychoses). In addition to examining the presence of specific facets of the various anxiety disorders, the ADIS–IV–L collects information on situational and cognitive cues for anxiety, making it particularly useful in cognitive–behavioral treatment settings. In contrast to the SCID, the ADIS–IV–L collects extensive information on anxiety symptoms from all individuals, including those who do not meet full diagnostic criteria. Although this allows for a more thorough evaluation, ADIS–IV–L interviews can often be quite lengthy. For more detailed information concerning the reliability of structured interviews used for the diagnosis of social anxiety disorder, the reader is referred to Hart, Jack, Turk, and Heimberg (1999).

ADDITIONAL ASSESSMENTS REQUIRED

Self-report questionnaires can be helpful in both research and clinical settings as a quick assessment of the extent to which an individual experiences social anxiety. Hart and colleagues (1999) described the most frequently used self-report measures for social anxiety in detail, a brief review of which follows. The Social Interaction Anxiety Scale (SIAS; Mattick & Clarke, 1998) assesses the degree to which an individual becomes anxious while interacting with others, either in groups or dyads. Social interaction situations, however, are not always the sole focus of anxiety; therefore, the Social Phobia Scale (SPS; Mattick & Clarke, 1998), which measures anxiety about being observed by others and fears that others will notice one's anxiety symptoms, is often administered in conjunction with the SIAS. The Social Phobia and Anxiety Inventory (SPAI; Turner, Beidel, Dancu, & Stanley, 1989) is an extensive questionnaire assessing somatic, cognitive, and behavioral responses to a wide variety of social and performance situations. The SPAI generates a large amount of information regarding the central components of social anxiety in a wide range of situations; however, the length of the questionnaire (a total of 109 responses are required) may be prohibitive in some settings. Although extremely useful assessment tools, the exclusive reliance on self-report questionnaires for the diagnosis of social anxiety disorder is not recommended.

Behavioral assessment tests (BATs) are a particularly relevant form of assessment for social anxiety disorder. Clinicians typically use informal observation during initial interviews and treatment to gain a better understanding of the ways in which an individual's social anxiety may manifest to others. More systematic and standardized assessment of social behavior can provide important information that may be helpful in guiding assessment and treatment. For example, it may be important to know that despite claims of complete incompetence in social interactions with peers, an individual with social anxiety disorder performs quite well during a role-played "cocktail party" conversation. Although the content of BATs may vary depending on the specific concerns of the client and the questions that the clinician wishes to address, they typically involve role-played exposures to feared social situations in a controlled setting. The BATs allow for direct observation of social performance, anxiety symptoms, subtle avoidance and escape behaviors, and the individual's anxiety immediately prior to, during, and after exposure to feared situations.

Comprehensive and thorough assessment is particularly helpful in the diagnosis of social anxiety disorder. Because individuals with social anxiety disorder may fear negative evaluation from the clinician, they may be less likely to report their symptoms or they may underestimate the pervasiveness of their anxiety unless probed directly about specific situations and concerns. Furthermore, individuals with social anxiety disorder may overestimate the extent to which their social skills are impaired because of their negatively biased interpretation of their own behavior or because avoidance is so pervasive that they have little experience on which to base judgments of their ability.

Although essential for diagnosis, detailed assessment can also be a helpful component of ongoing treatment. Self-monitoring of negative thoughts, physical sensations of anxiety, and avoidance behavior is key to fully understanding the nature and extent of an individual's social anxiety. A helpful device is a daily log of social anxiety in which the client may record situations in which anxiety occurred along with any negative thoughts, physical symptoms, or problematic behavior (e.g., avoidance, disengagement) in the situation. Individuals with social anxiety disorder may show particular difficulty in recalling accurately the degree of anxiety they experienced in situations occurring between therapy sessions, tending to remember these situations as more distressing than was actually the case at the time; daily self-monitoring allows them to more objectively and accurately report their anxiety. Self-monitoring techniques are further illustrated in the case description.

CASE ILLUSTRATION

Presenting Complaints

Michael was a 32-year-old single White male who was employed full-time at a bank. During administration of the ADIS–IV–L, Michael reported significant difficulties with social anxiety in social settings such as parties, speaking with unfamiliar people, dating situations, and initiating and maintaining conversations; performance situations such as participating at meetings and formal public speaking; and situations that require assertiveness, such as refusing unreasonable requests and asking others to change their behavior. Michael reported that these concerns, present since grade school, caused him considerable problems socially and professionally. In particular, he reported having great difficulty saying "no" to unreasonable requests, disagreeing with others, and asking others for help. This last concern revolved around Michael's difficulty asking his housemate to contribute his fair share of the housework. In addition, Michael had never had a romantic relationship and reported significant anxiety doing the things necessary to initiate dating relationships (e.g., speaking with someone he found attractive, asking someone out on a date). Finally, Michael reported that his social anxiety was associated with difficulty concentrating at work and carrying out the tasks that his job required. He frequently worried about what others thought of him; when others asked him a question or requested his assistance, he immediately dropped whatever he was doing, leaving a trail of incomplete tasks in his wake. Michael reported that he frequently felt detached from his surroundings and feared crying uncontrollably in anxiety-provoking situations. Physiological symptoms such as accelerated heart rate and chest pain accompanied his social anxiety.

History of the Disorder

Michael reported that his social anxiety began when he entered kindergarten at the age of 5. He stated that, although he did not recall being singled out and ridiculed, he remembered feeling shy around and avoidant of his preschool peers. However, as a child and adolescent, Michael was repeatedly ridiculed by his brother and male classmates for not acting or appearing masculine. He also recalled specific incidents in which his grammar-school girlfriend and classmates ridiculed him. By his early 20s, Michael's social anxiety had reached the point at which it created significant interference and distress. Michael completed college, but believes that his school performance was adversely affected by his social anxiety. He also stated that he pursued jobs that required only limited interaction with coworkers. Subsequent to the onset of his social anxiety, episodes of major depression, symptoms of generalized anxiety, and questions about his sexual preference emerged, all of which led him to seek treatment.

Medical History

At the time of the initial assessment, Michael reported having received a diagnosis of anemia and experiencing a childhood bout with chickenpox. Michael reported no current physical conditions that appeared relevant to his social anxiety.

Family History

Michael was the younger of two boys. At the time of the assessment, his parents were in their late 50s and married—his mother worked as a realtor and his father was a landscape architect. Michael reported that he felt closer to his mother, recalling having spent a significant amount of time in her company as a youngster. He experienced his father and older brother as overcontrolling, stern, and aloof. Michael stated that he had difficulty relating to both his father and brother.

Michael reported that his mother suffered from social anxiety but had never received a formal diagnosis of social anxiety disorder. He added that she had also experienced an episode of depression, which lasted for approximately 1 year and for which she received psychopharmacological treatment. Michael added that, to his knowledge, no other family member suffered from significant psychological distress or impairment.

Sexual History

Michael was not married, nor had he ever been involved in a serious romantic relationship, although he reported that he had been on several dates with women. As previously described, Michael's sexual history was complicated by questions about his sexual preference. Although Michael believed that he was not gay and had never had any romantic or sexual contact with a man, he questioned his sexual preference in light of thoughts that other people thought he was gay. Aside from leading Michael to question his sexual preference, these thoughts led him to doubt that women would find him attractive.

Mental Status Examination

Michael's mental status was unremarkable.

Prior Treatment

At the time of assessment, Michael was receiving no treatment; however, in the past he had received both psychotherapy and pharmacotherapy. Previously, he had seen two psychotherapists, one for 4 1/2 years and one for 6 years, to address his social anxiety, depression, and questions about his sexual preference. In addition, for his social anxiety, Michael had been prescribed 30 mg of BuSpar (buspirone) daily for several months in 1991, 20 mg of Prozac (fluoxetine) daily for 2 years from 1995 to 1996, and 20 mg of Paxil (paroxetine) daily for several months in 1997. He reported that none of these medications had been effective in ameliorating his social anxiety or depression. For Michael, the failure of these medications was a factor that complicated treatment initially as he reported a markedly diminished expectancy for a positive treatment outcome.

CASE CONCEPTUALIZATION

Modeling and Learning

Most accounts of social anxiety disorder assume a biological predisposition toward viewing social situations as threatening (the *diathesis*). Early learning experiences are presumed to provide the specific stimulus (the *stress*) for the development of heightened anxiety. Michael reported several early learning experiences that may have contributed to the development and worsening of his social anxiety. As a child, he experienced his father as stern and frightening, overcontrolling and rule bound. Michael reported that he was eager to please his father, but believed that his father did not acknowledge his achievements. On the contrary, Michael stated that his father harshly and often loudly pointed out his shortcomings. According to Michael, the tension between him and his father was most salient in the domain of athletics. Michael reported that his father's propensity to point out Michael's lack of athletic prowess was often coupled with remarks about the fact that his brother was very skilled athletically. Michael recalls feeling humiliated by the criticisms that his father would shout from the sidelines during his Little League games. Over time, Michael grew less hopeful that he would ever be able to please his father. Although Michael's father and brother spent a great deal of time together, Michael felt increasingly excluded by them.

These and other experiences of humiliation and ridicule from his father, brother, and peers during childhood and adolescence (see Life Events, following) may have contributed to his retreat into spending most of his time with his mother. Although he described his relationship with his mother as "close," we speculate that it might have been better characterized as "safe." However, her social anxiety may have had negative consequences for Michael's fragile sense of safety outside this relationship.

Life Events

Against a backdrop of a diathesis for social anxiety disorder and early learning experiences that may serve as catalysts for the development of social anxiety disorder, negative life events may further entrench incipient maladaptive beliefs. Michael recounted numerous events in which he experienced criticism, ridicule, and rejection from his brother, his peers, and a childhood girlfriend. One incident in particular continued to trouble Michael. When he was in second grade, he "got (his) first girlfriend," about whom he was extremely excited. After a few weeks of going to the movies together and to each other's house, his brother and his male classmates began to criticize and harass them. Presumably embarrassed by this negative attention, Michael's girlfriend made fun of him one day in front of their classmates. Michael recalled feeling shocked and humiliated by her rejection and violation of trust. He attributed his increasing avoidance of and shyness around his peers, particularly girls, to this incident.

Thus, Michael's early learning history may have contributed to his social anxiety in a number of ways. First, his early experience of his father and older brother as critical and unforgiving and their derisive comments about his lack of masculinity and athletic prowess may have influenced the development later in life of his beliefs about the expectations others held for him. That is, he came to believe that others held exacting standards for him, that women did not find him attractive because he was not masculine enough, and that others believed he was gay. Because of these beliefs, Michael feared that others would condemn him and even beat him up. Second, Michael spent the greatest amount of time with his socially anxious mother. Possibly to control her own social anxiety, Michael's mother created few opportunities for him to interact with peers or learn that social interactions are not necessarily as dangerous as his interactions with his father, brother, and peers may have suggested to him. She further communicated to him in her own behavior and affect that she did not consider social interactions to be "safe" for either Michael or herself. This environment may have begun training Michael to be vigilant for the harm that may come from social interaction. Furthermore, it provided few opportunities to develop a template for how acquaintanceships develop into friendships.

Genetics and Temperament

Proband and twin studies suggest that a general predisposition to interpret social situations as dangerous may be conferred genetically and account for at least a portion of the variance of social anxiety disorder. That Michael's mother exhibited symptoms of social anxiety is consistent with a possible genetic component to his social anxiety disorder. Michael also reported that he was shy around and avoided his peers when he was in preschool and early grade school. His description of his behavior is consistent with that of behavioral inhibition, a temperamental characteristic of infants and children that has been associated with the later development of social anxiety disorder.

Finally, persons with social anxiety disorder may have inherited a more extreme predisposition to fear biologically determined cues of danger such as anger, criticism, and social disapproval, particularly from members of society perceived to be more powerful. In such a scenario, perceived threats may elicit submission, escape, avoidance, and less dominance on the part of the socially anxious individual. In fact, Michael was particularly sensitive to cues of anger, criticism, and social disapproval and worked hard to avoid situations in which they might be experienced. During the course of treatment, Michael admitted that he had difficulty completing homework assignments that focused on the theme of becoming more assertive in interactions with others because he was concerned that the persons to whom he needed to assert (and who he perceived to be threatening, aggressive, and powerful) would retaliate against him and he would not be able to stand their negative reactions to him. Not surprisingly, he saw the negative consequences of asserting to these persons as greater than the cost of not doing so (i.e., facing his therapists, whom he perceived to be less threatening, aggressive, and powerful).

Physical Conditions

Michael evidenced no physical condition that has a demonstrated association with social anxiety disorder.

Drugs

Michael reported having never used drugs of abuse. He did pursue psychophar-macological treatment with Paxil (paroxetine) during the course of psychother-apy treatment for social anxiety disorder, the details of which are described in Role of Pharmacotherapy in the Case.

Socioeconomic and Cultural Factors

Michael's socioeconomic and cultural background is consistent with the de-mographic profile of a large percentage of persons with social anxiety disorder, and is further unremarkable with regard to case conceptualization.

Overall Conceptualization

Michael may have inherited a general tendency to become anxious in novel situations. His mother's social anxiety and overprotectiveness as well as several early negative social experiences may have contributed to his anxiety becoming focused exclusively on social situations and the negative consequences that may follow. Thus, an initial biological vulnerability was exacerbated by the conditions in which Michael was brought up and his specific developmental experiences.

Typical of persons with social anxiety disorder, Michael's social anxiety was created and maintained on a foundation of fear of negative evaluation in social and performance situations, which led to the development of beliefs that social interactions are dangerous. We now examine Michael's experience of social anxiety at a church party through the lens of our cognitive–behavioral theory (Rapee & Heimberg, 1997).

After receiving an invitation and up until the time he arrived the party, Michael reported that he thought almost exclusively about the other people who would attend the event and the threat each of them represented to him. For instance, he wondered whether a woman in whom he was interested would be there and who the other party guests (who might overhear and ridicule any conversations that he might have with this woman) would be. In addition, Michael brought to this party certain cognitive biases. For example, he expected that many of the guests would be critical of him such that he would be judged negatively, and he anticipated that the conversations that would take place at this party would be competitive events in which there would be a winner and a loser. Of course, his anticipatory anxiety and projection of this negative future increased his belief that he would be the one to lose.

At the party, his initial impressions of the reactions of the other guests were combined with information from past similar situations (e.g., criticism from his brother and peers, rejection by his grade-school girlfriend) and internal (e.g., palpitations) and external (e.g., a conversation partner excused himself to speak with someone else) cues to determine how the guests were likely to view him. That is, he constantly monitored his behavior and the behavior of others to determine whether there was any potential for negative evaluation. Ironically, Michael's allocation of his attentional resources to multiple factors (e.g., scanning the environment for evidence of negative evaluation, monitoring his performance for evidence of inadequacy, attending to thoughts about being evaluated negatively) made it harder to pay attention to dialog with other party guests and gave Michael a subjective sense of being overwhelmed and unable to handle the unpredictable social demands of the party.

As is common in all social situations, there is much information that can be collected by the person about how he or she is doing. However, like other persons with social anxiety disorder, Michael weighed more heavily evidence confirming that he was not doing well at the party than he did evidence to the contrary. For example, sweating, forgetting his train of thought, and a brief response by a woman to whom he was speaking were all interpreted by Michael as evidence that he was performing poorly and being evaluated negatively. However, he was apparently oblivious to the other people at the party who seemed to like him very much.

Michael took the biased data he had collected to heart and concluded that he had failed to live up to the expectations that he believed the other guests held for him. On the basis of this conclusion, he projected a future of continuing social rejection and unending loneliness and isolation. He also took this outcome, which he wholeheartedly believed to be true, as evidence in support of his negative beliefs about himself ("I am not masculine enough," "They think I am gay") and others (other people have high standards, are critical, and will reject me).

As the party progressed, Michael's distorted and negative internal dialog, his desire to escape (i.e., leave the party early), and his physical arousal all worsened. As these symptoms of anxiety elevated, they became further sources of distorted information about how his appearance and behavior were perceived by others. Thus, by the time he did leave the party, he was more thoroughly convinced than ever that he could not handle social situations and believed that the next party would be an even worse experience than this one had been. This vicious cycle of social anxiety increased the probability that Michael would judge the social situation as a failure, as he did. A collection of similar experiences strengthened maladaptive beliefs and lowered his expectations for success in future situations.

Diagnostic Assessment

Michael was examined by a trained interviewer using the ADIS–IV–L, at which time he reported that his primary problem was social anxiety. Michael clearly met criteria for social anxiety disorder, but he also reported several other concerns. First, he described several episodes in his life during which he experienced depressed mood, markedly diminished motivation, excessive self-blame, and impaired concentration. Thus, he also received a diagnosis of major depressive disorder. His episodes were occasionally marked by suicidal ideation; however, Michael denied ever intending to act on a formulated plan. His depression complicated his social anxiety because it contributed to a lack of motivation to expose himself to feared situations and doubts that anyone would ever want to date him or that life would ever be enjoyable.

Second, Michael endorsed many of the symptoms of generalized anxiety disorder, the diagnosis of which was subsumed under the diagnosis of major depressive disorder in accordance with the specifications of *DSM–IV*. Interestingly, many of his worries were exacerbated by a perceived inability to be assertive and a lack of belief in his efficacy at work. He worried that people would think that he was incompetent, that he was being taken advantage of by his brother, that people would beat him up if they believed that he was gay, and about whether he really was gay. In addition, he worried that his health would fail. Michael's worries contributed to chronic physiological symptoms such as restlessness, fatigue, concentration difficulties, and muscle tension.

Michael also reported some difficulty with obsessive thoughts, but these were not deemed sufficient to warrant a diagnosis of obsessive–compulsive disorder. His history was negative for alcohol or substance abuse. Following the assessment, he was assigned a principal diagnosis of social anxiety disorder and an additional diagnosis of major depressive disorder, recurrent.

Behavioral Assessment

During his initial assessment, Michael participated in two standardized behavioral assessment role-plays. In the first, he was asked to present a 4-minute impromptu speech to a male and a female role player. Michael's self-reported anxiety was consistently high in the few minutes before he began his speech. He remained anxious throughout the speech, although he reported a slight drop in the last minutes of the speech. After the role-play, Michael reported that he experienced negative thoughts throughout such as "I'm rambling" and "I'm boring them," and his assessment of his ability to communicate during the speech was very low. Although he appeared somewhat anxious at the start of the speech, he was actually quite eloquent in his presentation and the small audience felt that they had a good understanding of the points he was trying to convey.

In his second role-play, Michael interacted with the same two individuals in a staged "cocktail party" conversation. He again reported high anxiety throughout the anticipatory period; however, his anxiety gradually decreased to the moderate range during the conversation. He reported thoughts such as "I don't know how to stand comfortably" and, toward the end of the interaction, "This isn't so bad." Nonetheless, he judged his performance harshly, again rating his ability to communicate as quite low. Again, the perception of the role players was very different. To them, Michael was a poised and skilled conversationalist.

Prioritization of Targets for Treatment

As demonstrated in Michael's diagnostic assessment, although he experienced depression and excessive worry, social anxiety was perceived to be the most interfering and distressing concern, and therefore became the first priority for treatment. If Michael's depression had been more severe or if the therapists believed that, despite its lesser severity, it would interfere significantly with treatment of his social anxiety, treatment of his depression might have been the first order of business. In Michael's case, the therapists believed that despite the presence of a mild depressive disorder, he was reasonably motivated to begin treatment of his social anxiety disorder at that time. Nonetheless, the therapists were vigilant for increasing depressive symptoms and prepared to modify the treatment plan accordingly.

Despite the selection of social anxiety for initial intervention, the significant overlap between the thoughts that drive both anxiety and depression provided the therapists with opportunities to address these two concerns simultaneously. They encouraged Michael to challenge thoughts such as "I can't do this" or "This is hopeless," particularly when these thoughts seemed to be getting in the way of active engagement with treatment. In addition, if behavioral exposures did not appear to be addressing Michael's lessened activity and interest adequately, the clinician might have considered encouraging other forms of behavioral activation, such as getting involved in activities that do not involve a great deal of social interaction and limiting the number of hours spent in bed.

Finally, Michael reported that worries outside of social situations were bothersome, but not severely impairing; therefore, they were not initially a target of treatment. However, reevaluation of the presence of excessive worry after successful treatment of his social anxiety was necessary in order to determine whether they continued to pose a problem for Michael.

Selection and Prioritization of Treatment Strategies

Given the primacy of Michael's social anxiety disorder, this was the initial focus of treatment. The empirical literature for the treatment of social anxiety disorder supports the use of CBT as well as several medications. Because of Michael's less than satisfactory response to several pharmacological agents, an initial trial of cognitive–behavioral group therapy was recommended.

In the first few sessions, the cognitive–behavioral model of social anxiety disorder was explained to Michael. He completed homework assignments in which he self-monitored his anxiety (physical symptoms, thoughts, triggers, etc.). He and other group members were taught to identify negative cognitions or automatic thoughts, examine the relationship between negative cognitions and anxiety, challenge logical errors in their thoughts, and come up with rational alternatives. After Michael mastered these concepts, he completed in-session exposures to increasingly difficult feared situations while applying his newly learned cognitive skills. He and his therapists determined that it would be best for him to work first with situations that were mildly feared, such as having casual conversations with women in situations that would not lead to further contact, before moving on to conversations with women in more social environments, asking for dates, handling situations that arise on dates, and then on to situations that involve conversation with men, first in casual settings, then in sports settings, and finally in conflict situations that arise on the job. As he confronted and addressed these situations in his group therapy, he progressively exposed himself to more and more difficult situations in real life.

Dealing with Complicating Factors

Complicating factors for Michael included the subtlety of his avoidance mechanisms, obsessive thoughts, and panic symptoms. Michael possessed sophisticated social and interpersonal skills and an attractive self-presentation, and these would eventually become assets in his battle against social anxiety. However, to his detriment, his social skills enabled him to rely on subtle avoidance mechanisms to control his anxiety. Michael reported that, while in conversation with women, he would steer the conversation to safe places and could do so in a manner that did not appear awkward for his conversation partner. For instance, when unfamiliar topics were raised, he would guide the conversation onto more familiar ground rather than admit his ignorance; when points of view were expressed with which he disagreed, Michael either agreed or again changed the topic. In this way, he avoided anxiety-provoking aspects of these situations so deftly that it was difficult for his conversation partner or an observer to notice. In fact, until role-played exposures were conducted in his therapy group, Michael's therapists had not identified this subtle pattern of avoidance. Without the benefit of behavioral assessment, they might have missed it altogether. However, having identified it, exposure exercises were designed that specifically instructed Michael to avoid these avoidance behaviors.

The fact that Michael experienced obsessive thoughts was first noted during the diagnostic interview. He experienced repeated self-derogating thoughts about his sexual preferences, such as "you are a faggot," that occurred during social interactions or "whenever anyone looked at me." He also experienced blasphemous thoughts and curses that occurred when he was at church. These thoughts were particularly disturbing to Michael because he believed that they interfered with his ability to date women and maintain friendships with fellow Christians. He struggled with the question of whether his belief that others thought he was gay meant that he really was gay or whether it served only as an avoidance mechanism. In addition, he wondered whether his blasphemous thoughts meant that he was a hypocrite and a poor Christian. Indeed, these thoughts did interfere in dating and friendship situations and, more generally, kept people at arm's length. Although these thoughts were extremely disturbing to Michael, they occurred relatively infrequently (i.e., once or twice a day for less than a half-hour), and therefore did not meet criteria for obsessive–compulsive disorder.

Michael's obsessive thoughts were not determined to be a primary target of treatment; however, they were relevant because his thought process was characterized by thought–action fusion, a phenomenon most commonly observed among persons with obsessive–compulsive disorder who may believe something is true or likely to happen simply because they think the thought. Thought–action fusion may render an individual less willing to entertain alternative ways of viewing situations. In Michael's case these thoughts inevitably occurred when he confronted his most anxiety-evoking situations. This was taken into account in treatment by working first with less difficult situations and undermining some of the beliefs that were associated with Michael's obsessions. For instance, he was able to learn that he could have successful conversations with women in casual settings before the therapists asked him to work on asking someone on a date, and dating was addressed before dealing with conflict situations with men in positions of authority. However, had the obsessive thoughts become so overwhelming that they seemed to warrant direct intervention, the therapists might have pursued exposure and response prevention exercises focusing directly on these thoughts (e.g., instructing Michael to think these feared thoughts without engaging in any kind of reassurance behavior).

Finally, Michael experienced physiological symptoms when anxious, including accelerated heart rate and chest pain. At times Michael would experience full-blown panic attacks. However, the attacks were always expected and occurred only in social situations; therefore, he did not meet criteria for a diagnosis of panic disorder. Michael's tendency to become physiologically aroused decreased as a result of cognitive–behavioral interventions for social anxiety disorder. The therapists specifically targeted for cognitive restructuring those thoughts that contributed to increased arousal, such as "My heart's beating so fast that I'm going to have a heart attack," or "I get so anxious I can't breathe." The therapists might also have considered applied relaxation or breathing retraining to help Michael decrease his baseline arousal. In addition, if Michael continued to demonstrate significant fear of physiological symptoms, they might have considered interoceptive exposure exercises in which Michael would be asked to induce physical symptoms both in the therapy session and in real-life situations. Interoceptive exposure can also be considered as a component of behavioral exposures during the group sessions. For example, the clinician could have asked Michael to run up several flights of stairs before giving a speech as an exposure exercise.

Role of Pharmacotherapy in the Case

During cognitive–behavioral group treatment for social anxiety disorder, Michael began a course of a larger dose (40 mg/d) of Paxil (paroxetine), at which time he experienced marked improvement in his social anxiety and depression. Similar to other patients receiving concurrent psychotherapy and medication, Michael initially attributed all of his improvement to the medication, disregarding the fact that Paxil typically takes 4–6 weeks to achieve maximum effect and disqualifying any personal accomplishments that he made during the course of psychotherapy treatment. The relative contributions of psychotherapy and pharmacotherapy to Michael's improvement are unknown; however, to the extent that the Paxil was effective, the improved functioning of the serotonin and other neurotransmitter systems (e.g., norepinephrine, dopamine) may have been implicated in the improvement of his symptoms. However, clinical experience with Michael and many other patients suggests that it is important for the maintenance of gains that they learn to attribute the changes in their behavior and emotions to themselves rather than solely to their medication.

Managed Care Considerations

Michael successfully completed 12 sessions of cognitive–behavioral group therapy for social anxiety disorder while receiving a concurrent trial of 40 mg/d of Paxil (paroxetine). Similar to 80% of patients who complete 12 sessions of cognitive–behavioral group therapy for social anxiety disorder without concurrent pharmacotherapy, Michael achieved significant improvement in his social anxiety symptoms. It is currently under investigation whether concurrent pharmacotherapy increases the percentage of persons realizing treatment gains within 12 weeks or increases the speed with which gains are realized such that additional sessions become less necessary. Finally, although little published data support the use of group treatment over individual treatment for social anxiety disorder, group treatment has been the preferred form of treatment for social anxiety disorder for several reasons. First, it gives patients an opportunity to begin exposing themselves to social situations with other patients in session. Second, group treatment is more cost effective because it allows for treatment of patients in greater numbers (6–7 patients is ideal) within the same time frame.

SUMMARY

Michael was typical of many treatment-seeking persons with social anxiety disorder. His fears were generalized across several domains. He exhibited marked avoidance of some situations (e.g., dating situations, assertiveness) and endured others with significant distress (e.g., interacting with individuals at work and at church). Despite Michael's above-average intelligence and social presentation, he chose to work at a job that was not commensurate with his abilities and failed to incorporate positive responses from individuals, particularly women, with whom he interacted. Indeed, Michael fully endorsed the beliefs that he was incompetent, that women found him unattractive, and that he was not masculine enough.

Because many patients with social anxiety disorder present with similarly negative and rigid beliefs about themselves and the world, it is important to share with them the handful of empirically demonstrated predictors of treatment outcome. Based both on clinical observation and empirical data, probably the most influential predictors of outcome are outcome expectancy, rigidity of beliefs, trust, and homework compliance. Michael began treatment with markedly low expectancies that anything good would come from his investment of effort in treatment. Similar to other patients, he reported several previous unsuccessful attempts at treatment, and had come away with the belief that his problem was intractable. In addition, like other persons with social anxiety disorder, Michael held rigidly to his belief that he lacked skill in social and performance situations. Fortunately, Michael was inclined to trust his therapist, complied well with assigned homework in most instances, and quickly learned to consider alternative perspectives with regard to himself and treatment. It is important that patients with social anxiety disorder be made aware that they can influence the course of their treatment negatively via pessimism, lack of trust, rigid thinking, and failure to complete important homework tasks.

REFERENCES

American Psychiatric Association. (1994). *Diagnostic and statistical manual of mental disorders* (4th ed.). Washington, DC: Author.

DiNardo, P. A., Brown, T. A., & Barlow, D. H. (1994). *Anxiety Disorders Interview Schedule for DSM–IV: Lifetime version (ADIS–IV–L)*. San Antonio, TX: The Psychological Corporation.

First, M. B., Spitzer, R. L., Gibbon, M., & Williams, J. (1996). *Structured Clinical Interview for DSM–IV Axis I Disorders–Patient Edition* (SCID-I/P, Version 2.0). New York: New York State Psychiatric Institute.

Hart, T. A., Jack, M. S., Turk, C. L., & Heimberg, R. G. (1999). Issues for the measurement of social anxiety disorder. In H. G. M. Westenberg & J. A. Den Boer (Eds.), *Social anxiety disorder* (pp. 133–155). Amsterdam: Syn-Thesis Publishers.

Heimberg, R. G. (1996). Social phobia, avoidant personality disorder and the multiaxial conceptualization of interpersonal anxiety. In P. M. Salkovskis (Ed.), *Trends in cognitive and behavioural therapies* (pp. 43–61). Chichester: John Wiley & Sons Ltd.

Magee, W. J., Eaton, W. W., Wittchen, H. U., McGonagle, K. A., & Kessler, R. C. (1996). Agoraphobia, simple phobia, and social phobia in the National Comorbidity Survey. *Archives of General Psychiatry, 53,* 159–168.

Mattick, R. P., & Clarke, J. C. (1998). Development and validation of measures of social phobia scrutiny fear and social interaction anxiety. *Behaviour Research and Therapy, 36,* 455–470.

Rapee, R. M., & Heimberg, R. G. (1997). A cognitive–behavioral model of anxiety in social phobia. *Behaviour Research and Therapy, 35,* 741–756.

Schneier, F. R., Johnson, J., Hornig, C. D., Liebowitz, M. R., & Weissman, M. M. (1992). Social phobia: Comorbidity and morbidity in an epidemiologic sample. *Archives of General Psychiatry, 49,* 282–288.

Turner, S. M., Beidel, D. C., Dancu, C. V., & Stanley, M. A. (1989). An empirically derived inventory to measure social fears and anxiety: The Social Phobia and Anxiety Inventory. *Psychological Assessment, 1,* 35–40.

8

Obsessive–Compulsive Disorder

Paul M. G. Emmelkamp
and Patricia van Oppen
University of Amsterdam

DESCRIPTION OF THE DISORDER

According to the *DSM–IV*, either recurrent obsessions or compulsions have to occur for a diagnosis of obsessive–compulsive disorder (OCD). Essential for the diagnosis of OCD is that the complaints cause marked distress, are time consuming (take more than an hour), or interfere with social or work functioning. The content of the obsession or compulsion must be unrelated to any other Axis I disorder. *Obsessions* are repetitive, recurring thoughts, ideas, images, or impulses that are experienced as intrusive, and also as senseless or repugnant—the client attempts to ignore or suppress them. The client recognizes that the obsessions are the product of his or her own mind. *Compulsions*, however, are repetitive, apparent, and purposeful behaviors that are performed according to certain rules or in a stereotyped fashion. Compulsions have the function of neutralizing or preventing discomfort and/or anxiety.

Clinical Picture

Rituals or compulsions mostly accompany obsessions. Most clients with OCD have obsessions as well as compulsions. A minority of such clients suffers from obsessions only, most often harming obsessions. Clients with harming obsessions are afraid of harming others (e.g., by strangling) and avoid ropes and sharp objects (such as knives, scissors, or pieces of glass) or being alone with young children or helpless elderly people. A few are concerned only about harming themselves (e.g., by committing suicide). Clients with only rit-uals are seen very rarely. Generally, the obsessions are anxiety inducing and the performance of compulsions leads to anxiety reduction. The most com-mon compulsions involve cleaning and checking. Less common complaints are compulsive slowness, orderliness, hoarding, buying, and counting. A client, who suffers from compulsive hoarding collects all kinds of things and may have cupboards full with old bills, notes, hundreds of pairs of shoes, and un-derwear. These objects are not used, but the client is afraid of throwing them away because they may come in handy one day. *Compulsive buying* implies that the client has a strong inclination to buy a wide variety of items. Compul-sive counting often accompanies checking and washing. In some patients, such counting is the main problem. In a number of clients, neutralizing thoughts have the same function as rituals; that is, the undoing of the harmful effects of the obsession. Two types of avoidance behavior are distinguished: active and passive avoidance. The obsessive–compulsive client avoids stimuli that might provoke anxiety and discomfort (passive avoidance). Active avoidance refers to the motor component of obsessive–compulsive behavior (e.g., cleaning and washing) in case the passive avoidance failed. Examples of passive avoidance are clients with checking compulsions who avoid situations that provoke their rituals, such as being alone, driving a car, using matches, or being the last one going to bed. Individuals with a cleaning or washing obsession take many pre-cautions to avoid contamination. When obsessions are related to death, clients avoid all kinds of situations that suggest the notion of death, such as reading papers (obituaries), watching television, or going to a funeral (Emmelkamp, Bouman, & Scholing, 1993).

It is important for treatment planning to establish the exact nature of the content of the obsession. Obsessive thoughts can be either anxiety inducing or anxiety reducing. When obsessions are anxiety inducing, they may be ac-companied by rituals to reduce anxiety. Obsessional clients often engage in neutralizing thoughts (anxiety-reducing obsessions) in order to undo the pos-sible harmful effects of their obsession. For example, one obsessional client repeatedly thought: "I will strangle you," which was immediately followed by the thought: "I love you." The thinking of the neutralizing thought "I love you" led to temporarily relief of anxiety provoked by the aggressive thought. The neutralizing thoughts presumably serve the same function as the checking or washing rituals of other obsessive–compulsive clients (i.e., to produce anxiety reduction).

Throughout the 1990s, an increasing number of studies have focused on be-liefs and cognitive processes characteristic of obsessive–compulsive clients, including inflated responsibility, thought–action fusion, indecisiveness, mag-ical thinking, aversion to risk taking, pollution of the mind, and guilt. There is some evidence that specific beliefs are associated with specific obsessive-compulsive behaviors. For example, beliefs related to contamination (e.g., pollution of the mind) play an important part in washing but not in other obsessive–compulsive behaviors. Thought–action fusion appeared to be important in washing and checking, but not in impulses, precision, and rumination. Guilt was found to be related to rumination and checking, but not to other obsessive–compulsive behaviors (Emmelkamp & Aardema, 1999).

Comorbidity and Differential Diagnosis

There exists considerable comorbidity between OCD and other disorders. There is a considerable overlap between OCD and other *anxiety disorders*. Over half of the obsessive–compulsive clients have a lifetime prevalence of simple phobia, social phobia, or panic disorder. Furthermore, general anxiety disorder (GAD) is a comorbid disorder in 20% of the OCD clients (Abramowitz & Foa, 1998). The worrying in GAD and the obsessive concern with one's own health in *hypochondriasis* should not be diagnosed as OCD (van Rijsoort, Emmelkamp, & Vervaeke, 2000).

Depression is a frequent complication of OCD. Studies of comorbidity suggest that one third of obsessive–compulsive clients report major depression. An additional number of clients also qualify for the diagnosis of dysthymia. The obsessive–compulsive symptoms often worsen during the depressed mood, and severe depression may have a detrimental influence on the prognosis. Transition from OCD to depression occurs three times more often than transition from depression to OCD. Thus, in most cases, the depression is secondary to the OCD, which is not surprising, considering the severity of the complaints. When obsessive thoughts are part of a depressive episode and disappear when the depression subsides, the diagnosis of depression is more appropriate than the diagnosis OCD (Emmelkamp & van Oppen, 2001).

The frequency of *personality disorders* among obsessive–compulsives is high (van Velzen & Emmelkamp, 1999). The diagnosis of obsessive–compulsive personality disorder is given in 25% of clients, which is not more than in other anxiety disorders. Obsessive–compulsive personality traits are differentiated from OCD in that they are egosyntonic, rarely provoke resistance, and are seldom accompanied by compulsions. In OCD clients, symptoms are egodystonic and usually provoke resistance; compulsions are very common.

Clients with tics are diagnosed with *tic disorder*. Tics are seen as involuntary behaviors, whereas compulsions are intentional behaviors. Recent studies suggest that 10–30% of OCD clients also have a tic disorder.

Obsessions as part of a *psychotic episode* are not classified as OCD. Hallucinations and delusions must be differentiated from obsessions. The main diagnostic question here is whether the client recognizes that his or her thoughts or ideas are unreasonable. Previously, many investigators suggested that OCD and schizophrenia were related; however, longitudinal studies have not found an increased incidence of schizophrenia either in obsessive–compulsive clients or in their relatives (Emmelkamp & van Oppen, 2001).

Prevalence, Course, and Prognosis

Community surveys have shown a relatively high prevalence rate of OCD. The mean lifetime prevalence of OCD is 2.2%. In these community surveys, the prevalence of OCD was slightly higher among females than among males. Checking, however, is more prevalent among males, whereas washing and cleaning are more common among females. Mean age of onset is 20–25 years, with 10% starting before age 10 and 9% starting after age 40. Age at onset for males (20 years) is earlier than for females (25 years). Given the fact that most cleaners are women, it does not come as a surprise that cleaners have a later age of onset than checkers. Sometimes onset of OCD is immediate; typically, however, problems arise insidiously over several years (Emmelkamp & van Oppen, 2001).

If obsessive–compulsive clients do not get adequate treatment, the disorder tends to have a chronic and fluctuating course. Treatment of choice consists of behavior therapy; namely, in vivo exposure plus response prevention. Where this treatment is given, approximately 75% of clients displayed improvement and about 25% of clients remained unchanged on self-ratings of obsessive–compulsive symptoms, anxiety, and depression (Emmelkamp, in preparation). Recent studies suggest that cognitive therapy (van Oppen et al., 1995) and pharmacotherapy (i.e., tricyclic antidepressants and selective serotonine reuptake inhibitors; Pigott & Seay, 1998) are also promising, but long-term studies are needed before more definite conclusions are warranted.

METHODS TO DETERMINE DIAGNOSIS

Semistructured Interviews

Apart from the SCID-I, described in Chapter 2, clinicians can use semistructured interviews that have been developed specifically for the assessment of anxiety disorders (ADIS–R) or OCD (Y–BOCS).

- *Anxiety Disorders Interview Schedule–Revised* (ADIS–IV; DiNardo, Brown & Barlow, 1994). The ADIS–IV is a semistructured interview aimed primarily at the diagnosis of anxiety disorders departing from *DSM* criteria. Interrater reliability of OCD is good (Taylor, 1998).
- *Yale–Brown Obsessive–Compulsive Interview (Y–BOCS)*. The Y–BOCS is a semistructured interview to assess OCD symptomatology (Goodman

et al., 1989). Using a 64-item checklist, the interviewer asks the patient whether items referring to obsessions, compulsive behavior, and avoidance behavior have been present. Formal assessment is based on five items (independent of symptom content) assessing the (a) duration/frequency, (b) interference in social and occupational functioning, (c) distress, (d) resistance, and (e) perceived control for obsessions and compulsions, respectively. Interrater reliability is good and concurrent validity is satisfactory, but discriminant validity is poor. The Y–BOCS is sensitive to treatment effects (Taylor, 1998; van Oppen, Emmelkamp, & van Balkom, 1995).

ADDITIONAL ASSESSMENTS REQUIRED

Behavioral Measures

Although direct behavioral assessment has been highly valued by behavior therapists, in the area of OCD few studies have evaluated in vivo behavioral measures. There are a number of drawbacks that preclude the use of standardized behavioral measures, such as Behavioral Avoidance Tests (BAT) and direct behavioral observation with clients who are obsessive–compulsives. First, the problems OCD patients have are highly idiosyncratic, which makes a standardization and comparison across patients rather difficult, if not impossible. Second, the content of the obsession and the associated rituals may change in the course of time, thus limiting the use of such measures to evaluate treatment outcome. Third, given the numerous situations that are avoided by OCD patients, the use of a single-task BAT may not be representative of the variety of OCD problems they have. Although this problem may be circumvented partly by using multiple tasks, use of the BAT may interfere with the treatment to be evaluated: The more tasks that are needed to assess the target behaviors reliably, the more exposure patients receive during the assessment phase.

Less-structured behavioral assessment, however, can provide important information. For example, it makes sense to have a patient with an extensive washing ritual demonstrate how he or she washes. In some instances, rehearsal in role-play of certain situations that evoked anxiety can also reveal important information. One patient suffered from harming obsessions every time he had a quarrel. Repeated questioning about the course of these quarrels yielded little information. The course the quarrel takes becomes clearer when it is rehearsed in role-playing. One of the patient's colleagues criticizes him. The patient becomes furious but does not say anything, and when the tension becomes unbearable he finally goes to the manager and says, "If he doesn't shut up, I'll skewer him on a pitchfork!" Such diagnostic role-playing gives important information about the stimuli that gave rise to the patient's obsession.

In summary, whereas standardized behavioral tests are of little avail, behavioral observation, either in vivo or in role-playing, may add to the information gathered in the interview.

Self-Monitoring

A patient's self-registration can be valuable for insight into obsessive–compulsive problems and OCD-related anxiety. During the admission interview, the information is gathered retrospectively, and therefore is subject to distortion of memory, selective perception, social desirability, and so on. As soon as the therapist, in consultation with the patient, has determined one or more target behaviors, it make sense to have the patient keep a structured diary. It is important for the patient to fill out the diary regularly throughout the day. In doing so, not only can the frequency and intensity of obsessions and compulsive behavior be asessed, but the conditions under which this behavior occurs can be monitored as well.

Self-Report Measures

There are a number of self-report assessment devices available of which The Padua Inventory and The Maudsley Obsessive–Compulsive Inventory are most widely used.

The Maudsley Obsessive–Compulsive Inventory. The Maudsley Obsessive–Compulsive Inventory (MOCI; Hodgson & Rachman, 1977) consists of 30 items. The questionnaire can be used to give a total obsessionality score as well as four factor scores. High score on the checking subscale indicates that a great deal of time is spent every day checking things over and over again. The obsessional cleaning subscale includes items with respect to excessive concerns about germs and cleanliness, worries about contamination, and items concerning excessive washing. High score on the obsessional slowness scale indicates that the person adheres to a strict routine and often counts when doing a routine task. Finally, persons scoring high on doubting–conscientiousness have a strict conscience and usually have serious doubts about simple, everyday events rather than obsessive–compulsive tendencies. Reliability and validity of the MOCI was investigated by Emmelkamp, Kraaijkamp, and van den Hout (1999), who found that the internal consistency was high for the total score and moderate for the Checking and Cleaning subscales. Furthermore, the MOCI was found to have a high test–retest reliability. Thus, the total MOCI scale and the Checking and Cleaning subscales are reliable and use of the subscale slowness should be discouraged. As to validity, concurrent validity between the MOCI and several other measures of obsessional and compulsive behavior is satisfactory. Further, the Checking and Cleaning subscales could differentiate between checkers and washers in a reliable fashion. Thus, clients who were categorized as Checkers or Cleaners on the basis of their questionnaire score were usually assigned to the respective categories by clinicians.

Discriminant validity between OCD clients and normals is rather good. There is a clear cutoff point differentiating both groups: 97.5% of the normals have a score below 10 points and 89.9% of the obsessive patients have a score of 10 or more points. Furthermore, the MOCI was found to discriminate reliably among obsessional clients, clients with anorexia, and anxious clients. However, this questionnaire was unable to differentiate obsessives from depressives. Given the relationship between obsession and depression, the last finding is not surprising.

Obvious advantages of the MOCI are its easy administration, its discrimination of obsessives from other neurotic clients, and validation of two of the subscales (Checking and Washing). Although the MOCI may be used to evaluate effects of treatment, simple ratings of anxiety–discomfort for target obsessional problems on scales of 0–8 appeared to be a more sensitive index of change than the MOCI (Emmelkamp, Kraaijkamp, & van den Hout, 1999). It should be noted that currently a revised version (MOCI–R) is under development at the University of British Columbia, Vancouver, but psychometric data on clinical groups are still lacking.

The Padua Inventory–Revised.   The Padua Inventory (PI) was originally developed by Sanavio (1988) and the revised version (PI–R) was developed by van Oppen, Hoekstra, and Emmelkamp (1995a). The PI-R results in a total obsessionality score and has five subscales: (a) impulses, (b) washing, (c) checking, (d) rumination, and (e) precision. In contrast to the original, the PI–R was investigated psychometrically in large clinical groups. The internal consistencies are good to excellent. The PI–R was shown to have a robust factor structure across samples of OCD, clients with other anxiety disorders, and persons considered to be normal. The PI–R has been shown to discriminate obsessive–compulsives from clients diagnosed with panic, social phobia, and normal controls. Concurrent validity with related measures of OCD is good (van Oppen et al., 1995a).

The Self-Report Yale–Brown Obsessive Compulsive Scale.   A self-report version of the Yale–Brown Obsessive Compulsion Scale (Y–BOCS; Steketee, Frost, & Bogart, 1996). was developed and investigated. These data suggest that the self-report Y–BOCS may also be a promising questionnaire for assessing OCD symptoms. Before definite conclusions can be drawn, further research on clinical samples is needed.

Although the PI–R is sensitive to assess treatment change, both the PI–R and the Y–BOCS have been found to be less sensitive to change than the anxiety–discomfort scale (van Oppen, Emmelkamp, van Balkom, & van Dyck, 1995b). If improvement was evaluated in terms of clinical significance, different measures led to different results. There is only 57% overlap in clients who are rated as clinically significantly improved on all three measures.

It should be noted that another revised version of the PI is on the market in the United States in which all items that assess worry have been deleted (Burns, Keortge, Formea, & Sternberger, 1996). In doing so, the authors may have thrown out the good as well as the bad (van Rijsoort, Emmelkamp, & Vervaeke, 2000). Furthermore, psychometric data on clinical groups of this revised version of the PI are lacking; therefore, this version is not recommended for clinical use. The advantage of the PI–R is that it measures a broad range of obsessive–compulsive symptoms, but this is at the expense of assessing the severity of these symptoms. Another advantage is that it is easy to administer. In contrast to the PI–R and the MOCI, the Y–BOCS investigates the severity of OCD rather than the range of obsessive–compulsive symptoms. Furthermore, the Y–BOCS is relatively time consuming because it consists of a structured interview.

CASE ILLUSTRATION

Presenting Complaints

Maria, a 23-year-old emotionally neglected woman, was referred to our department for treatment of her obsessive–compulsive disorder. She also met *DSM–IV* criteria for agoraphobia, social phobia, and dysthymic disorder. Her Obsessive–compulsive complaints consisted of a whole range of rituals and concomitant obsessive thoughts. She experienced these obsessions as egodystonic (meaning "not fitting her,") and for a long time she thought she was "mad."

History of the Complaint

Maria's obsessive complaints started (without any immediate cause) when she was 9 years old and regularly visited a (student) neighbor. The obsession to wash after she had come home gradually developed ("Not that the student was very dirty, but just because · · ·"). After she washed her hands at the tap ("that had to run gently"), she did not allow herself to touch anything (e.g., doorknob) with her hands. Also during that time she started to wash her entire body ("until I looked raw and white as a sheet"), which often took an hour. This obsessive–compulsive washing behavior lasted for 6 months and then spontaneously disappeared. Next there came a period of well over 6 months in which she suddenly woke up at night and felt the urge to make her bed. This usually occurred at the beginning of the night and could recur six or seven times a night. This obsession also spontaneously disappeared, and thereafter she remained free of complaints for several years. At age 16, alternate obsessive themes began to occur.

Medical History

Maria has not been treated for any serious disease, so there appear to be no medical complications.

Family History

As Maria learned later in her life, she was a child born out of wedlock. Although her mother told her who her biological father is, she does not feel the need to have any contact with him. She is the youngest in a family with two brothers. When Maria was attending her first year of elementary school, her parents divorced, and her legal father left the parental home. The family was an incoherent entity in which everyone looked after himself or herself.

There was no evidence that her mother suffered from OCD. However, she apparently had borderline personality traits and antisocial personality traits. There was no information with respect to possible psychiatric disorders of her biological father. One brother was a compulsive gambler; the other suffered from severe alcohol dependency.

Sexual History

Maria's first sexual contact occurred with her present partner at the age of 16. She is satisfied with their current sexual relationship, although obsessive thoughts often interfere during sexual intercourse. When she is depressed, she does not want to have any sexual contact. Her partner is accepting of this.

Mental Status Examination

Maria's mental status is normal. There was no evidence that her basic orientation for time and place, attention, perception, or memory were disturbed. Although her obsessions were at times bizarre, they were experienced as egodystonic. Therefore, no formal screening test for mental status was required.

Prior Treatment

Maria was prescribed tranquilizers by her general practitioner for her OCD, and, together with her partner, had received 10 sessions of supportive psychotherapy at a community mental health center. Neither pharmacotherapy nor supportive psychotherapy had led to an improvement of her obsessions and compulsions. Because this community mental health center did not specialize in OCD, she was referred to our department.

CASE CONCEPTUALIZATION

Modeling and Learning

After her parents divorced, her mother frequented the pub daily and did not look after the children. They were dirty and untidy and got little to eat. For this reason, they were pestered by other children and were called "antisocials." Because of this, the mother placed them in another school; however, this was no improvement. Subsequently, the mother decided to keep the children at home. The result was that Maria attended elementary school for only 2 years. From age 7 to age 13, Maria did not attend any school and she got into mischief with her two brothers.

Between ages 13 and 16, Maria regularly visited a "clubhouse," in which she learned how to read and write, and where (together with her brothers) she got fed. In that period, she regularly (for several months in a row) lived with other people (e.g., social workers) because her mother wanted to put her in an institution. After the clubhouse period, she lived with her mother at home (from age 16 to 18). One brother was a compulsive gambler and needed money for his habit, and he obtained it by stealing and selling a stereo and other goods belonging to Maria. Her other brother became an alcoholic.

Maria blames her mother for having been so unloving earlier and for the bad way she was raised and parented. She attributes a great part of her present misery to her mother. On several occasions she accused her mother of this, which led to major fights.

In sum, there was no evidence of modeling of obsessive–compulsive behavior. Furthermore, although there were many traumatic experiences in the past, it is difficult to interpret these in terms of classical conditioning. As we have seen, Maria suffered from different obsessions that were unrelated to each other. Theoretically, one should find several traumatic experiences, each related in time to the onset of the specific obsessional theme. However, the content of the obsession changed without any environmental event occurring that would fit into a classical conditioning interpretation. It is more plausible that operant conditioning plays an important role. Maria seemed to have learned that performing rituals leads to anxiety reduction, thus reinforcing the obsession and avoidance behavior (e.g., rituals).

Finally, there is some evidence that obsessive–compulsive behavior is related to a lack of warmth and rejection by the parents of the patients (Hoekstra, Visser, & Emmelkamp, 1989). It is tempting to assume that such lack of warmth and rejection also played an important role in the development of obsessive–compulsive behavior in Maria. It is hypothesized that rituals may also serve the function of avoiding painful emotions related to the past.

Life Events

As noted previously, Maria had experienced many life events, but there was no one-to-one relationship between a specific life event and development of the OCD.

Genetics and Temperament

Studies showed that relatives of obsessive–compulsives have an increased risk of developing an anxiety disorder (Black, Noyes, Goldstein, & Blum, 1992; McKeon & Murray, 1987) but did not show that relatives of OCD patients have an increased risk of getting OCD. More recently, Pauls, Alsobrook, Goodman, Rasmussen, and Leckman (1995) found evidence for elevated risk of obsessive–compulsive disorder in probands of clients with OCD. Thus, results with respect to a genetic contribution in OCD are inconclusive.

In the present case, it is likely that she was vulnerable for development of a psychiatric disorder, given the fact that both her mother and her brothers were all presumably psychiatric cases. Interestingly, there was no evidence that anxiety disorders, including OCD, run in the family, but information on her biological father is lacking. If anything, the disorders in the family were in the areas of substance abuse and antisocial personality and/or borderline disorder. Surprisingly, none of the features of these disorders was evident in Maria. Despite the severe disorders she suffered from, she impressed observers as a rather strong personality.

Physical Conditions

Maria presented with no medical conditions that affected the OCD, agorapobia, social phobia, or dysthymia.

Drugs

From age 18 on, Maria has regularly used medication (mainly sleeping pills and other tranquilizers). Initially she took these pills to combat her obsessive complaints on prescription of her physician; later she also took these pills to "be away from it all for a while." She is not suicidal, however; when the medication was finished, she did not dare to ask for more and stopped taking it, which resulted in withdrawal symptoms. After some weeks, her condition improved.

Socioeconomic and Cultural Factors

It is clear that in this case, socioeconomic factors play an important role. Maria learned to survive for better or worse in an environment that was lacking any warmth or affection. It is surprising to see that she managed to stay in a relatively stable mutual satisfactory relationship. The relationship with her friend, whom she has known for 10 years and with whom she has lived for 6 years (from age 18) is described as rather good. She speaks highly of this man's qualities, perseverance, and prospects. She finds it incomprehensible that "that boy wants to have a hussy coming from such a family and who is unable to do anything."

She has hardly any contact with her brothers, sister, and mother, and the very occasional visits often end in a fight. She has no contact with either her legal father or her biological father. She has no further social contacts.

Maria has resolved to carry out an extensive plan to catch up and compensate for her missed opportunities. For this reason, she is now attending school in order to finish the elementary education program.

Overall Conceptualization

The problem analysis shows that a number of problem areas can be distinguished. Drawing on four interview sessions and the information from the questionnaires, the therapist constructed the following conceptualization of the case: Cumulative negative experiences in her childhood (i.e., unwanted child, divorced parents, being pestered, interrupted elementary education, and emotional neglect by her mother) led to a negative self-image, resulting in tension and uncertainty. This tension manifests itself in many situations and results in obsessive complaints, agoraphobia, and social phobia. As a result of these complaints, Maria has become depressed. This case conceptualization is pictured in Fig. 8.1.

Diagnostic Assessment

In the first session, Maria completed the ADIS. Apart from the OCD, Maria also fulfilled the criteria for a number of other *DSM–IV* disorders as discussed in the following:

- *Agoraphobia and Social Phobia.* Maria is afraid of fainting when leaving home and then making "a fool of herself." She has few social contacts and shudders to think of visiting the clinic or her physician. Sometimes she dares neither leave home nor cancel her appointment. In that case, she simply does not show up at all or her partner must accompany her.

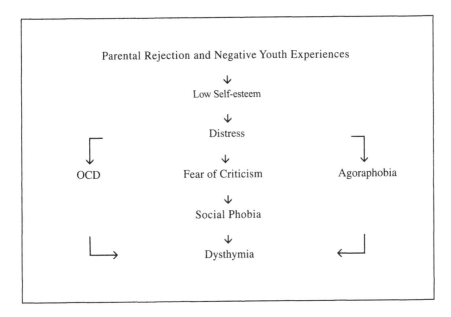

FIG. 8.1.   Case conceptualization for Maria.

She hardly ventures out of doors, and if she does, she keeps looking down to make sure not to look anybody in the face (she is afraid that people will look at her and think something negative about her; however, she says she does not care because "I don't know all those people"). The social fear is most notable when she has to go somewhere and arrives at the destination; she states that she does not to know what to do and is frightened to do something wrong. Because of her avoidance behavior, the specific cognitions that appear in fear-inducing situations remain unclear. Although panic attacks have occurred in the past, the last one occurred nearly a year ago.

• *Dysthymia.* Maria describes having had depressive moods several days a week for quite some time. She does not enjoy anything and detests life. Her depression often grows as the day progresses. Until recently, she would have asked for medication for these gloomy moods, but now she does not dare to ask her physician for any more.

Additional Assessments.   Her score on the MOCI is 22, which is more than 1 *SD* higher than the average of clients with an obsessive disorder (Emmelkamp, Kraaijkamp, & van den Hout, 1999). Her score on the Zung Depression Questionnaire is 67, confirming that she is rather depressed, according to Dutch norms. Her score on the SCL–90, a multidimensional psychopathology measure, is 273, which is high compared to Dutch norm scores of psychiatric outpatients. Her scores on the SCL–90 subscale for agoraphobia is high, and her score for interpersonal sensitivity (social anxiety) is very high. The Inventory of Interpersonal Situations (IIS), Van Dam-Baggen & Kraaimaat, 1999 shows that Maria rarely if ever passes criticism, demands attention, or makes the first move toward contact.

Behavioral Assessment

Rather than performing a formal behavioral assessment procedure, a very detailed list of present obsessive complaints was made. When Maria takes a shower, she has to watch carefully how she puts the shower gel onto the sponge. As long as she does not have any threatening thoughts, she can continue to shower; if she has "bad thoughts," she must carry out the previous action once more. "Bad thoughts" especially relate to the fact that her friend may get in an accident. When she washes her hair (four times a week), she has to make sure not to think of anybody having an accident; if she does, she must wash her hair once more. This may sometimes go on until the bottle is finished. Her friend must put the shampoo into her hands for the final washing, and, she is not allowed to watch his legs while he does so, lest he have an accident. She may start brooding about washing her hair 2 hours in advance. Once the ritual has begun, there is no way back and she must finish it.

A few times a day she changes her clothes, especially when she goes out. When stepping into bed, she must make sure not to see her friend's legs. If she does catch a glimpse, however, she must get up (not walk around, just stand still) and get into bed again.

When cleaning the windows (which she does almost every day), she must put the cloth into the water about 10 times and squeeze it out again, until she has a "good feeling." Curtains must be hung straight, also until she has a "good feeling." The same goes for cleaning the toilet, floors, and cutlery (four times through the washing-up process).

When ironing trousers, she must do the legs very quickly, before she gets unlucky thoughts again, causing her to carry out obsessive actions. When disturbing thoughts appear ("losing legs because of an accident"), she must perform the action once more and avoid having these bad thoughts. The same goes for folding and sewing clothes and picking up things.

In all the previously mentioned examples, the obsession is that the client begins an action that must be carried out in a particular way (without the obsessive thoughts). Once begun, she must carry on until no unlucky thoughts occur. It seems that she cannot resist this ritual as such.

Priorization of Targets for Treatment

In consultation with Maria, the therapist decided first to focus on the obsessive complaints, which dominate her the entire day. Treatment then was directed at the social phobia and agoraphobia when OCD complaints were no longer controlling her behavior all day long. Treatment for her depressed mood, was postponed because it was expected that her mood would improve substantially as a result of successful treatment of OCD, agoraphobia, and social phobia.

Selection and Priority of Treatment Strategies

To deal with the OCD, exposure and response prevention is the treatment of choice. Although cognitive therapy may also be considered, in Maria's case this option was believed to be less therapeutically helpful, given her socioeconomic background and lack of education. Furthermore, it was decided that Maria would try to carry out the exposure exercises on her own (self-controlled exposure). For the same reason, self-controlled exposure was chosen as the treatment for her social phobia and agoraphobia. Indeed, there is considerable evidence that this procedure is effective in social phobic and agoraphobic patients.

Initially, Maria tended to postpone carrying out exposure exercises, but after having made clear agreements about time and duration of the exercises, she managed not to give way to the impulses to carry out her compulsive rituals. Although her obsession had not yet disappeared after 15 sessions, it was decided in consultation with her to focus treatment attention on her social fear as well. Initially, the social phobic situations were also dealt with using exposure in vivo exercises. The exercises were an uphill struggle, however, and Maria regularly canceled therapy sessions.

Treatment was then adapted so that she did not have to perform exposure exercises in social situations. However, the elementary social situations were be practiced by using role-play so that Maria would feel more confident in social situations. After seven role-play sessions, Maria and the therapist were satisfied about the progress, and the exposure program was resumed. Because it appears rather difficult to practice the social situations because her fear in the street and in the bus had not declined, exposure was initially directed to her agoraphobia. Maria was now able to come to the clinic by bike or bus by herself, so after several weeks it was decided to extend exposure to social situations. After this part of the therapy was completed satisfactorily, it was followed by a number of sessions in which the treatment was again directed at the obsessive–compulsive behavior. Finally, an exposure in vivo session with the therapist took place in Maria's house in order to deal with the last remnents of obsessive–compulsive behavior.

In total, the therapy required 43 sessions. Maria is now free of complaints, and her depressive moods have disappeared. Meanwhile, she has passed her driving test, which she considers to simplify success of the therapy.

Dealing with Complicating Factors

In the course of the treatment, Maria's brother died because of a traffic accident resulting from his alcohol abuse. Although this led to an increase in depressed mood, she managed to continue with the exposure exercises for her compulsions. Therefore, there was no need to adapt the treatment program. Unexpectedly, however, the exposure exercises for her social phobia were rather difficult for Maria and so the strategy to treat it were adapted using role-plays with the therapist rather than real in vivo social situations.

Role of Pharmacotherapy

Maria periodically used sleeping pills in difficult periods (e.g., when her brother died and she had to confront her family). The use of serotonergic antidepressants was considered in advance as a possible additional treatment option, but it was not necessary to prescribe such medication in the course of the treatment.

Managed Care Considerations

Although this was a rather severe case, we believed it to be worthwhile to start treatment on an outpatient basis. There is considerable evidence that severe OCD clients can be treated as outpatients even when there are a number of comorbid disorders. Furthermore, most of the treatment consisted of self-controlled exposure in vivo, which is much more cost effective than therapist-controlled exposure in vivo. Although serotonergic antidepressants may enhance treatment effects in a few individual cases, there is no evidence that combined pharmacotherapy and behavioral treatment is generally more effective than behavioral treatment alone. Given the fact that most OCD clients relapse when they stop taking serotonergic antidepressants, prescribing such a pharmacological agent would presumably mean that the client would have to take the medication on a continuous basis, which would be rather expensive.

SUMMARY

In sum, most OCD clients have obsessions as well as compulsions. Research indicates that a number of specific cognitive processes are characteristic of OCD clients. There is a considerable overlap between OCD and other anxiety disorders. If obsessive–compulsive clients do not get adequate treatment, the disorder tends to have a chronic fluctuating course. The preferred form of treatment is behavior therapy, namely exposure in vivo plus response prevention. Other promising treatments are cognitive therapy and pharmacotherapy. Assessment instruments such as the Y–BOCS, structured diaries, MOCI, and PI–R, help on the one hand to classify obsessive–compulsive problems and on the other hand to evaluate the effects of treatment.

REFERENCES

Abramovitz, J. S., & Foa, E. B. (1998). Worries and obsessions in individuals with obsessive-compulsive disorder with and without comorbid generalized anxiety disorder. *Behaviour Research and Therapy, 36*, 695–700.

Antony, M. M., Downie, F., & Swinson, R. P. (1998). Diagnostic issues and epidemiology in obsessive–compulsive disorder. In R. P. Swinson, M. M. Antony, S. Rachman, & M. A. Richter (Eds.), *Obsessive–compulsive disorder: Theory, research, and treatment* (pp. 3–32). New York: Guilford.

Black, D. W., Noyes, R., Goldstein, R. B., & Blum, N. (1992). A family study of obsessive–compulsive disorder. *Archives of General Psychiatry, 49*, 362–368.

Burns, G. L., Keortge, S. G., Formea, G. M., & Sternberger, L. G. (1996). Revision of the Padua Inventory for obsessive compulsive disorder symptoms: Distinctions between worry, obsessions, and compulsions. *Behaviour Research and Therapy, 34*, 163–173.

Dam-Baggen, C. M. J. van & Kraaimaat, F. W. (1999). Assessing social anxiety: The Inventory of Interpersonal Situations (IIS). *European Journal of Psychological Assessment, 15*, 25–38.

DiNardo, P. A., Brown, T. A., & Barlow, D. A. (1994). *Anxiety Disorders Interview Schedule for DSM–IV.* San Antonio, TX:Psychological Corporation.

Emmelkamp, P. M. G. (in press) Behavior therapy with adults. In S. Garfield & A. Bergin (Eds.), *Handbook of psychotherapy and behavior change* (5th Ed.). New York: Wiley (in preparation).

Emmelkamp, P. M. G., & Aardema, A. (1999). Metacognition, specific obsessive–compulsive beliefs and obsessive–compulsive behaviour. *Clinical Psychology and Psychotherapy, 6*, 139–145.

Emmelkamp, P. M. G., Bouman, T. K., & Scholing. A. (1993). *Anxiety Disorders: A Practitioners Guide.* Wiley, Chichester.

Emmelkamp, P. M. G., Kraaijkamp, H. J. M., & van den Hout, M. A. (1999). Assessment of obsessive–compulsive disorder. *Behavior Modification, 23*, 269–279.

Emmelkamp, P. M. G., & van Oppen, P. (2001). Anxiety disorders. In: V. van Hasselt & M. Hersen (Eds.), *Advanced abnormal psychology.* Kluwer Academic, pp. 285–306, Plenum, New York.

Goodman, W. K., Price, L. H., Rasmussen, S. A., Mazure, C., Fleischmann, R. L., Hill, C. L., Heninger, G. R., & Charney, D. S. (1989). The Yale-Brown Obsessive Compulsive Scale: I. Development, use, and reliability. *Archives of General Psychiatry, 46*, 1006–1011.

Hodgson, R. J., & Rachman, S. (1977). Obsessional–compulsive complaints. *Behaviour Research and Therapy, 15*, 389–395.

Hoekstra, R. J., Visser, S., & Emmelkamp, P. M. G., A social learning formulation of the etiology of obsessive–compulsive diorders. In: P. M. G. Emmelkamp, W. T. A. M. Everaerd, F. Kraaimaat & M. van Son (Eds.), *Fresh Perspectives on Anxiety Disorders*, Swets, Amsterdam/Berwyn, 1989, pp. 115–124.

McKeon, P., & Murray, R. (1997). Familial aspects of obsessive–compulsive neurosis. *British Journal of Psychiatry, 151*, 528–534.

van Oppen, P., Emmelkamp, P. M. G., van Balkom, A., & van Dyck, R. (1995b). The sensitivity to change for measures of obsessive–compulsive disorder. *Journal of Anxiety Disorders, 9*, 241–248.

van Oppen, P., Hoekstra, R., & Emmelkamp, P. M. G. (1995a). The structure of obsessive–compulsive symptoms. *Behaviour Research and Therapy, 33*, 15–23.

van Oppen, P., de Haan, E., van Balkom, A. J. M. L., Spinhoven, P., Hoogduin, C. A. L., & van Dyck, R. (1995). Cognitive therapy and exposure in vivo in the treatment of obsessive–compulsive disorder. *Behaviour Research and Therapy, 33*, 379–390.

Pauls, D. L., Alsobrook, J. P., Goodman, W., Rasmussen, S., & Leckman, J. F. (1995). A family study of obsessive compulsive disorder. *American Journal of Psychiatry, 71*, 124–135.

Pigott, T. A., & Seay, S. (1998). Biological treatments for obsessive–compulsive disorder: Literature review. In R. P. Swinson, M. M. Antony, S. Rachman, & M. A. Richter (Eds.), *Obsessive–compulsive disorder: Theory, research, and treatment* (pp. 298–326). New York: Guilford.

Steketee, G., Frost, R., & Bogart, K. (1996). The Yale–Brown Obsessive Compulsive Scale: Interview versus self-report. *Behaviour Research and Therapy, 34*, 675–684.

Taylor, S. (1998). Assessment of obsessive–compulsive disorder. In R. P. Swinson, M. M. Antony, S. Rachman, & M. A. Richter (Eds.), *Obsessive–compulsive disorder: Theory, research, and treatment* (pp. 229–257). New York: Guilford.

van Dam-Baggen, C. M. J., & Kraaimaat, F. W. (1999). Assessing social anxiety: The Inventory of Interpersonal Situations (IIS). *European Journal of Psychological Assessment, 15*, 25–38.

van Rijsoort, S., Emmelkamp, P. M. G., & Vervaeke, G. (2000). Assessment of worry and OCD: How are they related. *Personality and Individual Differences* (in press).

van Velzen, C., & Emmelkamp, P. M. G. (1999). The relationship between anxiety disorders and personality disorders: Prevalence rates and co-morbidity models. In J. Derksen, H. Groen, & C. Maffei, (Eds.), *Treatment of personality disorders* (pp. 129–153). New York: Plenum.

Posttraumatic Stress Disorder

Joanne L. Davis and Ron Acierno
Medical University of South Carolina

DESCRIPTION OF THE DISORDER

Shell shock, battle fatigue, combat neurosis (Tomb, 1994), and *battered wives' syndrome* are well-known lay descriptors of negative emotional responses to trauma. The first edition of the *Diagnostic and Statistical Manual of Mental Disorders* (*DSM*; American Psychiatric Association, 1952) categorized such reactions as *gross stress reaction*, and the *DSM–II* (APA, 1968) used the term *transient situational disturbance* (Tomb, 1994). The *DSM–III* (APA, 1980) was the first to refer to these symptoms as *posttraumatic stress disorder* (PTSD), and required that the traumatic event be an experience "outside the range of usual human experience" (p. 236). However, recent research on posttraumatic stress reactions resulted in several changes in the conceptualization of PTSD in the *DSM–IV* (APA, 1994; Kilpatrick, Saunders, Veronen, Best, & Von, 1987; Breslau, Davis, Andreski, & Peterson, 1991; Resnick, Kilpatrick, Dansky, Saunders, & Best, 1993b). First, the definition of a stressor thought to cause negative reactions was altered. Instead of requiring an unusual or rare experience, the *DSM–IV* now requires that the initial stressor include (a) confrontation with an event or events that involve actual or threatened death or serious injury, or a threat to the physical integrity of self or others; and (b) a response involving intense fear, helplessness, or horror. The definition also includes a caveat for children that allows for reactions involving disorganized or agitated behavior. Such definitional changes have several important implications for the diagnosis. Specifically, the *DSM–IV* (APA, 1994) allows for inclusion of nonrare experiences (e.g., severe reactions to minor traumas) as well as indirect experiences of trauma (e.g., a child witnessing parental violence). Furthermore, this new definition places greater emphasis on an individual's perception of threat at the time of the trauma.

The PTSD diagnosis is composed of three symptom categories: reexperiencing, avoidance, and hyperarousal. One or more of the following reexperiencing symptoms is required: recurrent and intrusive recollections of the event, recurrent distressing dreams of the event, acting or feeling as if the event is recurring, intense psychological distress at exposure to a reminder of the event, or a physiological reaction to a reminder of the event. Three or more of the following avoidance symptoms are required: efforts to avoid thoughts, feelings, or conversations related to the event; efforts to avoid people, places, or things that are reminders of the event; inability to recall an important aspect of the event; decreased interest in previously enjoyed activities; feeling detached or estranged from others; restricted range of affect; or a sense of foreshortened future. Two or more of the following symptoms are required from the hyperarousal category: difficulty falling or staying asleep, irritability or outbursts of anger, difficulty concentrating, hypervigilance, or an exaggerated startled response. Criteria for posttraumatic responses in children are somewhat different from criteria for adults (see Schwarz & Perry, 1994, for a description of PTSD in children).

Other features associated with PTSD should be considered during assessment and treatment. In addition to specific PTSD criteria, individuals with the disorder may also report difficulties in interpersonal relationships; problems with modulation of affect; "survivor guilt"; self-destructive and impulsive behaviors; dissociative symptoms; somatic complaints; feelings of shame, despair, and hopelessness; and social withdrawal. Furthermore, PTSD is associated with higher rates of panic disorder, agoraphobia, obsessive–compulsive disorder, social phobia, specific phobia, major depressive disorder, somatization disorder, and substance-related disorders (APA, 1994). The temporal relationship of onset among these disorders is unclear, however; that is, traumatic events may increase the risk for multiple types of mental health problems, developing PTSD may create a vulnerability to other forms of psychological difficulties, and/or the presence of other psychopathology may create a vulnerability to PTSD. These hypotheses warrant additional investigation.

Overall, population prevalence estimates of past-year PTSD range from 2.3% to 4.2%, and estimates of lifetime PTSD range from 7.8% to 12.3% (Breslau et al., 1991; Kessler et al., 1995; Resnick et al., 1993b). Variability of estimates depends on the population sampled, methods of PTSD and trauma assessment used, and specific diagnostic definitions. Helzer, Robins, and McEvoy (1987) used data from the Epidemiologic Catchment Area Survey and the Diagnostic Interview Schedule (DIS; Robins, Helzer, Croughan, & Ratcliff, 1981) and estimated the prevalence of lifetime PTSD to be 1% of the total population. This study, however, did not use sensitive methodology for trauma detection, particularly sexual assault. Breslau and coworkers (1991) used a version of the DIS that was revised to be more sensitive to traumatic stress and found lifetime prevalence in the general population to be 9%. The lifetime prevalence rate among the subset of individuals exposed to a traumatic event was estimated to be 23%.

Women typically report higher rates of PTSD than men (Breslau et al., 1991; Norris, 1992), and the primary index events differ between men and women. Specifically, combat and witnessed violence are the most common precipitating events for men, whereas sexual and physical assaults are the most common precipitating events for women (Kessler et al., 1995; Kilpatrick & Resnick, 1993). The type of event experienced appears to influence risk of developing PTSD. Overall, sexual assault, physical assault, and motor vehicle accidents appear to be responsible for most cases of PTSD (Norris, 1992). Other risk factors include being of non-white ethnicity (Kulka et al., 1990; Norris, 1992), personal or familial history of psychopathology (Breslau et al., 1991; Davidson, Smith, & Kudler, 1991), and younger age 18–39 (Norris, 1992).

Theories proposed to explain reactions to exceptionally stressful or traumatic events draw from both psychological and biological realms. Learning theorists (e.g., Becker, Skinner, Abel, Axelrod, & Cichon, 1984; Kilpatrick, Veronen, & Resick, 1982; Kilpatrick, Veronen, & Best, 1985) posit that through classical conditioning, salient stimuli or cues (conditioned stimuli) present during the traumatic event are associated with dangerous stimuli (unconditioned stimuli; e.g., rape) and result in the conditioned response of fear and other negative affect. For example, the sound of gunshots, shrapnel wounds, and seeing friends killed are unconditioned stimuli that initially elicit feelings of fear and terror. Other salient contiguous stimuli (e.g., people, places, time of day, odors, tastes) also become able to elicit the fear response. In attempts to obviate the negative affect associated with the traumatic event, individuals often begin avoiding places, people, or situations that remind them of the trauma (i.e., conditioned stimuli) and elicit the fear response. Thus, a veteran may not watch war movies, go near military bases, or be involved in any activities that include loud noises (e.g., fireworks); a rape victim may stop dating, leaving her house after dark, or boarding elevators with men present. Escaping and subsequently avoiding reminders of the trauma results in a reduction of anxiety, which negatively reinforces avoidance behaviors.

In addition to learning theory, information processing theory highlights the role of cognitive appraisal and the meaning of the event for the individual who develops PTSD. Research findings support the notion that perception of threat is a better predictor of subsequent PTSD symptoms than is the actual injury involved in the traumatic experience (Kilpatrick, Saunders, Amick-McMullan, Best, Veronen, & Resnick, 1989). This theory proposes that individuals who experience trauma develop certain patterns of thinking and feeling about the world that are called *fear structures*. These fear structures consist of memory information related to stimuli associated with the traumatic event (e.g., the rapist was a tall man driving a green van), responses to the trauma (e.g., feelings, thoughts, behaviors), and the meaning of the trauma (e.g., how the individual perceives the trauma to have affected his or her life) (Chemtob, Roiblat, Hamada, Carlson, & Twentyman, 1988; Foa, Steketee, & Olasav-Rothbaum, 1989; Freedy & Donkervoet, 1995). Many stimuli that are not inherently dangerous (e.g., loud noises) are nonetheless incorporated into the fear structure. When an individual is confronted with stimuli that are in some way associated with the trauma (dangerous or not), the fear network is activated. Due to avoidance behaviors, which include avoiding thoughts of the trauma, little opportunity is available for exposure to corrective information to modify the fear structure. Obviously, this theory shares several aspects of learning theory.

Another information processing theory holds that traumatized individuals sometimes develop problematic mental representations or belief systems called *schema*. Schema is defined as a way of thinking about oneself, others, and the world (McCann, Sakheim, & Abrahamson, 1988; Resick & Schnicke, 1993). These schemata influence the way people think and feel, as well as how they respond to stimuli in their environment. McCann et al. (1988) identified five schemata that are vulnerable to distortion by traumatic events, including safety, trust, intimacy, power, and esteem. More recent research suggests that religious beliefs may also be distorted or altered by traumatic experiences (Falsetti, Resick, & Davis, in submission). Resick and Schnicke (1993) stated that the common responses following trauma are related to difficulties incorporating trauma experiences into existing belief systems. When individuals experience or encounter a schema-incongruent event (one that does not fit with their previous conceptualizations of the world), the experience and its accompanying emotions may be overwhelming. At this point, the individual must either alter the information to fit the schema (assimilation) or alter the schema to fit the information (accommodation). For example, if a woman's rape schema includes only the notion of a woman being raped by a stranger, and she is subsequently raped by an acquaintance, she may assimilate, or alter, the information by convincing herself that she was not raped. She might label the event as a miscommunication, or perhaps think that she did or said something that the offender misconstrued. By contrast, if the rape victim were to accommodate the information, she might change her schema to incorporate the possibility that someone known and trusted can be dangerous and can perpetrate an assault.

Resick and Schnicke (1993) noted another phenomenon in their work with rape victims that involves problematic accommodation. *Overaccommodation* involves an extreme distortion in schema. For example, instead of changing one's schema to include the possibility that some trusted individuals can be dangerous, the victim of acquaintance rape may change her schema to suggest that all men are dangerous and cannot be trusted. Overaccomodation may result in dichotomized thought processes and restrict the cognitive flexibility with which individuals interpret and evaluate future information.

METHODS TO DETERMINE DIAGNOSIS

A comprehensive PTSD assessment includes not only specification of symptoms but also collection of information on the nature of the trauma.

Assessing the Trauma

A primary difficulty in studying PTSD involves assessment of the traumatic event. Oftentimes, researchers and clinicians consider only the trauma that brought a client into treatment. However, recent studies indicate that experiencing multiple traumas may have an additive negative impact on an individual's functioning (Mullen, Martin, Anderson, Romans, & Herbison, 1996; Wind & Silvern, 1992) and the effect of each trauma should be considered. As discussed previously, certain trauma characteristics (e.g., threat of death or physical injury, actual physical injury) also affect the victim's response and are thus relevant areas for assessment (Kilpatrick, Saunders, Amick-McMullan, Best, Veronen, & Resnick, 1989; Wilson, Smith, & Johnson, 1985). Finally, assessment of traumatic events, particularly violence, should also cover such basic areas as frequency, duration, number of incidents, relationship to the perpetrator (for interpersonal violence), type of trauma, fear of injury, and extent of actual injury.

Several instruments are available to assess the type and nature of traumatic events. Resnick, Best, Kilpatrick, Freedy, and Falsetti (1993a) developed the Trauma Assessment for Adults (TAA), which is available as a self-report measure or clinician-administered interview. The TAA measures 14 types of traumatic events as well as age at first and last occurrence, duration, frequency, fear of physical injury or death, actual physical injury, and relationship to the perpetrator if appropriate. The TAA also uses behaviorally specific questions that bypass cultural or language barriers to psychometric sensitivity.

Assessing the Symptoms

Several clinician-administered interviews, are available to assess PTSD criteria. The PTSD module from the *Structured Clinical Interview for DSM–IV–Patient Edition* (SCID; First, Spitzer, Gibbon, & Williams, 1995) provides specific prompts and follow-up inquiries intended to be read verbatim to respondents to assess presence or absence of each PTSD symptom listed in the

DSM–IV. Symptom presence is rated on a 3-point confidence scale based on the interviewer's interpretation of victim's responses to prompts. Respondents are asked to rate symptoms in terms of their "worst" trauma experience. Although specific instructions for probe questions and guidelines for response interpretation are provided, the instrument is intended for use by clinicians and highly trained interviewers.

In contrast to the SCID–IV, the Diagnostic Interview Schedule (DIS; Robins, Helzer, Cottler, & Goldring, 1988) was designed specifically for use by nonprofessional interviewers. The DIS also differs from the SCID in that it allows the PTSD diagnosis to be made with reference to three specific Criterion A events, whereas the SCID considers only the "worst" event. Diagnosis is assigned on the basis of responses to specific questions relating to each PTSD symptom defined in the *DSM–III–R.*

The Clinician Administered PTSD Scale (CAPS; Blake et al., 1990) was designed specifically to yield both continuous (i.e., severity) and dichotomous (i.e., diagnostic) information exclusively for PTSD. The CAPS is intended for use by professionals and trained paraprofessionals, and addresses the 17 symptoms of PTSD that compose the *DSM–IV* diagnosis. Thirteen additional questions target associated symptoms not part of the formal PTSD diagnosis, as well as functional impact of symptoms on social and vocational spheres. Separate ratings of frequency and intensity of each symptom are made on 5-point (0–4) scales that use specific behavioral reference anchors to maximize standardization and consistency of interviews. Both previous-month and lifetime presence of the disorder are measured.

In addition to structured clinical interviews, several PTSD self-report measures are widely used. The PTSD Symptom Scale–Self-Report (PSS–SR; Foa, Riggs, Dancu, & Rothbaum, 1993a) includes 17 items that correspond directly to the *DSM–IV* symptoms. As such, this self-report scale permits diagnosis of the disorder. The PSS–SR is intended for use with individuals who have a known history of assault, and should thus be accompanied by a trauma screen when assessing individuals for whom basic background information is lacking. For all items, symptom frequency over the preceding 2 weeks is reported on a 4-point scale. A total score is obtained by summing each symptom rating. Subscale scores are calculated by summing symptoms in the reexperiencing (four items), avoidance (seven items), and arousal (six items) clusters.

The Modified PTSD Symptom Scale–Self-Report (MPSS–SR: Resick, Falsetti, Resnick, & Kilpatrick, 1991) is a modification of the PTSD Symptom Scale developed by Foa and coworkers (1993a). This scale includes a measure of the severity of each of the 17 items. Severity of PTSD symptoms is rated on a 5-point scale from "not at all distressing" to "extremely distressing." Similar to the PSS–SR, the measure MPSS–SR permits diagnosis of PTSD.

The Impact of Events Scale (IES; Horowitz, Wilner, & Alvarez, 1979) has a longer history of use than the PSS–SR, but provides relatively less diagnostic specification. The IES is a 15-item self-report measure constructed to assess intrusion and avoidance symptoms of PTSD experienced over the previous week. Symptoms are phrased in the first person and respondents rate their frequency on a 4-point scale. The scale focuses on cognitive PTSD symptomatology (as opposed to somatic arousal) and is an excellent indicator of subjective distress. Although the IES does not permit diagnosis of PTSD along with criteria defined by the *DSM–IV*, severity cutoff scores have been used to predict diagnostic status.

ADDITIONAL ASSESSMENTS REQUIRED

As discussed previously, PTSD often presents with a variety of other psychological difficulties and disorders. Experiencing a traumatic event may induce symptoms that are not captured adequately by the PTSD diagnosis. Other diagnoses and conditions associated with experiencing trauma include additional anxiety disorders (e.g., panic disorder), mood disorders (e.g., depression), substance use disorders, sexual dysfunction (e.g., sexual aversion disorder), and interpersonal problems (e.g., difficulty trusting others). Traumas occurring in early childhood (e.g., childhood sexual and physical abuse) have also been associated with personality disorders; however, causality has not been well studied. Falsetti and Resnick (2000) also suggest including assessments of social support, cognitions, and causal attributions and describe various assessment tools for use in these areas. A comprehensive assessment of the client's current and recent functioning is necessary in order to ascertain the full extent of the individual's difficulties and inform and guide treatment decisions.

CASE ILLUSTRATION

Presenting Complaints

Lynn is a 21-year-old unmarried African American woman who reported that she was raped repeatedly by her maternal uncle over the course of a summer approximately 6 years ago. Lynn became pregnant as a result of the rape and had a son at the age of 16. She presented to the outpatient counseling clinic with symptoms of anxiety, depression, social isolation, and irritability. Lynn believed that her distress was directly related to the rapes by her uncle.

History of the Disorder

Lynn reported that when she was 15 years old, her 24-year-old uncle came to stay with her family for a summer. The sexual abuse began soon after he moved in. He began by asking her to massage him and "accidently" exposed himself on several occasions. She grew increasingly uncomfortable being alone with him, and the abuse quickly escalated to vaginal, oral, and anal rape. Lynn stated that her uncle made her believe the abuse was her fault, and threatened that her family would kill him or he would kill her if she told anyone. Physical force was used during the abuse and included restraining her, pulling her hair, and slapping her.

In the fall following the abuse, Lynn went to see a doctor, who informed her that she was pregnant and subsequently informed her mother. Lynn told her mother that the father of the child was a boyfriend. During the intake interview, Lynn reported that she had been afraid to tell her mother about the assaults by her uncle because she felt guilty and embarrassed, and believed her mother would be angry with her. When she informed her uncle of the pregnancy, her uncle beat her in an attempt to abort the baby. When this failed and she refused to have an abortion, her uncle moved out of the house and out of the state. She disclosed the abuse and the true identity of the father to her mother approximately 2 weeks before coming to the clinic, 5 years after the rapes occurred.

Lynn reported experiencing significant anxiety that has become progressively worse since the abuse began. She reported nightmares about the abuse and the perpetrator almost every night. During the day, she has flashbacks of abuse incidents and her uncle's voice. Specifically, she would hear him calling her a whore and telling her to shut up when she would beg him to leave her alone. She stopped socializing with her friends, as they were interested in dating and Lynn was not interested in men at all. In fact, she had increasing difficulties even being around men, including classmates and professors. She reported experiencing significant anxiety that often developed into feelings of intense fear and various physiological symptoms, including sweating, trembling, shortness of breath, nausea, and chest pains (e.g., panic attacks) if a man approached her or tried to talk to her. She also began having panic attacks even when men were not around. She was afraid that others would treat her differently because of the rape, and felt increasingly distant from other people, including her family. She did not feel close to her son, frequently yelled at him, and believed that she should feel more positive and nurturing toward him than she did. She also reported depression that began soon after initiation of the abuse incidents and increased significantly following the birth of her son.

Lynn completed high school and began attending the local community college, but was not involved in any extracurricular activities. Her mother helped take care of her child during the day while she was in school. She reported that many evenings and weekends she was unable to take care of her child because she was too distressed, fatigued, or apathetic. She reported significant difficulty concentrating on schoolwork or focusing on any specific task. She was too tired in the evenings and on weekends to try to catch up on her schoolwork, and was subsequently failing several courses. She was unable to articulate plans for the future, including whether she planned to finish college.

Medical History

Lynn's medical history was unremarkable. She carried her son to term and the birth was uncomplicated. She was unaware of significant medical concerns in her family.

Family History

Lynn is the second of four children. She has one older brother, who was in jail for drug-related charges at the time of the intake, and two younger brothers in middle school. Her parents' relationship was quite abusive, and they separated when Lynn was 6 years old. Her father was an alcoholic and was involved infrequently with the family, even when he and Lynn's mother were still together. Lynn reported that she has not seen her father in approximately 15 years, although he would occasionally call and speak with her and her brothers. The family was very poor and lived in public housing when Lynn began treatment. Lynn's mother was not close to her own extended family, and the sexual assault became a significant source of friction among family members. On several occasions, family members stated that they did not believe that Lynn was raped; rather, they believed that the sexual involvement between Lynn and her uncle was consensual. These interactions augmented Lynn's own feelings of guilt and belief that she was at fault for the assaults, as her uncle had told her.

Sexual History

Lynn denied being sexually active prior to or since the rapes by her uncle. She reported being very nervous about sexual matters and had no interested in becoming sexually involved with anyone for a long time, if ever. She had gone to see her doctor after the assault because she was concerned about possibly having contracted a sexually transmitted disease (STD). Although she tested negative for all STDs, she continued to feel "dirty and unclean."

Mental Status Examination

At the time of the initial interview, Lynn was dressed casually and appeared her stated age. She was cooperative and pleasant throughout the interview. Her eye contact was good, except when she was discussing the rapes, at which time she lowered her head and stared at the floor. She was alert and appeared to have no difficulties with attention and concentration. She was oriented to person, place, and time. Her speech was unremarkable as to tone, rate, and volume. Her mood was sad and anxious, and her affect was congruent with the topic. She reported no abnormal perceptions. Her thought processes were goal directed and coherent. She denied suicidal and homicidal ideation. Although no formal evaluation was conducted, Lynn appeared to be of average intelligence. Her judgment and insight into the cause of her problems were somewhat limited.

Prior Treatment

Lynn had not previously sought counseling, either inpatient or outpatient, for any reason, and stated that she was quite apprehensive about what would happen in therapy.

CASE CONCEPTUALIZATION

Modeling and Learning

Children learn how to cope with life stressors through several pathways. They may be biologically predisposed to respond in particular ways. They also learn through observing the behaviors and coping styles of those around them. For example, children whose parents are alcoholics may be predisposed to abuse alcohol due to genetics and/or as a learned strategy to reduce stress. Lynn's brother learned from his father that substance use was a viable strategy for dealing with problems. In Lynn's case, she witnessed the destructive nature of her father's substance use and was determined not to use this as a coping strategy. Instead, she adapted her mother's method of coping: withdrawal. Lynn would retreat from friends, family, and activities during periods of anxiety or depression. This method was an effective albeit maladaptive strategy that temporarily reduced anxiety, but ultimately exacerbated her depression.

Life Events

As a young child, Lynn witnessed severe violent acts her father perpetrated on her mother. She was exposed to the negative influence of her father's alcoholism on the family, which included episodes of violence, frequent loss of jobs, and subsequent financial insecurity. She also witnessed significant violence in her community, as her neighborhood was in the middle of the "drug district" and her older brother became involved in a gang, subsequently using and dealing drugs.

Genetics and Temperament

Although not causally established, research has indicated a possible biological link in vulnerability to depression. Twin studies find a 76% concordance rate for affective disorders in monozygotic twins compared to a 19% rate in dizygotic twins. When monozygotic twins are reared apart, the concordance rate falls to 67%. Thus, there appears to be evidence supporting both biological and environmental components of depression (Kaslow, Doepke, & Racusin, 1994). Lynn also appeared to have both components contributing to her depression. First, Lynn's mother had been diagnosed previously with major depression, suggesting a potential biological connection. Second, as described previously, Lynn learned her coping style of withdrawing from activities and social supports from her mother.

Physical Conditions

The physical symptoms of pregnancy served to increase Lynn's depression. The nausea, abdominal pains, and headaches were cues not only of the trauma itself, but of the result of the trauma: her pregnancy. Furthermore, Lynn attended school until shortly before she delivered. She suffered significant harassment from her classmates due to her pregnant state. Throughout her pregnancy and for sometime afterwards, Lynn hated her body; she could not look at herself without the thought of a baby growing inside of her that she did not want and that was conceived in such horrific conditions.

Drugs

Lynn denied a history of substance use; however, due to the alcohol use by her father and drug use by her brother, she may have a propensity for using substances to cope with stress.

Socioeconomic and Cultural Factors

Lynn's family had always struggled financially, and their situation became even more precarious when her father left the family. Her family was also socially isolated. They had moved away from family and friends and did not have access to resources in the community. In terms of cultural factors, there is equivocal evidence regarding the effects of race on one's response to trauma or stress. Many studies have failed to find differential rates of PTSD for crime-related and general trauma based on race (Breslau et al., 1991; Cottler, Compton, Mager, Spitznagel, & Janca, 1992; Kilpatrick et al., 1989; Norris, 1992; Weaver & Clum, 1995), whereas other studies have found that African

Americans evidenced greater rates of PTSD (Green, Grace, Lindy, Gleser, & Leonard, 1990) and report more subjective distress (Norris, 1992). More research is needed examining the effect of race on response to trauma before firm conclusions can be drawn.

Overall Conceptualization

Many of the factors discussed previously may have increased Lynn's vulnerability to posttraumatic stress. She grew up in an environment surrounded by violence, both within and outside of her home. She witnessed the devastating impact of substances on her neighborhood and on her own family. Her family struggled financially for years and was never able to move out of the drug-infested neighborhoods to a safer residence. When Lynn's uncle moved in and the assaults began, she felt trapped, believing that there was no one she could turn to who could end the abuse. Although they were close, Lynn had watched her mother struggle unsuccessfully within an abusive relationship. For years, Lynn tried to cope on her own with the assault. At the time she began treatment, only her mother knew what had happened. She was very supportive but had difficulty coping with what happened, in part because she was also raped by a family member as a teenager and had never received treatment. Overall, when she started treatment, Lynn was a strong individual who was overwhelmed by a variety of stressors. The lack of social support combined with financial strains on the family exacerbated her difficulties. Furthermore, she had to contend with a significant reminder of the rape on a daily basis: her son. She reported that she loved him, but had difficulty not seeing her uncle when she looked at him. She was concerned that her difficulties bonding with him would affect his development.

Diagnostic Assessment

The initial part of the assessment involved a clinical interview in which demographic and background information were gathered and Lynn described the trauma and her responses. The therapist was fairly certain at this point that Lynn probably met criteria for PTSD and some form of depression. A structured clinical interview and self-report measures were used to determine Lynn's diagnosis. She was administered the PTSD, panic disorder, and mood disorders portions of the Structured Clinical Interview for *DSM–IV*. Results from the interview indicated that she met the criteria for PTSD, chronic; Panic Disorder without Agoraphobia; and Major Depressive Disorder, recurrent, moderate.

An assessment of previous traumatic events was conducted next using the Trauma Assessment for Adults (Resnick, Best, Kilpatrick, Freedy, & Falsetti, 1993a). In addition to the sexual assault incidents perpetrated by her uncle, Lynn reported being in a natural disaster (a hurricane) and witnessed her father physically abusing her mother, leaving her mother seriously injured. The Trauma Symptom Inventory (Briere, 1995) was administered to assess for trauma symptoms. The three validity scales were within normal limits, suggesting that she responded in a straightforward manner. She endorsed one critical item, "wishing you were dead," and scored at clinical elevations on 8 of the 10 clinical scales, including anxious arousal, depression, anger/irritability, intrusive experiences, defensive avoidance, dissociation, sexual concerns, and impaired self-reference. A profile analysis revealed a classic posttraumatic presentation, with the highest elevations on intrusive experiences, dissociation, defensive avoidance, and anxious arousal. She scored in the moderate range of depression on the Beck Depression Inventory (BDI; Beck, Ward, Mendelson, Mock, & Erbaugh, 1961).

During the clinical interview, Lynn reported significant sexual concerns, although she was not sexually active at the time. She denied engaging in substance use. Finally, she did not appear to meet criteria for a personality disorder.

Behavioral Assessment

During the assessment period and throughout treatment, Lynn completed daily monitoring records of PTSD symptoms. For each panic attack, she completed a monitoring form that included information regarding attack severity, symptoms, duration, people present, whether it was a stressful event, and whether there were any trauma cues present.

Prioritization of Targets for Treatment

The results of a comprehensive assessment should provide the therapist with a thorough understanding of the factors that contributed to the development and maintenance of the client's difficulties. Furthermore, at this point the therapist should have a clear conception of which symptoms or difficulties appear to be causing the most severe functional impairment. It will likely be necessary to target these symptoms first in treatment; otherwise they may prevent progress in other areas.

A necessary step when prioritizing targets for treatment is to consider the impact of any comorbid diagnoses on the client's functioning. The Expert Consensus Guidelines Series (Foa, Davidson, & Frances, 1999b) issued guidelines specific to PTSD that may be useful for the clinician when determining how to prioritize the course of treatment. For example, a common comorbid condition with PTSD is substance use disorders. The guidelines recommend use of anxiety management for patients with PTSD and substance abuse or dependence. Other resources recommend treating the substance disorder prior to beginning trauma-focused treatment because substance use may be used as an inappropriate coping strategy, limit one's ability to use social supports, and increase one's risk of further victimization.

In Lynn's case, the depression appeared to be causing the most significant immediate impairment. During the initial part of treatment, she missed many sessions and had difficulty completing and bringing her homework to session. Her depression was targeted first in order to increase her attendance and compliance with treatment as well as to provide her with a sense of hope. The manner in which the depression was handled is described below in the section entitled Dealing with Complicating Factors.

Selection of Treatment Strategies

Prior to describing strategies utilized in Lynn's treatment, we present a brief description of the different treatment strategies for PTSD and a summary of the current status of research on the efficacy of PTSD treatments in general, and specifically for sexual assault. The majority of treatments involve exposing the patient, imaginally or in vivo, to stimuli that are typically avoided. Exposure allows for extinction of the learned fear response, as evidenced by a decrease in physiological arousal and subjective fear in the presence of target stimuli. Through repeated exposure, patients learn that the stimuli that were associated with the traumatic event are not dangerous, or in conditioning terms, the fear response is extinguished, and avoidance of the stimuli decreases.

Prolonged Exposure.   Prolonged exposure (PE; Foa & Rothbaum, 1998) involves repeated imaginal exposure to the traumatic event through having the client repeatedly recount, in great detail, the trauma in a safe environment (e.g., the therapist's office). Through experiencing the conditioned stimulus repeatedly (e.g., memories and associated stimuli of the event), extinction of the fear response is achieved. To further increase the benefits of exposure and decrease the amount of time required to extinguish fear responses to the recounted event, clients also audiotape sessions and review the tapes between sessions. Treatment may also include in vivo exposure, in which the client is asked to expose themselves to actual safe situations, people, or places they have avoided unnecessarily.

Stress Inoculation Training.   Stress Inoculation Training (SIT) is a cognitive–behavioral treatment originally developed by Meichenbaum (1974) and later used with rape victims (Kilpatrick, Veronen, & Resick, 1982). SIT involves three phases: education, skill building, and application. The education phase involves teaching information regarding the development of the fear response, identifying cues that trigger the fear, and instruction in progressive muscle relaxation. The skill-building phase consists of teaching diaphragmatic breathing, thought stopping, covert rehearsal, guided self-dialog, and role-playing. In the application phase, clients integrate and apply skills specifically to assist in confronting feared and avoided behaviors/events.

Cognitive Processing Therapy.   Cognitive processing therapy (CPT) combines elements of exposure therapy and cognitive restructuring (Resick, 1992; Resick & Schnicke, 1993). The exposure component involves writing detailed accounts about the traumatic event and reading these accounts for homework and in session. The cognitive aspects include helping the client recognize and experience emotions related to the rape, as well as identifying and modifying distorted cognitions related to beliefs about oneself, others, and the world. Education and homework assignments target the identification and evaluation of the impact of trauma on safety, trust, power, esteem, and intimacy. Throughout treatment, time is spent discovering and modifying a client's "stuck points" (i.e., conflicts between one's schema and new information related to the trauma).

Multiple Channel Exposure Therapy.   Multiple Channel Exposure Therapy (MCET; Falsetti, 1997) is a 12-week manualized treatment developed to treat individuals suffering from both PTSD and panic attacks. MCET combines components of cognitive processing therapy (Resick & Schnicke, 1993) and panic control treatment (Barlow & Craske, 1988). The treatment includes education about traumatic events and correlates of trauma, education about causes and responses to panic attacks and PTSD, breathing retraining, cognitive exposure, in vivo exposure, and cognitive restructuring to address distorted thinking related to the trauma or panic attacks (Falsetti, 1997).

Eye Movement Desensitization and Reprocessing.   Eye-movement desensitization and reprocessing (EMDR) is a controversial treatment for PTSD developed by Shapiro (1989). The treatment involves asking the patient to imagine the traumatic event and hold the image while visually tracking a rapidly moving object (e.g., the therapist's fingers, a light). The defining feature of EMDR is the eye movements; however, there has been significant controversy in the field regarding the necessity of the saccadic movements. Overall, research suggests that eye movements are not necessary (Devilly, Spence, & Rapee, 1998) and that the exposure component of this treatment is the "active" ingredient.

Outcome Studies.   This section briefly summarizes several reviews of PTSD treatments. Prolonged exposure is effective in treating combat veterans (Keane, Fairbank, Caddell, & Zimering, 1989) and victims of sexual assault (Foa et al., 1999a). Research demonstrates that both PE and SIT (without the in vivo exposure component) produced significant improvements at the posttreatment assessment. The SIT group reported significantly fewer PTSD symptoms immediately following treatment, but the PE group showed more improvements at the 3-month follow-up (Foa, Rothbaum, Riggs, & Murdock, 1991). One study (Foa et al., 1999a) compared SIT, PE, and a treatment that combined SIT and PE. The investigators found that in the intent-to-treat sample (clients who did not complete the treatment), PE produced greater improvement on specific outcome measures, including anxiety, global social adjustment, depression, and PTSD severity than SIT (without the exposure component) and a combination of PE and SIT. In the sample that completed treatment, all three active treatments produced superior improvements to a wait-list control group, and improvements were maintained at follow-up. The active treatments did not differ from each other, however.

Multiple Channel Exposure Therapy has not yet been compared to other treatments; however, data suggests that this innovative treatment is effective in reducing symptoms of both PTSD and panic attacks compared to a wait-list control group (Falsetti & Resnick, 2000). Case studies and controlled outcome studies found equivocal results regarding the effectiveness of EMDR. One study (Devilly & Spence, 1999) comparing cognitive–behavioral treatment and EMDR found that both treatments reduced PTSD symptoms; however, CBT was superior in terms of clinical gains, tolerance of treatment, and maintenance of treatment gains. Overall, the effectiveness of EMDR remains unclear and does not appear to provide therapeutic benefits beyond standard exposure-based treatments. For a review of studies using EMDR, the reader is referred to Cahill, Carrigan, and Frueh (1999).

Priority of Treatment Strategies

The specific type of treatment and treatment strategies the clinician chooses to use with their clients largely depends on the type of trauma experienced, the severity of PTSD symptoms, comorbid diagnoses, and available coping strategies. For the case discussed here, we chose MCET because of the prominence of both PTSD and panic symptoms. Initially, the plan with Lynn was to begin by targeting PTSD and panic symptoms; however, in light of her level of depression and its subsequent interference in her attendance and compliance with homework assignments (in combination with her desire to avoid trauma-related issues), an appointment with a psychiatrist was made to assess the appropriateness of an antidepressant to help alleviate her depression. (For more information on medication issues, see the sections on complicating factors and the role of pharmacotherapy)

The core of exposure therapy, confronting trauma cues and the negative affect associated with them, is quite difficult for most people. Many clients do not have adequate strategies to cope with the discomfort associated with exposure therapy. Thus, it is often important to bolster such skills prior to beginning exposure-based work, especially with clients who also have comorbid diagnoses, such as panic disorder. We were concerned about conducting exposure treatment without first providing Lynn with some coping strategies to reduce her panic symptoms. Using the MCET treatment, initial sessions focused on education about PTSD and panic disorder and the role of trauma in their development. Treatment also involved identifying conditioned cues for the fear response, writing about the meaning of the trauma, learning coping skills (e.g., diaphragmatic breathing), and reducing panic (e.g., through interoceptive exposure techniques). This work enabled Lynn to begin experiencing some mastery of her symptoms and allowed her to be more hopeful about her situation.

Next, Lynn was taught to identify some of her distorted cognitions. One of her prominent distorted thoughts focused on blaming herself for the rapes. This thought was targeted in several exercises designed to modify distorted cognitions. At this point, she was ready to confront the trauma. She completed several writings about the traumatic events and read them in session and at home while monitoring her anxiety. Through this exercise, more distorted cognitions were identified (e.g., "Any man interested in me only cares about sex") and challenged.

In vivo exposure exercises involved developing a hierarchy of events or situations that Lynn continued to avoid because of the traumatic event. She choose to target her fear of going places with family members, going places alone, and being alone with a man. A hierarchy of activities was developed for each targeted fear, and she began to complete these as homework assignments. For example, Lynn's hierarchy targeting her fear of being alone with a man involved six steps, including standing at the elevator watching people get on and off, ride the elevator with one or more women, ride with women and at least one man, ride alone with a man for one floor, and ride alone with a man for several floors. Lynn progressed rapidly through these exercises and was soon able to ride elevators with men, sit in the therapist's office with a male therapist, go for walks on her own, play in the park with her younger brothers and son, and go out to eat with family members. The last phase of treatment focused on five specific areas affected by the trauma: trust, intimacy, esteem, power/competence, and safety. Education was provided on the impact of trauma on each of these areas, and Lynn completed homework assignments in which she identified distorted congnitions related to each area.

Dealing with Complicating Factors

Due to the severity of Lynn's depression and her desire to avoid any reminders of the trauma, including therapy, it took several attempts for her to become invested in and attend treatment regularly. In fact, she had only been seen four times in the first 3 months that her case was opened. We opted to initiate a behavioral contract for attendance of therapy sessions. Specifically, we conducted a session that had three goals: (a) the therapist and Lynn developed and signed a contract that required her to attend three of every four sessions in order to continue to be seen at our clinic, (b) the rationale for the therapy was reviewed, and (c) she was given information about the discomfort associated with exposure therapy. The therapist forecast for Lynn that her desire to avoid sessions would increase and that her symptoms would likely worsen before they diminished. Next, a session was held with the psychiatrist, resulting in alleviating her concerns about taking an antidepressant medication. (This process is discussed in more detail later.) The contract was quite effective in increasing Lynn's attendance, compliance with homework assignments, and medication compliance. She progressed quite well through the remainder of the treatment.

Role of Pharmacotherapy in the Case

The study of pharmacotherapy for PTSD has increased. Investigations are complicated by the use of a combination of drugs to deal with different aspects of the disorder and the comorbid disorders that are so frequently observed. Medications used to treat PTSD include tricyclic antidepressants, benzodiazepines, monoamine oxidase inhibitors (MAOI), serotonin-specific reuptake inhibitors (SSRI), and medications with anticonvulsant and mood-stabilizing properties (Van Etten & Taylor, 1998). One (Sutherland & Davidson, 1994) meta-analysis found that attrition rates in the drug therapies were greater than attrition rates for psychological treatments and control conditions. Drop-out rates did not differ by type of drug. Among the drug treatments, SSRIs were the most effective. Unfortunately, whether treatment effects continue following withdrawal of the medications could not be evaluated. Overall, studies suggest that drugs with serotoninergic action achieve positive effects (Sutherland & Davidson, 1994); however, in light of the high drop-out rates associated with medications, a combined approach may be most appropriate.

As discussed previously, Lynn was encouraged to see a psychiatrist due to her depression and the role that depression (as well as avoidance) was playing in her difficulty attending treatment regularly. Next, we held a joint session with the psychiatrist and thoroughly reviewed her concerns about the medications and the potential obstacles to her being compliant with taking the medicine as prescribed. Lynn's primary concern about the medication was related to difficulty tolerating the side effects. She agreed to take the medication for 1 month, at which time she would again meet with the psychiatrist to discuss any difficulties or concerns. She also agreed to report any concerns or problems to the therapist. The psychiatrist increased the length of graduation of the dosage so that Lynn was able to get used to smaller levels of the side effects before the dosage increased. Lynn complied with the medication regime and began reporting less depression soon after reaching a therapeutic dosage.

Managed Care Considerations

This patient was covered by Medicaid insurance. However, managed care directives are becoming increasingly relevant to psychologists. Initially, the primary outcome of managed care involvment in psychological services was to reduce the quantity of treatment sessions offered. Ironically, this had the effect of forcing therapists and personnel directors to increasingly adopt the most effective, efficient, and empirically supported interventions. Therefore, although limiting the overall quantity of services patients can obtain, managed care may have indirectly increased the quality of services delivered.

SUMMARY

Research and treatment for PTSD have expanded tremendously in the past two decades. Several theories have been proposed to explain symptom manifest as a response to trauma and currently, several treatments are available to target these symptoms, as well as other difficulties (e.g., cognitive distortions) that may accompany the disorder. A manualized treatment, MCET, has also been developed to target PTSD and one of the common cooccurring diagnoses, panic attacks. MCET was used in Lynn's case, as described previously. She attended a total of 18 weekly individual therapy sessions. The initial four sessions focused on assessment and targeting Lynn's depression in an effort to increase her compliance and provide her with a sense of hope. Twelve sessions focused on symptoms of PTSD and panic attacks and followed the MCET protocol. Finally, two booster sessions following treatment focused on maintenance of treatment gains and relapse prevention.

Immediately on completing the MCET protocol, Lynn reported having one panic attack in the previous month, in contrast to the three or four per week that she reported at the beginning of treatment. She denied intrusive experiences, including nightmares. On two occasions following treatment, she reported experiencing unpleasant interpersonal interactions. She found herself beginning to avoid the individuals involved, but quickly identified her avoidance and used skills she learned in treatment to decrease her avoidance. Although no longer hypervigilant, Lynn reported that she believed she would always be more cautious than she had prior to the rapes. She was determined that the trauma would no longer control her life.

During the latter part of treatment, as part of her in vivo exposure homework, Lynn began to socialize with her friends. At the second and final booster session, she reported that she had been on three dates with a man she met through a mutual friend. Her family situation improved as well during this time. She was able to continue with school and started a part-time job in the evenings, which helped with the family's financial situation. She enrolled in a parenting class through the community college and reported improved relations with her son. She was still taking the antidepressant medication at the second booster session, and discussed her recent meeting with her psychiatrist and the plan to taper the medications.

Several issues were discussed in the two booster sessions to help Lynn maintain treatment gains and plan for potential future obstacles. Information about the effect of trauma on intimacy was reviewed, and issues related to sexuality in general and the effects of trauma on sexuality in particular were discussed. Various potential risk factors were identified that might lead to a resurgence of her symptoms, including revictimization, life stressors, and handling her son's questions about his father. Lynn engaged in appropriate problem solving in sessions related to these potential difficulties, and appeared to have gained sufficient self-confidence and assertiveness to identify and use community resources, if necessary.

REFERENCES

American Psychiatric Association (1952). *Diagnostic and statistical manual of mental disorders.* Washington, DC: Author.

American Psychiatric Association (1968). *Diagnostic and statistical manual of mental disorders–2nd Ed.* Washington, DC: Author.

American Psychiatric Association (1980). *Diagnostic and statistical manual of mental disorders–3rd Ed.* Washington, DC: Author.

American Psychiatric Association (1987). *Diagnostic and statistical manual of mental disorders–3rd Ed.–Revised.* Washington, DC: Author.

American Psychiatric Association (1994). *Diagnostic and statistical manual of mental disorders–4th Ed.* Washington, DC: Author.

Barlow, D. H., & Craske, M. G. (1988). *Mastery of anxiety and panic manual.* Albany: Center for Stress and Anxiety Disorders.

Beck, A. T., Ward, C. H., Mendelson, M., Mock, J. E., & Erbaugh, J. K. (1961). An inventory for measuring depression. *Archives of General Psychiatry, 4,* 561–571.

Becker, J. V., Skinner, L. J., Abel, G. G., Axelrod, R., & Cichon, J. (1984). Sexual problems of sexual assault survivors. *Women and Health, 9,* 5–20.

Blake, D. D., Weathers, F. W., Nagy, L. M., Kaloupek, D. G., Klaumizer, G., Charney, D., & Keane, T. M. (1990). A clinician rating scale for assessing current and lifetime PTSD: The CAPS-1. *The Behavior Therapist, 13,* 187–188.

Breslau, N., Davis, G. C., Andreski, P., & Peterson, E. (1991). Traumatic events and posttraumatic stress disorder in an urban population of young adults. *Archives of General Psychiatry, 48,* 216–222.

Briere, J. (1995). *Professional manual for the Trauma Symptom Inventory,* Odessa, Florida: Psychological Assessment Resources.

Cahill, S. P., Carrigan, M. H., & Frueh, B. C. (1999). Does EMDR work? And if so, why?: A critical review of controlled outcome and dismantling research. *Journal of Anxiety Disorders, 13* (1–2), 5–33.

Chemtob, C., Roiblat, H. L., Hamada, R. S., Carlson, J. G., & Twentyman, C. T. (1988). A cognitive action theory of posttraumatic stress disorder. *Journal of Anxiety Disorders, 2,* 253–275.

Cottler, L. B., Compton, W. M. III, Mager, D., Spitznagel, E. L., & Janca, A. (1992). Posttraumatic stress disorder among substance users from the general population. *American Journal of Psychiatry, 149*, 664–670.

Davidson, L. M., Smith, R., & Kudler, H. (1991). Familial psychiatric illness in posttraumatic stress disorder. *Comprehensive Psychiatry, 30*, 338–345.

Devilly, G. J., & Spence, S. H. (1999). The relative efficacy and treatment distress of EMDR and a cognitive–behavior trauma treatment protocol in the amelioration of posttraumatic stress disorder. *Journal of Anxiety Disorders, 13* (1–2), 131–157.

Devilly, G. J., Spence, S. H. & Rapee, R. M. (1998). The clinical and statistical efficacy of Eye Movement Desensitization and Reprocessing: Treating PTSD within a veteran population. *Behavior Therapy, 29*, 435–455.

Falsetti, S. (1997). The decision-making process of choosing a treatment for patients with civilian trauma–related PTSD. *Cognitive and Behavioral Practice, 4*, 99–121.

Falsetti, S. A., Resick, P. A., & Davis, J. L. (manuscript under review). *Changes in religious beliefs following trauma.*

Falsetti, S. A., & Resnick, H. S. (2000). Treatment of PTSD using cognitive and cognitive behavioral therapies. *Journal of Cognitive Psychotherapy, 14*(3), 261–285.

First, M. B., Spitzer, R. L., Gibbon, M., & Williams, J. B. (1995). Structured Clinical Interview for DSM–IV Axis I Disorders-Patient Edition (SCID–I/P, Version 2). New York: Biometrics Research Department, New York State Psychiatric Institute.

Foa, E. B., Dancu, C. V., Hembree, E. A., Jaycox, L. H., Meadows, E. A., & Street, G. P. (1999a). A comparison of exposure therapy, stress inoculation training, and their combination for reducing posttraumatic stress disorder in female assault victims. *Journal of Consulting and Clinical Psychology, 59*, 715–723.

Foa, E. B., Davidson, J. R. T., & Frances, A. (1999b). The Expert Consensus Guideline Series: Treatment of posttraumatic stress disorder. *The Journal of Clinical Psychiatry, 60* (Supplement 16), 6–76.

Foa, E. B., & Rothbaum, B. O. (1998). *Treating the trauma of rape: Cognitive behavioral therapy for PTSD.* New York: Guilford Press.

Foa, E. B., Riggs, D. S., Dancu, C. V., & Rothbaum, B. O. (1993a). Reliability and validity of a brief instrument for assessing posttraumatic stress disorder. *Journal of Traumatic Stress, 6*, 459–473.

Foa, E. B., Rothbaum, B. O., & Steketee, G. S. (1993b). Treatment of rape victims. *Journal of Interpersonal Violence, 8*, 256–276.

Foa, E. B., Rothbaum, B. O., Riggs, D. S., & Murdock, T. (1991). Treatment of posttraumatic stress disorder in rape victims: A comparison between cognitive behavioral procedures and counseling. *Journal of Consulting and Clinical Psychology, 59*, 715–723.

Foa, E. B., Steketee, G. S., & Olasov-Rothbaum, B. O. (1989). Behavioral/cognitive conceptualization of posttraumatic stress disorder. *Behavior Therapy, 20*, 155–176.

Freedy, J. R., & Donkervoet, J. C. (1995). Traumatic stress: An overview of the field. In: J. R. Freedy & S. E. Hobfoll (Eds.), *Traumatic stress: From theory to practice* (pp. 3–28). New York: Plenum Press.

Green, B. L., Grace, M. C., Lindy, J. D., Gleser, G. C., & Leonard, A. (1990). Risk factors for posttraumatic stress disorder and other diagnoses in a general sample for Vietnam veterans. *American Journal of Psychiatry, 147*, 729–733.

Helzer, J. E., Robins, L. N., & McEvoy, L. (1987). Post-traumatic stress disorder in the general population. *New England Journal of Medicine, 317*, 1630–1634.

Horowitz, M., Wilner, N., & Alvarez, W. (1979). Impact of Event Scale: Measure of subjective distress. *Psychosomatic Medicine, 41*, 209–218.

Kaslow, N. J., Doepke, K. J., & Racusin, G. R. (1994). Depression. In: V. B. Van Hasselt & M. Hersen (Eds.), *Advanced abnormal psychology* (pp. 235–252). New York: Plenum Press.

Keane, T. M., Fairbank, J. A., Caddell, J. M., & Zimering, R. T. (1989). Implosive (flooding) therapy reduces symptoms of PTSD in Vietnam combat veterans. *Behavior Therapy, 20*, 245–260.

Kessler, R. C., Sonnega, A., Bromet, E., Hughes, M., & Nelson, C. B. (1995). Posttraumatic stress disorder in the National Comorbidity Survey. *Archives of General Psychiatry, 52,* 1048–1060.

Kilpatrick, D. G., & Resnick, H. S. (1993). Posttraumatic stress disorder associated with exposure to criminal victimization in clinical and community populations. In: J. R. T. Davidson & E. B. Foa (Eds.), *Posttraumatic stress disorder: DSM–IV and beyond.* Washington, DC: American Psychiatric Press.

Kilpatrick, D. G., Saunders, B. E., Amick-McMullan, A., Best, C. L., Veronen, L. J., & Resnick, H. S. (1989). Victim and crime factors associated with the development of crime-related posttraumatic stress disorder. *Behavior Therapy, 20,* 199–214.

Kilpatrick, D. G., Saunders, B. E., Veronen, L. J., Best, C. L., & Von, J. M. (1987). Criminal victimization: Lifetime prevalence, reporting to police, and psychological impact. *Crime and Delinquency, 33* (4), 479–489.

Kilpatrick, D. G., Veronen, L. J., & Best, C. L. (1985). Factors predicting psychological distress among rape victims. In: C. R. Figley (Ed.), *Trauma and its wake. Vol. 1. The study of and treatment of posttraumatic stress disorder* (pp. 113–141). New York: Brunner/Mazel.

Kilpatrick, D. G., Veronen, L. J., & Resick, P. A. (1982). Psychological sequelae to rape: Assessment and treatment strategies. In: D. M. Dolays & R. L. Meredith (Eds.), *Behavioral medicine: Assessment and treatment strategies* (pp. 473–497). New York: Plenum Press.

Kulka, R. A., Schlenger, W. E., Fairbank, J. A., Hough, R. L., Jordan, B. K., Marmar, C. R., & Weiss, D. S. (1990). *Trauma and the Vietnam War generation: Report of findings from the National Vietnam Veterans Readjustment Study.* New York: Brunner/Mazel.

McCann, I. L., Sakheim, D. K., & Abrahamson, D. J. (1988). Trauma and victimization: A model of psychological adaptation. *The Counseling Psychologist, 16* (4), 531–594.

Meichenbaum D. (1974). *Cognitive Behavior Modification.* Morristown, NJ: General Learning Press.

Mullen, P. E., Martin, J. L., Anderson, J. C., Romans, S. E., & Herbison, G. P. (1996). The long-term impact of the physical, emotional, and sexual abuse of children: A community study. *Child Abuse and Neglect, 20* (1), 7–21.

Norris, F. H. (1992). Epidemiology of trauma: Frequency and impact of different potentially traumatic events on different demographic groups. *Journal of Consulting and Clinical Psychology, 60,* 409–418.

Resick, P. A. (1992). Cognitive treatment of crime-related posttraumatic stress disorder. In: R. D. Peters, R. J. McMahon, & V. L. Quinsey (Eds.), *Aggression and violence throughout the life span* (pp. 171–191). Newbury Park, CA: Sage Publications.

Resick, P. A., Falsetti, S. A., Resnick, H. S., & Kilpatrick, D. G. (1991). *The Modified PTSD Symptom Scale–Self Report.* St. Louis: University of Missouri and Charleston, SC: National Crime Victims Research and Treatment Center, Medical University of South Carolina.

Resick, P. A., & Schnicke, M. K. (1993). *Cognitive processing therapy for rape victims: A treatment manual.* Newbury Park, CA: Sage Publications.

Resnick, H. S., Best, C. L., Kilpatrick, D. G., Freedy, J. R., & Falsetti, S. A. (1993a). *Trauma Assessment for Adults Self-Report.* Charleston: The National Crime Victims Research and Treatment Center, Medical University of South Carolina.

Resnick, H. S., Kilpatrick, D. G., Dansky, B. S., Saunders, B. E., & Best, C. L. (1993b). Prevalence of civilian trauma and PTSD in a representative national sample of women. *Journal of Consulting and Clinical Psychology, 61,* 984–991.

Robins, L., Helzer, J., Cottler, L., & Goldring, E. (1988). *NIMH Diagnostic Interview Schedule Version III Revised (DIS–III–R).* St. Louis: Washington University Press, Medical College of Pennsylvania.

Robins, L. N., Helzer, J. E., Croughan, J., & Ratcliff, K. (1981). National Institute of Mental Health Diagnostic Interview Schedule. *Archives of General Psychiatry, 38,* 381–389.

Schwarz, E. D., & Perry, B. D. (1994). The post-traumatic response in children and adolescents. *Psychiatric Clinics of North America, 17* (2), 311–326.

Shapiro, F. (1989). Eye movement desensitization: A new treatment for PTSD. *Journal of Behavior Therapy & Experimental Psychiatry, 3*, 211–217.

Sutherland, S. M., & Davidson, J. R. T. (1994). Pharmacotherapy for posttraumatic stress disorder. *Psychiatric Clinics of North America, 17* (2), 409–423.

Tomb, D. A. (1994). The phenomenology of posttraumatic stress disorder. *Psychiatric Clinics of North America, 17* (2), 237–250.

Van Etten, M., & Taylor, S. (1998). Comparative efficacy of treatments for posttraumatic stress disorder: A meta-analysis. *Clinical Psychology and Psychotherapy, 5*, 126–145.

Weaver, T. L., & Clum, G. A. (1995). Psychological distress associated with interpersonal violence: A meta-analysis. *Clinical Psychology Review, 15* (2), 115–140.

Wilson, J. P., Smith, W. K., & Johnson, S. K. (1985). A comparative analysis of PTSD among various survivor groups. In: C. R. Figley (Ed.), *Trauma and its wake: The study and treatment of posttraumatic stress disorder* (pp. 142–172). New York: Brunner/Mazel.

Wind, T. W. & Silvern, L. (1992). Type and extent of child abuse as predictors of adult functioning. *Journal of Family Violence, 7*, 261–281.

Generalized Anxiety Disorder

Robert Ladouceur
Université Laval, Quebec

Michel J. Dugas
Concordia University, Montreal

DESCRIPTION OF THE DISORDER

Anxiety may have affected human beings since the beginning of time, but only recently have attempts been made to examine its diverse forms more closely. In particular, anxiety, which is a general feeling of uneasiness experienced during several daily life situations, has been poorly understood. In the past, this type of anxiety has been called *existential*, *free-floating*, or *pervasive*. Currently, however, it is recognized as a specific disorder referred to as *generalized anxiety disorder* (GAD).

The definition of GAD remained vague and controversial for several years. Initially, authors referred to *free-floating anxiety* to describe an anxious reaction that they related to omnipresent factors in the environment. In 1980, however, GAD was officially recognized in the third edition of the *Diagnostic and Statistical Manual of Mental Disorders* of the American Psychiatric Association (APA, 1980). It was originally considered a residual diagnostic category, which meant that it could not be diagnosed in the presence of another disorder. The view of GAD as a residual category resulted in low diagnostic reliability and, above all, an inability to account for individuals who suffer from excessive worry about everyday concerns. It was not until the *DSM–III–R*(1987) was published that GAD became a primary diagnostic category. Manifestation of unrealistic or excessive anxiety and worry thus became the first diagnostic criterion of this anxiety disorder. Although GAD was mainly defined in terms of cognitive symptoms, the diagnosis also required presence of at least 6 of

18 somatic symptoms that were divided into three categories: motor tension, autonomic hyperactivity, and vigilance and scanning (APA, 1987). In spite of the fact that the *DSM–III–R* improved the diagnostic reliability of GAD, it remained relatively weak compared to other anxiety disorders.

In order to clarify the definition of GAD and improve its diagnostic reliability, the *DSM–IV* made many significant changes. The first diagnostic criterion for GAD became "Excessive anxiety and worry (apprehensive expectation), occurring more days than not for at least 6 months, about a number of events or activities (such as work or school performance)" (APA, 1994, p. 435). The worry must be difficult to control and lead to significant distress or impairment in important areas of functioning (e.g., social, occupational). The notion of unrealistic worry was not retained in the *DSM–IV* because of the difficulty in distinguishing cases in which worry was realistic or justified from cases in which it was not. As mentioned previously, the *DSM–IV* explicitly includes a criterion related to the control of worries and the distress or daily interference resulting from worry and anxiety. By determining the client's degree of control, the clinician can indirectly evaluate the excessive aspect of worries. Finally, in order to improve the diagnostic specificity of the somatic criteria, the *DSM–IV* changed the diagnostic criteria from 6 out of 18 to 3 out of 6 symptoms: (a) restlessness or feeling keyed up or on edge, (b) being easily fatigued, (c) difficulty concentrating or mind going blank, (d) irritability, (e) muscle tension, and (f) sleep disturbance. Although studies of the diagnostic reliability of GAD as defined by the *DSM–IV* are just beginning to appear, our clinical experience suggests that these changes in GAD criteria may lead to greater diagnostic agreement.

Given that excessive and uncontrollable worry represents the cardinal feature of GAD, the notion of worry must be clearly defined; for instance, how does worry differ from anxiety? Since the mid-1980s, researchers have attempted to distinguish *worry* from *anxiety* by defining these constructs specifically. Borkovec and colleagues (1983) first defined *worry* as a chain of thoughts and images that are difficult to control and charged with negative emotions. They added that *worry* represents an attempt to solve a problem, real or fictitious, whose outcome is uncertain and that may lead to negative consequences. Furthermore, they stated that people who suffer from generalized anxiety are experts at identifying possible problems and difficulties, but are less skilled when it comes to actually solving problems. This characteristic may be due to the fact that identification of potential problems focuses more on conceivable difficulties than on possible solutions.

Research has shown that worry generally focuses on the following themes: family, finances, work, disease, and interpersonal relationships. However, as this list is not exhaustive, it is important to clarify the precise themes that provoke worry for each individual. In one study (Dugas et al., 1998a) comparing worry themes of GAD patients to those of other anxiety disorder patients, we found that GAD patients reported more worry about unlikely outcomes. With regard to immediate or current problems, there were no significant differences between the two groups, possibly because worrying about current problems may be adaptive. However, worrying about hypothetical problems that may never occur is rarely adaptive. Normal worrying, which is aimed at the facilitation of problem solving, rarely involves distant concerns. Therefore, excessive worry about situations that are both distant and unlikely appears to be a characteristic of GAD.

How does worry manifest itself in the majority of GAD patients? It is interesting to note that worries often take the form of verbal–linguistic thoughts (internal monologs) rather than terrifying mental images. Research suggests that worries are experienced as thoughts in 70% of cases and that the remaining 30% correspond to images. Borkovec and Inz (1990) showed that over the course of a relaxation session, subjects with GAD experienced more thoughts and fewer images than nonanxious individuals. Moreover, all participants indicated that the proportion of thoughts increased during a worry period. Another revealing fact is that following a clinical intervention, clients with GAD indicated a decrease of thoughts and an increase of mental imagery! These results indicate that worries are intimately linked to a mental script, an internal monolog that individuals repeat to themselves, composing a never-ending story.

METHODS TO DETERMINE DIAGNOSIS

The differential diagnosis of GAD is often a considerable challenge for clinicians. Even though modifications introduced into the *DSM–IV* favor a more systematic diagnostic procedure, the fact remains that in some cases, it is difficult to differentiate GAD from other emotional disorders. This is especially true for social phobia, obsessive–compulsive disorder, and hypochondriasis.

Social phobia is characterized by a persistent and intense fear of one or more social situations. Because exposure to these social situations provokes an anxious reaction, the individual often attempts to avoid or to escape them. Although the main feature of GAD is presence of excessive and uncontrollable worry, social phobia is characterized by fear and anxiety that relate specifically to social situations. In our clinical trials, social phobia is the most frequent comorbid anxiety disorder found among GAD patients. This is not surprising, given that GAD worry may concern, among other things, social situations. The therapist must therefore determine if the patient's worry primarily focuses on being embarrassed or shy in social situations. If so, the clinician should make the appropriate diagnosis of social phobia. However, if the patient's difficulties cannot be conceptualized as being exclusively "social" in nature, the differential diagnosis becomes more difficult. For example, if in addition to social situations, the patient is preoccupied with the health of his or her children, professional responsibilities, and finances, the clinician should also consider a diagnosis of GAD. Furthermore, the clinician should determine whether the worry or fear of being embarrassed in public mark the simultaneous presence of social phobia. This scenario is relatively frequent, given that the worry and anxiety of individuals with GAD often encompass social themes.

The differential diagnosis of GAD in relation to obsessive–compulsive disorder (OCD) can also represent quite a challenge for the clinician. OCD involves presence of obsessions and/or compulsions. In the case in which the clinician observes that a person experiences marked overt compulsions, a diagnosis of OCD is warranted. When the patient also complains of excessive and uncontrollable worry concerning situations that are not related to their compulsions, the clinician should consider an additional diagnosis of GAD. However, 15% to 20% of patients suffering from OCD do not report overt compulsions; for these patients, the diagnosis of OCD rests on the presence of obsessions, which, like worries, represent a form of cognitive intrusion. In some cases, the distinction between these two types of intrusive thoughts is fairly clear. For example, the person conducting the assessment may easily distinguish an obsession that translates into an impulse (e.g., a parent who feels compelled to push their child down the stairs) from a worry about a minor daily event (e.g., imagining oneself arriving late for a meeting at work). However, intrusive thoughts that fall neatly into one of these two categories are quite rare. In most cases, patients experience cognitive intrusions that can be conceptualized as either an obsession or a worry. Consider the case of a person who has frequent cognitive intrusions concerning the accidental death of their child. Should these thoughts be seen as an obsession or a worry? The *DSM–IV* does not fully address this question.

In order to facilitate the differential diagnosis of GAD and OCD without overt compulsions, intrusive thoughts should be evaluated on several dimensions. Although the evaluation of any one dimension of an intrusive thought is not sufficient to differentiate an obsession from a worry, the evaluation of several dimensions can help the clinician to get an overall view and reach a more appropriate decision regarding the nature of the intrusive thought. The first dimension to consider is the form of the thought: an obsession frequently appears as a "flash" or mental image, whereas a worry usually corresponds to an internal monolog or mental narrative. The clinician can also consider the egosyntonic/egodystonic character of the intrusion: an obsession is typically more egodystonic than a worry. The intrusive thought should be further analyzed according to the following principle: an obsession is generally a static phenomenon (that is, the same image repeatedly reoccurs), whereas a worry is regularly reported as a dynamic and neverending scenario. Finally, the therapist should attempt to identify the function of the intrusive thought. Our clinical experience suggests that OCD patients tend to believe that their thoughts will end up provoking the feared outcome. For example, persons with OCD might believe that, if they think too often about their child being involved in a car accident, the feared event will occur. However, patients with GAD are more likely to believe that their worries will prevent a harmful event from occurring. Using the same example, individuals with GAD might believe that worrying about their child being involved in a car accident will somehow prevent such an event from occurring. Overall, despite the fact that the differential diagnosis between OCD without overt compulsions and GAD requires additional effort, the clinician can arrive at a satisfactory judgment by making a detailed and rigorous analysis of their patient's cognitive intrusions.

The final area to cover as to differential diagnosis is the relationship between GAD and hypochondriasis. *Hypochondriasis* can be defined as an excessive preoccupation with having a serious disease or illness. Such preoccupation usually rests on the erroneous interpretation of physical symptoms; a state that may persist despite numerous medical examinations that invalidate the basis of this preoccupation. Worries in GAD are also frequently related to concerns about the person's physical health. The clinician must therefore determine whether the client's preoccupations represent a worry that is characteristic of GAD or a fear that is typical of hypochondriasis. If the client's concerns are restricted to health, a diagnosis of hypochondriasis should be retained. However, when the client reports several excessive worries, including preoccupations with health, there is reason to question the pertinence of a comorbid diagnosis of hypochondriasis. First, it is important to determine whether the client's preoccupations result from an erroneous interpretation of physical symptoms. The more therapists observe the importance of this factor, the more likely they will be to retain a diagnosis of hypochondriasis. Second, one must question whether the number of the client's medical consultations is truly excessive. The more the client consults without any apparent reason, the more pertinent the diagnosis of hypochondriasis becomes. Finally, clinicians should ask their clients whether they believe they have already contracted a serious disease. The results of a study conducted by our research team indicates that hypochondriasis involves the conviction of being gravely ill; the client thus considers that the source of their preoccupation has already come true. The opposite is true for GAD; worry reflects the client's fear of contracting this illness in the near or distant future. By assessing these diverse dimensions carefully, the clinician should be able to distinguish between a fear related to hypochondriasis and a GAD-related worry.

The evolution of the diagnostic criteria of GAD since the 1980s has led to corresponding changes as to assessment. Given that GAD was originally considered a nonspecific disorder (i.e., free-floating or pervasive anxiety), it was assessed with general measures of anxiety. Although these measures remain useful, examination of the specific symptoms, particularly worry, now plays a central role in the assessment process. In our clinical work, we typically use two types of measures to establish the presence of GAD: a structured diagnostic interview and self-report measures of GAD symptoms.

Given the diagnostic subtleties outlined, use of a structured interview such as the Anxiety Disorders Interview Schedule for *DSM–IV* (ADIS–IV; Di Nardo, Brown, & Barlow, 1994) greatly facilitates the clinician's work. Administration of the ADIS–IV typically takes 1 to 2 hours and yields information on presence of Axis I disorders and includes severity ratings. The interview thoroughly assesses all anxiety disorders and screens for mood disorders, somatoform disorders, psychoactive substance use disorders, psychotic disorders, and medical problems. The section on GAD, which takes about 20 minutes to administer, allows the clinician to assess the extent, frequency, and seriousness of worry. Moreover, it examines the content of worry, the amount of time spent worrying on a daily basis, and the GAD somatic symptoms.

Subsequent to the structured interview, self-report questionnaires are administered in order to collect complementary data on diverse aspects of the disorder. The Worry and Anxiety Questionnaire (WAQ; Dugas, Freeston, Lachance, Provencher, & Ladouceur, 1995) is an 11-item self-report scale that assesses the *DSM–IV* diagnostic criteria for GAD. The WAQ discriminates accurately between GAD patients and nonclinical controls and shows good test–retest reliability over a 10-week interval (Dugas et al., 1995). Furthermore, the WAQ somatic subscale shows sensitivity to change over treatment. In one clinical trial (Ladouceur et al., in press), we found that scores on the WAQ somatic subscale significantly decreased following cognitive–behavioral therapy for GAD, whereas they remained unchanged in a wait-list control condition.

The Penn State Worry Questionnaire (PSWQ; Meyer, Miller, Metzger, & Borkovec, 1990) includes 16 items that measure the tendency to engage in chronic, excessive, and uncontrollable worry. The PSWQ is unifactorial and possesses high internal consistency and test–retest reliability; it also has adequate convergent and discriminant validity (Meyer et al., 1990). Like the WAQ, the PSWQ is sensitive to change over the course of treatment (Ladouceur et al., 2000).

ADDITIONAL ASSESSMENT REQUIRED

Our research shows that intolerance of uncertainty represents a key cognitive characteristic of patients with GAD (Dugas, Gagnon, Ladouceur, & Freeston, 1998). *Intolerance of uncertainty* may be defined as the excessive tendency of an individual to consider it unacceptable that a negative event may occur, however small the probability of its occurrence. Because intolerance of uncertainty plays such an important role in the etiology and maintenance of excessive and uncontrollable worry, it should also be assessed in GAD patients. To this end, our research team developed and validated a self-report measure of intolerance of uncertainty.

The Intolerance of Uncertainty Scale (IUS; Freeston, Rhéaume, Letarte, Dugas, & Ladouceur, 1994) includes 27 items relating to the idea that uncertainty is unacceptable; reflects badly on a person; and leads to frustration, stress, and the inability to take action. The IUS distinguishes GAD clients from nonclinical controls and from clients with other anxiety disorders (Ladouceur et al., 1999). The questionnaire has excellent internal consistency, as well as good criterion, convergent and discriminant validity (Freeston et al., 1994).

CASE ILLUSTRATION

Presenting Complaints

Tom is a 48-year-old man who is married and the father of a 22-year-old women. He works as an administrator for a large company that specializes in computers, a job that he has occupied for the last 15 years. During the previous 5 years, he has become increasingly worried and anxious following important policy changes at work. He is overwhelmed with worries for about 5 hours a day, and experiences the following physical symptoms: agitation, fatigue, concentration problems, and difficulty sleeping. The diagnostic assessment revealed that Tom suffered from severe GAD and mild panic disorder.

History of the Disorder

Tom felt that the state of his physical health had been quite stable until 5 years ago, when he began seeing his doctor once a year for a complete medical examination. In his early 40s, Tom consulted the doctor several times, believing he had a cardiac problem. His doctor assured him this was not the case and diagnosed him with panic disorder. After receiving treatment for panic disorder, Tom was better able to distinguish anxiety symptoms from symptoms associated with physical problems. He also reported having occasional headaches that he would usually attribute to overworking. However, when his headaches persisted for several hours, he began to fear that cancer was causing the headaches.

Family History

Tom is the oldest of three children. He reported that, as a child, his parents were demanding and often entrusted him with the responsibility of watching over his brother and sister. He also mentioned that his father worried about the family's financial situation and the future of his children. With the recent deterioration of his parents' health, Tom reported that he worries frequently about their physical and emotional well-being. Tom's relationship with his wife is satisfying and stable. He stated that he often discusses his worries with his wife, who frequently tells him that "he is worrying for no good reason." His 22-year-old daughter is a university student, and although Tom realizes that she has no major problems, he worries whenever he notices that she is tired or stressed because of her studies. He also recognizes that he resembles his own father in this regard and often worries about his daughter's future.

Sexual History

Tom's sexual development was normal. During adolescence, he had many friends and started dating at the age of 16. He met his wife when he was in college and they have been married for 24 years. He reported no particular problems in this area of his life.

Mental Status Examination

The mental status examination revealed no significant cognitive deficits. In fact, Tom's cognitive functioning appeared to be excellent.

Prior Treatment

Tom had never consulted a physician or mental health professional specifically for his tendency to worry. At 41 years of age, when his family doctor diagnosed panic disorder, Tom began taking anxiolytic medication (i.e., Xanax). He also participated in cognitive–behavioral therapy that helped him to reduce the frequency of his panic attacks. He stopped taking his anxiolytic medication at 43 years of age. At Tom's last medical examination, his doctor suggested that he resume taking his medication because he was reporting feeling anxious on a regular basis, although not to the extent of the panic attacks he had experienced a few years earlier. For the previous 8 months, Tom has been taking 0.5 mg of Xanax per day.

CASE CONCEPTUALIZATION

Modeling and Learning

When he was living at home with his parents, Tom was exposed to a father who worried a great deal about the family's financial situation. His father wanted his children to receive the higher education that he did not have the opportunity to obtain. Therefore, a source of modeling was his father's preoccupation about family finances and how this might affect the future of his children.

Life Events

A major problem situation was associated with Tom's excessive worries. Specifically, he had to cope with an anxiety-provoking situation at work: his company was in the process of a major reorganization. Although he did not believe that the reorganization was necessary, he also realized that he had to deal with it. He therefore spent countless hours trying to find ways of adapting to the changes in his company.

Genetics and Temperament

Tom's genetic heritage from his father was probably a predisposing factor for his excessive worries and anxiety. From a very young age, Tom showed signs of being quite withdrawn and anxious.

Physical Conditions

Tom worked long hours in the evening before a meeting in an attempt to foresee all the potential problems that might occur. Despite his efforts, he was unable to anticipate all possible difficulties, and his fatigue prevented him from reacting effectively to the unexpected events that did inevitably occur. He had the impression that the extra hours of preparation were improving his performance; unfortunately, they seemed to be having had opposite effect by leading to harmful fatigue. This excessive fatigue exacerbated his psychological vulnerability to worry.

Drugs

Apart from the Xanax he was taking for his anxiety, Tom was taking no other medication. Thus, no other drugs affected his psychological functioning.

Overall Conceptualization

Because GAD was clearly the primary disorder in this case, and panic disorder was not a major problem, the priority was to tackle Tom's worries. Given that our research has shown that intolerance of uncertainty is a key factor underlying worry, this was addressed right from the beginning of therapy. During the first treatment sessions, Tom attempted to convince us that the company's reorganization made no sense by bringing company memos announcing changes in priorities and downsizing policies with him to therapy. We emphasized that we believed Tom, and that it was not necessary to bring the memos to therapy. In fact, the memos were not useful because what was most important was to examine how Tom was dealing with the uncertainty of the situation at work. Tom explained that he had developed strategies aimed at reducing his stress, and although they did not produce the expected results, he continued to use them.

   We showed Tom that by taking all this time to prepare for his meetings, he was attempting to eliminate the uncertainty associated with his company's current situation. Unfortunately, not only was this a difficult undertaking, it also was not possible. Most of the uncertainty in this situation, as in many others, was inevitable. Having accepted this idea, Tom agreed to work on increasing his tolerance to the uncertainty he was experiencing in his job. We explained to him that in order to change his degree of tolerance, he would have to change some of his behaviors. It was suggested that he ask himself the following question: "If I were tolerant of uncertainty, what would I do in this situation?" Using the example of his extensive preparation on the evening before a meeting, Tom realized that he would reduce the amount of preparation time if he were more tolerant of uncertainty. We then helped him to select the files that actually required special attention for the next meeting. Although Tom agreed with the idea of reducing his preparation time, he felt anxious at not reviewing all of the files before the next meeting. We normalized his feeling of uneasiness by explaining that people often feel anxious when they adopt a new behavior. This is not necessarily a sign that the behavior is "wrong" or that it should not be repeated; on the contrary, it is normal to feel uneasy during the first few trials of any new behavior. However, it is important to order the behaviors according to an ascending degree of difficulty (a hierarchy), beginning with something small and realistic. For example, Tom began by decreasing his preparation for meetings with his staff. Later in therapy, he was able to limit his preparation when meeting with his superiors.

Behavioral Assessment

Because our treatment involves specific strategies for different types of worries, we present these worry types and their clinical implications before continuing with the treatment illustration. Our clients with GAD have described worries that concern (a) immediate problems that are "grounded in reality," and (b) improbable events that are not "grounded in reality." Examples of the first type of worry, which concern immediate problems, include worries about interpersonal conflicts, being on time for appointments, getting the car fixed, or making minor house repairs. Research shows that when faced with problems, GAD clients report initial cognitive, affective, and behavioral reactions (problem orientation) that are ineffective or counterproductive. Considering that worry is associated with poor problem orientation, problem-solving training with an emphasis on problem orientation should be applied to worries about immediate problems that are grounded in reality.

The second type of worry refers to improbable events that are not grounded in reality. Worries about the possibility of someday going bankrupt or becoming seriously ill (in the absence of immediate financial or health problems) are examples of this type of worry. These worries are not within the reach of problem-solving training because no problem actually exists. However, cognitive exposure can be applied to these worries. Research shows that the verbal content of worry represents avoidance of fear-provoking imagery and that worry is negatively reinforced by a decrease in aversive somatic activation. Thus, an account of the role of worry as avoidance of fearful images and the existence of a group of worries about problems that do not actually exist (and are not amenable to problem solving) suggest the use of functional cognitive exposure to fearful images.

Prioritization of Targets for Treatment

The main goal of the treatment is of course to decrease the tendency to worry and eliminate GAD. To do this, the intervention targets intolerance of uncertainty, erroneous beliefs about worry, poor problem orientation, and cognitive avoidance. As mentioned previously, the treatment begins by stressing the importance of dealing with uncertainty in everyday life. Because uncertainty is pervasive in everyday life, the treatment's goal is not to eliminate uncertainty, but rather to recognize, accept, and develop coping strategies when faced with uncertain situations.

Second, the treatment attempts to correct erroneous beliefs about worry. Compared to moderate worriers, high worriers believe that worry is more useful because it helps prevent negative outcomes from occurring and minimizes the negative effects (e.g., feelings of guilt or shame) if these outcomes should occur. High worriers also believe that worry is helpful because it motivates them, prepares them for the worst, and distracts them from emotional topics. Compared to nonclinical controls, GAD clients report that worrying is more effective in preventing negative outcomes and promoting positive ones (Dugas et al., 1998b).

Treatment also targets poor problem orientation. High levels of worry are related to poor problem orientation (the person's cognitive set when faced with a problem) and unrelated to knowledge of problem-solving skills per se. Furthermore, GAD clients have poorer problem orientation than other clients with anxiety disorders and nonclinical controls (Ladouceur et al., 1999). However, GAD clients have similar knowledge of problem-solving skills to the other two groups. Clearly, then, GAD clients appear to possess adequate knowledge of problem-solving skills, but they may have difficulty actually solving their problems because of a tendency to react to them in a nonproductive way. Such poor problem orientation includes seeing the problem as a threat to be avoided rather than a challenge to be met, and having poor confidence in one's problem-solving ability.

The final treatment target is cognitive avoidance. Borkovec and colleagues (1983) carried out most of the research to date on the avoidance function of worry. They have shown that worry is mostly made up of verbal–linguistic cognitive activity, which may suppress fear-related mental imagery. The avoidance of mental imagery appears to lead to an inhibition of the sympathetic autonomic system, which may in turn negatively reinforce worry. Because it is associated with avoidance of mental imagery and resulting physiological activation, worry may interfere with emotional processing.

Selection of Treatment Strategies

Returning to our treatment illustration, we presented the main features of our GAD model to Tom and defined worry as a cognitive process that concerns negative future events and that is accompanied by feelings of anxiety. We also explained the distinction between worries that are linked to immediate problems and worries that concern improbable events. Based on this information, Tom was asked to note his worries three times per day, evaluate the level of anxiety associated with each one, and classify them according to their type (current problem or improbable event). After 1 week, Tom noticed that his main worries concerned his professional tasks and responsibilities (current problem) as well as his financial situation (improbable event).

In the next phase of treatment, we focused on Tom's beliefs about the usefulness of worrying. He felt that his worrying was beneficial for several reasons. He stated that administrators like himself have numerous responsibilities, and that worrying about work allowed him to be better prepared, and therefore deal more effectively with crisis situations. Tom felt that if he worried less, he would be less effective when dealing with difficult situations. Using Socratic questioning, we helped him address the validity of this belief. Although he worried a great deal and he was often able to solve his problems, we emphasized that it was quite a leap to assume that reducing his worries would result in a decrease in his ability to deal with situations at work. Because Tom also confused effective planning (developing an appropriate plan of action) with worrying, he viewed his worries as beneficial. Although planning and preparing were useful and did help him perform well, the usefulness of his worrying had not been demonstrated. Therefore, we asked him to explain why he believed worrying was beneficial. Tom reported that there had been a time when he had not been very enthusiastic or worried about his job. During that time, a crisis at work developed that he had not been able to address effectively. According to Tom, this example proved that his worries were beneficial. However, he also realized that when he was feeling particularly enthusiastic about his work, he also worried less yet did a very good job of managing crisis situations. This new piece of evidence revealed an important point to Tom: discouragement about work, and not worrying less, had probably been the harmful element when it came to reacting to the difficult situation. Furthermore, Tom's belief that he needed to worry in order to be ready for a crisis made him feel that by worrying he was in some way reducing the uncertainty of potential problems. However, this same conviction led him to worry excessively and experience high levels of stress and anxiety. These observations eventually led him to conclude that he was paying a high price for believing that his worries were helpful, especially when he had no real proof that they were in fact doing any good.

The next step of the intervention involved helping Tom to become aware of his own problem-solving ability, using his performance at work as an example. Tom noted that after a period of anger, indecisiveness, and worry, he would often find solutions regarding a problem at work. Without exception, however, he would experience a period of stress, sometimes lasting several days, before solving the problem. Tom believed, and with reason, that he had good problem-solving skills, but said that he would sometimes get "bogged down" when faced with a problem. We explained that a negative problem orientation was preventing him from applying his problem-solving skills properly. For instance, Tom was not simply aiming for the best possible solution, he wanted to find the perfect solution. Given the kind of downsizing that had been taking place at Tom's work, ideal outcomes were very rare: when people lose their jobs, they are disappointed, to say the least. Nonetheless, Tom spent several days trying to find a nonexistent perfect solution, which led to him feeling very anxious and discouraged. When he was exhausted, he would end up making the most appropriate decision given the circumstances, an option that he had often identified but refused to accept at the beginning of the problem-solving process. Once he understood that the search for a perfect solution was preventing him from finding a realistic solution, he attempted to find, from the beginning of the problem-solving process, the best possible solution for the problem within the given context. This simple strategy, when strategically employed, was of great help.

The next phase of treatment addressed Tom's cognitive avoidance. Among his exaggerated preoccupations was the unlikely event of declaring personal bankruptcy. Certainly, this thought was linked to a legitimate feeling of insecurity regarding his work; however, he stated clearly that he knew it was unlikely that he would ever go bankrupt, even if he lost his job. When this worry intruded, he tried to reassure himself by saying: "It's impossible, it will never happen; so stop thinking about it." Yet, although Tom knew that this outcome was improbable, he also knew that it was not totally impossible. Not surprisingly, this strategy was not helpful in dismissing his worries about bankruptcy. At this point in therapy, we introduced him to the principles of avoidance, neutralization, and exposure. Tom came to understand that although avoidance and neutralization (subtle efforts to control or remove the thought) may be effective for decreasing anxiety in the short term, ultimately they lead to an increase in anxiety and fear in the longer term. He also learned that exposure would lead to considerable anxiety in the short term but would result in a decrease in anxiety and fear in the longer term. We then asked him to develop an imaginary scenario describing his bankruptcy, which he recorded on a looped-tape cassette. Tom then exposed himself to this scenario by listening to the tape every day for periods ranging from 20 to 50 minutes. After 3 weeks of daily exposure sessions, this worry diminished to a point where it no longer interfered with his daily life.

The final phase of the intervention concerned ways of helping Tom prevent an eventual relapse. This consisted of getting him to anticipate conditions that would be likely to reactivate his worrying. It also involved asking him to view his strengths and weaknesses in a realistic way. For example, he knew that in 2 months, he would be invited to participate in a series of meetings to redefine his tasks and responsibilities at work. Tom felt that this event would lead to a substantial increase in his worry and anxiety. Confident of the fact that he would be able to react adequately, he took the time to assess the key issues and then prepared himself to face the situation by applying the strategies that he had recently learned. Following treatment, Tom no longer met diagnostic criteria for GAD; his worries lasted less than 30 minutes per day, when they had initially taken up to 5 hours. In addition, Tom reported that he was very satisfied with his therapeutic progress. As an epilog to this case illustration, let us mention that Tom was able to master his fears and worries when he finally did debate, with his superiors, the nature of his job, and he claimed to be satisfied with his new role in the company.

Dealing with Complicating Factors

The first complicating factor that might arise during therapy relates to intolerance of uncertainty. Although clients can readily accept the importance of increasing tolerance to uncertainty in order to reduce their worries, they are sometimes resistant to the idea that this is best achieved through concrete actions. Even if patients know that their intolerance of uncertainty fuels their tendency to worry, they find it hard to change their threshold of tolerance by simply thinking about it. Clients should understand that it is difficult to increase their tolerance for uncertainty through cognitive means alone; they must also change their behavior. We have observed that concrete actions represent the most effective means of increasing one's tolerance for uncertainty. In fact, therapeutically effective actions often involve behaving in a novel way in a given situation. The therapist can therefore help the client identify a behavior to replace their habitual, maladaptive behavior. In Tom's case, one of the concrete actions used to improve his tolerance of uncertainty at work was to reduce the time he spent preparing before meetings. We helped him identify the files requiring special attention and suggested concrete strategies that would help him follow his new plan of action.

A second potential complication during treatment concerns cognitive exposure. Some clients experience difficulty applying cognitive exposure, often because of their beliefs about the consequences of anxiety. Fear of anxiety and its consequences may interfere with the client's efforts to engage in cognitive exposure. For example, the patient may fear that the anxiety experienced during exposure will provoke a cardiac arrest or lead to a total loss of control. If this should be the case, the therapist should first ask the client to think back to all the times that they experienced intense anxiety, and point out that the patient never experienced a cardiac arrest or a total loss of control. The therapist can then explain that the previously experienced anxiety is the same anxiety that is experienced during exposure; thus, exposure will not lead to disastrous consequences. The only difference is that the client chooses to experience the anxiety within the framework of a structured exercise. The notions of avoidance and neutralization also must be explained carefully so that the exposure exercises are fully effective. The client's understanding of how the anxiety associated with their threatening scenario varies according to how much they avoid thinking about the scenario, neutralize it, or fully expose themselves to it, is predictive of the success they experience with exposure. The therapist may wish to present cognitive exposure as an alternative to worrying excessively about improbable events for months or years. By using cognitive exposure, clients think about their worries intensely, once a day, for a few weeks, and reduce their worry or even eliminate it altogether.

Role of Pharmacotherapy in the Case

As previously mentioned, Tom was taking anxiolytic medication (Xanax, 0.5 mg, id) to help him deal with his anxiety. At the beginning of therapy, he decided to continue taking his medication, at least for the first half of therapy. He felt this would allow him to carry out the homework exercises without worrying about experiencing moments of intense anxiety. However, near the end of therapy, he felt much less anxious and decided, along with his physician, to reduce the dose and frequency of Xanax. The medication was gradually tapered until complete cessation.

SUMMARY

The treatment for GAD outlined in Tom's case description has been developed over many years and is based on clinical observations and later confirmed by empirical data. Recent data show that this cognitive–behavioral treatment, which targets excessive worry exclusively, also leads to a significant decrease in GAD somatic symptoms (see Ladouceur et al., 2000). These findings suggest that in many cases it may not be necessary to target the somatic symptoms of GAD clients direclty during treatment. It appears that by decreasing their level of worry, many GAD clients also manage to decrease the severity of their attendant somatic symptoms. Data from our clinical trials also indicate that the treatment described here leads to maintenance of therapeutic gains on a long-term basis.

To conclude, a cognitive–behavioral treatment that targets intolerance of uncertainty, erroneous beliefs about worry, poor problem orientation, and cognitive avoidance is effective for treating GAD. A final word for the clinician using this approach for treating GAD is required. That is, many patients have reported that distinguishing between two types of worries (worries that concern current problems and worries that concern improbable events) was very helpful in that it allowed them to feel in control of their worries and know how to handle each specific worry. Not trying to solve a problem that does not yet exist, and may never exist, is certainly an important step toward reducing excessive worry.

REFERENCES

Borkovec, T. D., & Inz, J. (1990). The nature of worry in generalized anxiety disorder: A predominance of thought activity. *Behaviour Research and Therapy, 28*, 153–158.

Borkovec, T. D., Robinson, E., Pruzinsky, T., & DePree, J. A. (1983). Preliminary exploration of worry: Some characteristics and processes. *Behaviour Research and Therapy, 21*, 9–16.

Di Nardo, P. A., Brown, T. A., & Barlow, D. H. (1994). *Anxiety Disorders Interview Schedule for DSM–IV (ADIS–IV).* San Antonio: Psychological Corporation.

Dugas, M. J., Freeston, M. H., Lachance, S., Provencher, M., & Ladouceur, R. (1995, July). *The Worry and Anxiety Questionnaire: Initial validation in nonclinical and clinical samples.* Poster session presented at the World Congress of Behavioural and Cognitive Therapies, Copenhagen, Denmark.

Dugas, M. J., Freeston, M. H., Ladouceur, R., Rhéaume, J., Provencher, M. D., & Boisvert, J.-M. (1998a). Worry themes in primary GAD, secondary GAD and other anxiety disorders. *Journal of Anxiety Disorders, 12*, 253–261.

Dugas, M. J., Gagnon, F., Ladouceur, R., & Freeston, M. H. (1998b). Generalized Anxiety Disorder: A preliminary test of a conceptual model. *Behaviour Research and Therapy, 36*, 215–226.

Freeston, M. H., Rhéaume, J., Letarte, H., Dugas, M. J., & Ladouceur, R. (1994). Why do people worry? *Personality and Individual Differences, 17*, 791–802.

Ladouceur, R., Dugas, M. J., Freeston, M. H., Léger, E., Gagnon, F., & Thibodeau, N. (2000). Efficacy of a new cognitive–behavioral treatment for generalized anxiety disorder: Evaluation in a controlled clinical trial. *Journal of Consulting and Clinical Psychology, 68*, 957–964.

Ladouceur, R., Dugas, M. J., Freeston, M. H., Rhéaume, J., Blais, F., Gagnon, F., Thibodeau, N., & Boisvert, J.-M. (1999). Specificity of generalized anxiety disorder symptoms and processes. *Behavior Therapy, 30*, 191–207.

Meyer, T. J., Miller, M. L., Metzger, R. L., & Borkovec, T. D. (1990). Development and validation of the Penn State Worry Questionnaire. *Behaviour Research and Therapy, 28*, 487–496.

11

Primary Insomnia

Michael T. Smith
Michael L. Perlis
University of Rochester School of Medicine and Dentistry

DESCRIPTION OF THE DISORDER

Epidemiological surveys estimate that insomnia afflicts approximately one third of the U.S. population, with 10 to 15% of adults reporting disturbed sleep as a serious and persistent problem (e.g., Ancoli-Israel & Roth, 1999). Far from being benign, persistent or chronic insomnia is associated with a number of serious individual and societal consequences. Insomnia has been linked consistently to increased medical and psychiatric morbidity and is associated with decreased quality of life, impaired job performance, increased absenteeism, and life-threatening accidents (e.g., Ford & Kamerow, 1989) (Kupperman, Lubeck, & Mazonson, 1995).

Broadly defined, *insomnia* refers to problems initiating and/or maintaining sleep or the complaint of nonrestorative sleep that occurs at least three nights a week and is associated with daytime distress or impairment (World Health Organization, 1992). The term *primary insomnia* is used to distinguish insomnia that is considered to be a distinct diagnostic entity from insomnia that is a secondary symptom of an underlying medical and/or psychiatric condition. Within the American Academy of Sleep Medicine's nosology [the International Classification of Sleep Disorders–Revised (ICSD–R)], *primary insomnia* is referred to as *psychophysiologic insomnia*. The ICSD–R definition is more directly tied to the etiologic underpinnings of the disorder. Although we do not use this term throughout this chapter, it has the advantage of describing the disorder in terms that suggest how insomnia is initiated and maintained.

Psychophysiologic insomnia is described as "a disorder of somatized tension and learned sleep-preventing associations that results in the complaint of insomnia and associated decreased functioning during wakefulness" (American Sleep Disorders Association, 1990, p. 28).

Somatized tension refers to either the client's subjective sense of, or objective measures of, somatic and/or cognitive hyperarousal while attempting to sleep. Somatic arousal is characterized by increased peripheral nervous system activity, such as increased muscle tension, rapid heart rate, and sweating. Cognitive arousal is characterized by the increased occurrence of central nervous system mediated activity, such as intrusive presleep cognitions, racing thoughts, and rumination. Learned sleep-preventing associations refers to a pattern of presleep arousal that appears to be learned or classically conditioned to the bedroom environment. A common report that suggests conditioned arousal is the patient who states, "I was feeling exhausted, but the minute I got into bed it was like my mind ignited with worries about not sleeping." Such patients often report sleeping better when away from home or in a different bedroom. For example, many are able to fall asleep on the couch, but suddenly find themselves wide awake when retiring to bed.

Patients with primary insomnia usually have a normal preferred sleep phase (i.e., between 10:00 PM and 8:00 AM), take between 30 and 120 minutes to fall asleep, awaken 2–4 times per night, and obtain between 4 and 6 hours of sleep a night. This pattern usually occurs on more than 3–4 nights per week and has persisted for a period of time ranging from months to years. Insomnia lasting less than 1 month is generally considered acute and is often associated with clearly definable precipitants, such as stress, acute pain, or substance abuse. Although the complaint of persistent insomnia may have a clear antecedent, patients often report that their sleep problems seem "to have a life of their own" and that they occur throughout the week (i.e., not only on weekdays). Substantial deviations from these general parameters may be suggestive of other sleep disorders.

METHODS TO DETERMINE DIAGNOSIS

Rule Out Secondary Insomnia

As a secondary disorder or as a symptom of other disorders, the inability to fall asleep (initial insomnia), stay asleep (middle insomnia), or the tendency to awaken early in the morning (terminal insomnia) may be related to a variety of factors, including primary medical or psychiatric conditions, drug use or abuse, or other extrinsic or intrinsic sleep disorders. A careful clinical history is required to determine if any of these factors may account for the patient's symptoms. Typical medical exclusions include untreated or unstable gastrointestinal disorders [e.g., gastroesophageal reflux disease (GERD)], cardiopulmonary disorders (e.g., heart disease), and neuroendocrine disorders (e.g., estrogen deficiency). Typical psychiatric exclusions include untreated or unstable affective and/or anxiety disorders. Typical drug use or abuse exclusions include the use of medications and/or recreational drugs that have insomnia as a direct or withdrawal effect. Typical sleep disorders exclusions include other intrinsic sleep disorders (e.g., sleep apnea), circadian rhythm disorders (e.g., shift-work sleep disorder), and extrinsic sleep disorders (e.g., inadequate sleep hygiene). Table 11.1 contains an abridged list for each of these categories. Figure 11.1 provides a schematic that characterizes the differential diagnostic process. Table 11.2 contains a complete list of intrinsic, circadian, and extrinsic sleep disorders as they are defined by the ICSD-R nosology (ASDA, 1990).

Distinguish Fatigue from Excessive Daytime Sleepiness

Perhaps the most fundamental distinction for sleep disorder complaints pertains to the subtle difference between daytime sleepiness and daytime fatigue. Often, patients use the terms interchangeably. *Fatigue* refers to physical and/or mental weariness; the patient clearly indicates that their performance is compromised and attributes this to being "worn out." *Sleepiness*, however, may or may not include fatigue, but is characterized by the patient clearly indicating that "they are fighting to stay awake" or that they cannot resist falling asleep. Daytime fatigue is characteristic of primary insomnia. Excessive daytime sleepiness is characteristic of patients with intrinsic sleep disorders such as obstructive sleep apnea or nocturnal myoclonus.

ADDITIONAL ASSESSMENTS REQUIRED

In addition to the clinical interview, behavioral sleep medicine specialists often use a number assessment tools to gather more precise diagnostic information. A typical intake assessment battery of assessments includes a general sleep/medical history questionnaire; a screen for psychopathology, which most often includes symptom inventories for both depression and anxiety severity [e.g., the Beck Depression Inventory (BDI), Beck, Ward, Mendelson, Mock, & Erbaugh, 1961; the Beck Anxiety Inventory (BAI), Beck & Steer, 1990], a screen for excessive daytime sleepiness [e.g., the Epworth Sleepiness Scale (ESS), Johns, 1991], and a retrospective sleep questionnaire [e.g., the Pittsburgh Sleep Quality Index (PSQI), Buysse, Reynolds, Monk, Berman, & Kupfer, 1989]. In addition, behavioral sleep medicine specialists use daily

TABLE 11.1
Common Factors That Contribute to Insomnia

Medical Illness
   Head injuries
   Hyperthyroidism
   Chronic obstructive pulmonary disease
   Asthma
   Hypertension
   Coronary artery disease
   Arthritis
   Fibromyalgia
   Headache and low back pain
   Seizures
   Gastroesophageal reflux disease
   Parkinson's disease
   Alzheimer's disease
Psychiatric Illness
   Major depression
   Generalized anxiety disorder
   Posttraumatic stress disorder
   Panic disorder
   Bipolar disorder
   Schizophrenia
Acute Effects of Medication
   Alcohol
   Amphetamines
   Caffeine
   Reserpine
   Clonidine
   SSRI antidepressants
   Steroids
   L-dopa
   Theophyline
   Nicotine
   Nifedipine
   Beta agonists (albuterol)
Effects of Withdrawal from Medication
   Benzodiazepines
   Barbiturates
   Alcohol
Other Sleep Disorders
   Obstructive sleep apnea
   Narcolepsy
   Nocturnal myoclonus (periodic limb movement disorder)
   Restless legs syndrome
   Phase advance sleep disorder
   Phase delay sleep disorder
   Sleep state misperception disorder

(*Table continues on next page*)

TABLE 11.1 (*Continued*)

Nightmare disorder
Parasomnias
Poor Sleep Environment
Noise
Ambient temperature
Light
Sleeping surface
Bedpartner
Poor Sleep Habits
Extended time in bed
Naps
Irregular schedule
Situational Factors
Life stress
Bereavement
Unfamiliar sleep environment
Jet lag
Shift work

Adapted from Perlis, M. L., and Youngstedt, S. (2000). The diagnosis of primary insomnia and treatment alternatives. *Journal of Comprehensive Therapy*, 26 (4), 298–306. Reprinted with permission. © American Society of Contemporary Medicine and Surgery.

sleep diaries to monitor sleep complaints prospectively. Sleep diaries typically gather information on time to bed, wake time, sleep latency (SL), frequency of nightly awakenings (FNA), wake time after sleep onset (WASO), total sleep time (TST), early morning awakenings (EMA), medication/substances taken before bed, daytime napping, and subjective assessments of sleep quality and daytime functioning. Sleep diaries are critical for the assessment of sleep–wake patterns, can be helpful in the differential diagnosis of circadian rhythm disorders, and are an integral component of the behavioral treatment process. Additional paper-and-pencil assessments that are often helpful in diagnosing and monitoring treatment outcome are self-report measures of presleep arousal and negative beliefs about sleep (e.g., Pre-Sleep Arousal Scale, Nicassio, Mendlowitz, Fussell, & Petras, 1985; Beliefs and Attitudes About Sleep Scale, Morin, 1993).

In clinical practice, assessment of primary insomnia does not require an in-laboratory, polysomnographic (PSG) study to substantiate the diagnosis. This is true for three reasons. First, there is enough of a correspondence between the subjective complaint and objective measures that PSG assessment is not required to verify the sleep continuity disturbances. Second, traditional polysomnography does not reveal or allow for the quantification of the underlying sleep pathophysiologies that presumably give rise to the client's complaints. Third, and most pragmatically, third-party payers will not reimburse for sleep studies on patients with likely primary insomnia. However, sleep studies, are

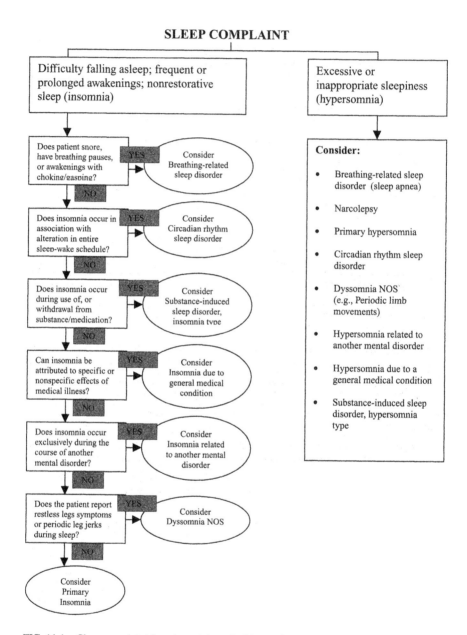

SLEEP COMPLAINT

Difficulty falling asleep; frequent or prolonged awakenings; nonrestorative sleep (insomnia)

Excessive or inappropriate sleepiness (hypersomnia)

Does patient snore, have breathing pauses, or awakenings with choking/gasping? — YES → Consider Breathing-related sleep disorder — NO

Does insomnia occur in association with alteration in entire sleep-wake schedule? — YES → Consider Circadian rhythm sleep disorder — NO

Does insomnia occur during use of, or withdrawal from substance/medication? — YES → Consider Substance-induced sleep disorder, insomnia type — NO

Can insomnia be attributed to specific or nonspecific effects of medical illness? — YES → Consider Insomnia due to general medical condition — NO

Does insomnia occur exclusively during the course of another mental disorder? — YES → Consider Insomnia related to another mental disorder — NO

Does the patient report restless legs symptoms or periodic leg jerks during sleep? — YES → Consider Dyssomnia NOS — NO

Consider Primary Insomnia

Consider:

- Breathing-related sleep disorder (sleep apnea)
- Narcolepsy
- Primary hypersomnia
- Circadian rhythm sleep disorder
- Dyssomnia NOS (e.g., Periodic limb movements)
- Hypersomnia related to another mental disorder
- Hypersomnia due to a general medical condition
- Substance-induced sleep disorder, hypersomnia type

FIG. 11.1. Sleep complaint flowchart. Adapted with permission from Buysse, D. J., and Perlis, M. L. (1996). The evaluation and treatment of insomnia. *Journal of Practical Psychiatry and Behavioral Health. March*, 80–93.

TABLE 11.2
DYSSOMNIAS

Intrinsic Sleep Disorders	Circadian Rhythm Sleep Disorders	Extrinsic Sleep Disorders
Psychophysiological insomnia	Time zone change (jet lag) syndrome	Inadequate sleep hygiene
Sleep state misperception		Environmental sleep disorder
Idiopathic insomnia	Shift work sleep disorder	Altitude insomnia
Narcolepsy	Irregular sleep–wake pattern	Adjustment sleep disorder
Recurrent hypersomnia	Delayed sleep phase syndrome	Insufficient sleep syndrome
Idiopathic hypersomnia	Advanced sleep phase syndrome	Limit setting sleep disorder
Posttraumatic hypersomnia	Non-24-hour sleep–wake disorder	Sleep-onset association disorder
Obstructive sleep apnea syndrome	Circadian rhythm sleep disorder NOS	Food allergy insomnia
Central sleep apnea syndrome		Nocturnal eating (drinking) syndrome
Central alveolar hypoventilation syndrome		Hypnotic-dependent sleep disorder
Periodic limb movement disorder		Stimulant-dependent sleep disorder
Restless legs syndrome		Alcohol-dependent sleep disorder
Intrinsic sleep disorder NOS		Toxin-induced sleep disorder
		Extrinsic sleep disorder NOS

Adapted from Perlis, M. L., and Youngstedt, S. (2000). The diagnosis of primary insomnia and treatment alternatives. *Journal of Comprehensive Therapy*, 26 (4), 298–306. Reprinted with permission. © American Society of Contemporary Medicine and Surgery.

indicated if the client fails to respond to treatment or demonstrates symptoms consistent with other intrinsic sleep disorders.

Use of additional objective devices in the diagnosis and treatment of insomnia can be particularly helpful in diagnostically ambiguous cases or when the clinician suspects a high degree of sleep state misperception. *Sleep state misperception* is a term (as well as disorder) used to describe a common finding among clients with insomnia—that there is often a discrepancy between a client's subjective impression of sleep parameters and what is measured via PSG recording. At the level of self-report, extreme values (gathered retrospectively or prospectively) may suggest that that this is a component of the disorder (i.e., sleep latencies of greater than 2 hours, wake after sleep onset of greater than 2 hours, or a total sleep time of equal to or less than 4 hours). In the absence of a PSG study, actigraphs can be used to obtain corroborating data. *Actigraphs* are wristwatch-like devices that use motion/movement detectors to estimate the traditional sleep continuity parameters (i.e., SL, WASO, FNA, and TST). The estimation is accomplished via well-validated algorithms that differentiate between sleep and wakefulness by the absence of movement per designated time interval.

CASE ILLUSTRATION

Identifying Information

(Identifying information has been altered to protect confidentiality). Mr. Simpson is a 59-year-old, married, European American male who works part-time as a financial consultant. He and his wife have a 29-year-old son and a 31-year-old daughter. He is 6′1″ and weighs 190 lbs (body mass index = 25).

Presenting Complaint

Mr. Simpson has had trouble falling asleep since college. It has become worse lately and he is afraid it will prevent him from returning to work full-time.

Sleep Continuity/Quality

In the previous 6 months, Mr. Simpson reported trouble falling asleep with a sleep latency of 90 to 120 minutes, 4 or more nights per week, including weekends. Although his sleep latency varies from night to night, he reports that he rarely falls asleep in less than 30 minutes. He indicated that he wakes up two to three times per night for about 30 to 60 minutes total, approximately 4 nights per week. He denied early-morning awakenings, and states that he often has trouble waking up on time and sleeps late into the morning. When attempting to fall asleep or return to sleep, Mr. Simpson reports that he ruminates and feels cognitively aroused ("can't turn my mind off") despite feeling tired and fatigued during the day. In addition, when he awakens in the middle of the night, he reports that he feels angry about his sleeplessness and is worried about his work performance the next day. When sleeping in novel environments (work-related travel or vacations), Mr. Simpson reports his insomnia is reliably less severe under these conditions.

Daytime Functioning/Symptoms

Mr. Simpson reportedly wakes up with a dry mouth and headaches 2 mornings per week. He stated that his daytime fatigue interferes with his ability to work and enjoy daily activities. He expressed a specific concern that his problems with insomnia might interfere with his plans to return to a full-time work schedule.

History of Presenting Complaint

Mr. Simpson first experienced insomnia when in college and has been in-termittently bothered by sleep initiation and maintenance problems since. He indicated that he tolerated his sleep difficulties, which flared periodically during times of stress, until 1996. At this time, his sleep initiation problem worsened in association with job-related turmoil (he was a corporate vice president in an organization that was in the midst of massive "downsizing"). In response to the demands of his job, he began working late into the night and attempted to cope with daytime fatigue by sleeping late on weekends (1:00 PM) and by drinking large quantities of caffeine (16 to 18 cups a day) during the week. In 1997, his contract was not renewed, reportedly because of the corporate restructuring. At this time, he gained 30 lbs (from 190 to 210 lbs) and his insomnia worsened to the point where it was a significant problem every night. He first sought evaluation and treatment for sleep disturbance at this time.

Prior Treatment for Sleep Disorders

In 1997, Mr. Simpson was evaluated by Dr. Pickwick at the Dickens' Sleep Disorders Center in Atlanta, Georgia. He sought help at this time at the urging of his wife, who complained that he was snoring excessively at night. In addition to trouble initiating and maintaining sleep, he reportedly experienced severe daytime sleepiness in addition to fatigue. He underwent a PSG study and the results indicated mild obstructive sleep apnea (respiratory disturbance index [RDI], 15 per hour). No evidence of other intrinsic sleep disorders was obtained. Treatment recommendations were to lose weight and use nightly CPAP (a form of ventilation that increases the patency of the oropharyngeal airway during sleep). Mr. Simpson lost 25 lbs, with noticeable improvement in snoring and daytime sleepiness, but he still reported trouble falling and staying asleep. He did not tolerate the CPAP device, which he stated exacerbated his insomnia.

After discontinuing CPAP, he sought treatment from his primary care physician (PCP) who worked with him to cut back on caffeine and attend to sleep hygiene principles. He no longer drinks coffee after noon and exercises regularly three times a week for 30 minutes. His PCP prescribed amitriptyline (20 mg, qhs). Mr. Simpson reported that this medication provided some benefit. He was able to fall asleep more quickly. He was less troubled by middle-of-the-night awakenings and according to his wife, the medication made his snoring less severe. Unfortunately, these gains were accompanied by anticholinergic effects, which were not tolerable for the patient. He discontinued the amitriptyline after 3 months. Mr. Simpson has since tried and benefited from temazepam and zolpidem. Neither he nor his PCP, however, wish to use these medications on a long-term basis. In January 2000, Mr. Simpson was re-referred to Dr. Pickwick for his problems with persistent insomnia. After a physical exam and a repeat PSG study that revealed that the RDI was within normal limits (5/hr), Dr. Pickwick referred the patient to the Behavioral Sleep Medicine Service for evaluation and treatment.

Medical History

The patient denied any perinatal complications, reportedly achieved all developmental milestones within the normal time frames and described himself as having a relatively healthy childhood with the exception of frequent throat infections that abated following a tonsillectomy (1950). The patient's adult medical history is significant for a closed head injury with loss of consciousness (1960); chronic lower back and lower extremity musculoskeletal pain (since high school; Mr. Simpson believes these problems are secondary to sports injuries sustained playing intramural basketball in high school and college); frequent heartburn [gastroesophageal reflux disease (GERD)], particularly after rich meals, without reported nocturnal sequelae (since 1975); moderate–chronic colitis (without findings on colonoscopy [since 1980]); and gall bladder disease (1989). His mild chronic pain condition is managed well with ibuprofen (prn). The GERD is treated with weekly doses of ranitidine. The colitis is a problem only during periods of stress and is not being treated currently. The gall bladder disease was treated successfully with a cholecystectomy (1990). The patient reported that he quit using tobacco 10 years ago. He had smoked a pack of cigarettes a day since the age of 21.

Psychiatric History

Mr. Simpson denied previous psychiatric or psychological treatment, including hospitalizations. He also denied a history of suicidal ideation, or attempts. Mr. Simpson denied any history of recreational drug use and reportedly drinks alcohol socially in moderation (1–3 beers, 3 times per month.). Based on his self-report, it is likely that he experienced a significant adjustment disorder with depressed mood after the loss of his corporate position in 1997 and with the diagnosis of his wife's cancer in 1998.

Current Medications

Mr. Simpson is currently taking ranitidine (Zantac, 75 mg, prn) 4 times/week for heartburn and ibuprofen (800 mg, prn) 2 days/week for back pain.

Family and Social History

The patient lives with his wife of 34 years. They have two children who are ages 29 (male) and 31 (female) and are healthy and independent young adults. Mr. Simpson is an only child. Both of his parents have been deceased for 10 years, having died from cardiovascular disease. The patient's father was a prominent attorney, described as a "workaholic" who frequently complained of insomnia but never sought treatment. His mother worked as a part-time nurse. Mr. Simpson denied any family psychiatric history, and stated that he enjoyed a relatively happy childhood with no reported history of physical or sexual abuse. He characterized himself as having been a hard-driving student as a teenager who was active in sports. He graduated at the top of is high school class before earning his BA and MBA degree from Oxford University. His wife was diagnosed with uterine cancer in 1998, which has remitted, status post hysterectomy.

Sexual History

Mr. Simpson's sexual history was non-contributory.

Mental Status Exam

The patient was a well-groomed, athletic, distinguished looking gentleman. He presented carrying a leather briefcase, wearing khaki pants and a button-down shirt and holding a cup of coffee. His speech was normal in volume, rate, and tone. He was pleasant and cooperative. His affect was euthymic, appropriate to content and full in range. He described his mood as "Okay, but somewhat irritable." He appeared to be mildly self-critical. He denied current and past suicidal/homicidal ideation, intent, or plan. His thought contents were focused on presenting his symptoms with no evidence of bizarre or delusional beliefs. He was oriented to person, place, and time. His thought processes were logical and goal-directed, with no distractibility noted, and there was no evidence of thought disorder. His insight, judgment, and impulse control appeared to be good. His intellect appeared to be well above average, although his IQ was not assessed formally.

CASE CONCEPTUALIZATION

Modeling and Learning

Mr. Simpson described several factors consistent with the potential role of modeling and classical conditioning in the maintenance of his insomnia. With respect to modeling, it appears that Mr. Simpson adopted an approach to work and life consistent with the model of role functioning provided by his father. He learned at an early age to place an extreme degree of importance on work and performance at the expense of maintaining a well-balanced lifestyle. His father (presumably his primary male role model) reportedly sacrificed a consistent daily routine and regular sleep/wake schedule to pursue career success.

As indicated previously, his father also suffered from insomnia. Although a chronic problem, Mr. Simpson's father did not seek medical attention, and this may have conveyed the message that sleeplessness was not to be considered a significant problem. Consistent with this conceptualization is that Mr. Simpson sought treatment only at the insistence of his wife, some 25 years after his problems first manifested.

With respect to the potential role of classical conditioning, his presentation is consistent with a number of factors that point to the possibility that conditioned hyperarousal may play a central role in maintaining his chronic insomnia complaint. Mr. Simpson noted that despite feeling fatigued during the day, he feels alert and ruminative when it is time for bed, suggesting that the bed and bedroom operate as conditioned stimuli eliciting cognitive arousal that interferes with sleep initiation and maintenance. Further evidence of a discriminative, learned association of arousal with his bed and bedroom is suggested by Mr. Simpson's observation that when he sleeps in a new environment, such as in a different room, he has less trouble sleeping. Additional information gleaned from a careful behavioral analysis would be useful to determine the extent to which Mr. Simpson spends time awake in bed or engages in cognitively arousing tasks in his bed or bedroom. Such activities would create the opportunity for a pairing of the bed and bedroom with wakefulness rather than sleep and relaxation. Mr. Simpson also described a common complaint among patients with primary insomnia, namely, presleep thought content focused on his inability to fall asleep and stay asleep and on the potential consequences of poor sleep on his career. Such negative cognitions can lead to performance anxiety and may become readily conditioned to the presleep state.

Life Events

The impact of life stressors appear to have played an important role in initiating Mr. Simpson's chronic sleep problems. His original acute episodes of insomnia were likely precipitated by stress associated with scholastic life and/or final exams in college. The insomnia, which is now chronic, is likely to have been precipitated (in part or whole) by the events that occurred in 1996 through 1998. As previously indicated, during this time Mr. Simpson experienced a significant increase in stress at work; development of poor sleep hygiene habits in association with work-related stress (i.e., working late into the night, increasing caffeine consumption, decreasing physical exercise, and extending his sleep period on weekends); significant weight gain; and ultimately the loss of his high-paying, high-status corporate vice presidency. The stress of his wife's cancer diagnosis may have also been a significant maintaining factor for the insomnia to the extent that it did not allow Mr. Simpson time to recover from the stressors of the previous 2 years.

Genetics and Temperament

Mr. Simpson described some traits that appear to make him particularly susceptible to physiologic hyperreactivity and/or hyperarousal. He described himself as having a hard-driving, perfectionistic, achievement-oriented personality style. He stated that he often overreacts to minor stressors and he generally has trouble physically "winding down" after becoming aggravated. He also described himself as "hyper" and joked that he must have the "metabolic rate of a chipmunk." Finally, he characterized himself as a "worrier." Each of these characterizations represent or correspond to forms of arousal that are likely to contribute to insomnia (as well as other stress-related conditions like gastritis, colitis, and chronic musculoskeletal pain).

Psychological Factors

Mr. Simpson indicated that his chronic insomnia significantly diminishes his quality of life and ability to cope. The psychological consequences of his insomnia include mood disturbance, attention, concentration and memory difficulties, and a negative impact on his self-concept. Although the underlying mechanisms by which chronic insomnia may influence psychological functioning is unknown, such disturbances are commonly reported by patients with insomnia, and may be seen not only as a consequence of the disorder, but also as a contributing factor to a vicious cycle that further perpetuates sleep continuity and quality disturbances.

Drugs

The patient reports taking ibuprofen and Zantac on an as-needed basis with presumably little impact on his sleep or psychological functioning. He has tried a number of hypnotics and over-the-counter medications, some with unwanted side effects (e.g., amitriptyline: daytime sedation, dry mouth). The patient made a conscious effort to discontinue medication in part due to discomfort with the notion of needing medication to sleep, fears related to dependency, and tolerance effects.

Socioeconomic and Cultural Factors

From a broad perspective, Mr. Simpson's complaint can be contextualized as growing out of a societal devaluation of the importance of sleep and the hypervaluation of productivity. It can be argued that these prevailing sentiments loom larger in the corporate climate where Mr. Simpson functioned as a top executive. In this environment, working late into the night is the norm; fatigue and the effects of sleep deprivation are routinely minimized and many of the compensatory behaviors used to ameliorate such effects (e.g., chronic use of stimulants, irregular sleep–wake schedules, the use of alcohol as a hypnotic), although romanticized, contribute directly to the development of chronic insomnia. In short, it is likely that the cultural backdrop, including Mr. Simpson's own family of origin's "subculture," have contributed substantially to the clinical course of his sleep disorder.

Overall Conceptualization

Mr. Simpson's chronic insomnia may be understood broadly from within the behavioral model proposed by Spielman, Caruso, and Glovinsky, (1987). As illustrated in Fig. 11.2, the model posits that insomnia occurs acutely in relation to both predisposing (trait) and precipitating (state) factors and occurs chronically in relation to perpetuating or maintaining factors. Thus, an individual may be prone to insomnia due to trait characteristics (e.g., automatic hyperreactivity), experience acute episodes because of precipitating factors (e.g., life events), and have chronic insomnia owing to a variety of perpetuating factors (e.g., irregular sleep–wake schedules).

Mr. Simpson exhibits a variety of characteristics that may be identified as predisposing factors, including hyperreactivity, somatic hyperarousal, and a

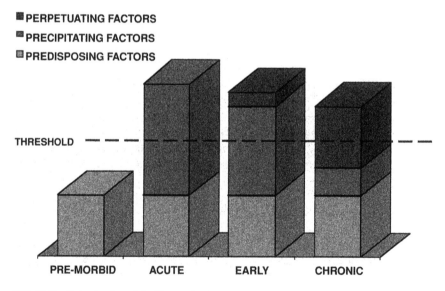

FIG. 11.2. Behavioral model of insomnia. Adapted with permission from Spielman, A. J., and Glovinsky, P. (1991). The varied nature of insomnia. In: P. J. Hauri (Ed.), *Case studies in insomnia* (pp. 1–15). New York: Plenum Press.

tendency toward worry and rumination. Each of these factors is likely to make Mr. Simpson vulnerable to insomnia, particularly during times of stress. He reported a variety of incidences that may have served as precipitating factors, including, although not limited to, the events that lead up to the loss of his job and his wife's illness. Finally, he engaged in a variety of behaviors that may be characterized as *perpetuating factors*, which are implemented to compensate for insomnia and daytime fatigue. Rather than correct the problem, however, these strategies serve to maintain the insomnia (in the absence of the original precipitating factors) and/or contribute to the development of conditioned hyperarousal that is characteristic of chronic insomnia. Mr. Simpson engaged in a number of maladaptive strategies, such as sleeping in on weekends, drinking excessive amounts of caffeine, and spending excessive time awake in bed in an effort to obtain more sleep. Each of these strategies disrupts the regularity of his circadian sleep–wake cycle and increases the opportunity for the bed and bedroom to become classically conditioned stimuli associated with wakefulness and arousal as opposed to sleep. Evidence for the presence of conditioned arousal in Mr. Simpson's case is suggested by his report of improved sleep when in a different environment (change in conditioned stimuli) as well as his reportedly experiencing an abrupt increase in cognitive arousal (mind racing, etc.) when he lies down to sleep.

Diagnostic Assessment

As indicated previously, the diagnosis of primary insomnia requires a thorough clinical history and assessment to rule out medical and psychiatric factors that commonly have insomnia as a secondary symptom. Ideally, clients with chronic insomnia are referred for treatment by a health care professional who has either ruled out or stabilized an underlying medical/psychiatric condition, such as endocrine abnormalities (e.g., hyperthyroidism) or an occult intrinsic sleep disorder, which may be responsible for the client's complaint of insomnia. Although most patients referred by primary care physicians have been evaluated medically, many clients with insomnia have not had either a psychiatric evaluation or been evaluated for the presence of an occult intrinsic sleep disorder, such as sleep apnea or nocturnal myoclonus (i.e., PLMs).

Medical Factors. Common medical illnesses that should be considered in ruling out the diagnosis of primary insomnia include insomnias secondary to chronic pain, cardiopulmonary diseases (e.g., chronic obstructive pulmonary disease), gastrointestinal disorders (e.g., GERD), renal disease, and neurologic conditions (e.g., dementia). In the instances in which such medical illnesses are not stable and/or well managed with treatment, the insomnia should be treated as a symptom of the parent disorder (see Table 11.1).

In Mr. Simpson's case, he describes himself as in relatively good physical health. Once it is verified that that Mr. Simpson is free from systemic illness, attention should be paid to the possibility that the client's problems with heartburn are contributing to the sleep maintenance component of his insomnia complaint. It is often the case that reflux disorders may disturb sleep and be associated with prolonged awakenings, even in the absence of heartburn-like sensations. A therapeutic trial with antacid medications (e.g., antacids, H_2 blockers, proton-pump inhibitors, prokinetic drugs) may be warranted if his middle insomnia fails to respond to treatment.

Psychiatric Disturbance.   Insomnia is a significant feature of the majority of psychiatric illnesses, particularly affective and anxiety disorders. Conversely, many patients with primary insomnia exhibit at least subsyndromal levels of psychiatric symptomatology (Ford and Kamerow, 1989). There is also a fair amount of evidence that the two classes of disorders may interact. For example, primary insomnia may be a risk factor for new onset and/or recurrent major depression, and may be a prodromal symptom of both (Perlis, Giles, Buysse, Tu, & Kupfer, 1997). In clinical practice, it is often difficult to distinguish the primacy or directionality of the relationship. That is, whether insomnia represents a subsyndromal form or a residual symptom of a psychiatric disorder, or if the insomnia is primary and the psychiatric symptomatology (e.g., mood disturbance, attention and concentration difficulties) is secondary to sleep loss. Although such distinctions may seem academic, identifying which disorder is primary has important treatment implications. As with medical illness, when the psychiatric illness is deemed primary, pharmacologic and/or nonpharmacologic strategies that target the psychiatric illness specifically should be the first line treatment. Alternately, if the insomnia is identified as primary, pharmacologic and/or nonpharmacologic strategies that target the insomnia specifically should be the first line treatment. In either case, both forms of symptoms should be monitored so as to allow a change in treatment strategy, as the clinical situation warrants.

In reviewing Mr. Simpson's self-report psychiatric history, it appears that he may have experienced an untreated adjustment disorder or major depressive episode after the loss of his job and when his wife was diagnosed with cancer. As part of his intake diagnostic evaluation, he was administered the BDI (Beck, Ward, Mendelson, Mock, & Erbaugh, 1961) and the BAI (Beck, & Steer, 1990) to evaluate systematically his current levels of depression and anxiety. He scored an 11 on the BDI and a 10 on the BAI. Although these scores do not suggest that the client is likely to meet the criteria for an affective or anxiety disorder, they nonetheless reflect clinically significant levels of depressive and anxiety symptomatology. Furthermore, it should be noted that these values are characteristic of patients with primary insomnia. Given these data, Mr. Simpson's insomnia would be treated as primary, but the hypothesis that there is a masked depression or a dysthymic disorder should be retained as a diagnosis to be ruled out should he fail to respond to treatment.

Other Intrinsic Sleep Disorders. The primary diagnoses to be ruled out within this domain are sleep apnea, narcolepsy, and periodic limb movement/restless legs syndrome. Each of these disorders may have insomnia as a chief complaint. When attempting to screen for these disorders during an intake interview, a useful consideration is whether the client reports excessive daytime sleepiness (EDS), which refers to the tendency to fall asleep at inappropriate times and places. As indicated previously, such a tendency should be discriminated clearly from the complaints of fatigue or anergia. Clients with primary insomnia often report fatigue and anergia, but less often complain or demonstrate excessive daytime sleepiness. In the absence of a formal assessment using PSG procedures like the Multiple Sleep Latency Test (MSLT; Association of Professional Sleep Societies, 1986), brief self-report measures, such as the ESS (Johns, 1991) can serve as rough guideline to determine whether one is dealing with disorders of excessive daytime somnolence (DOES) or disorders of initiation and maintenance (DIMS).

With respect to Mr. Simpson's case, he denied falling asleep inappropriately during the day, such as while driving, eating, or talking with others. His score on the ESS was 3, well below the usual cutoff of 10, which indicates clinically significant daytime sleepiness. With respect to symptoms of intrinsic sleep disorders other than insomnia, he endorsed some mild agitation in his limbs while trying to sleep, but this symptom impressed as more indicative of psychomotor agitation and/or somatic arousal rather than restless legs syndrome. He did not complain of paresthesias in his legs, and denied muscle cramping or twitching that interfered with his sleep. He denied cataplexy, sleep paralysis, or hypnogogic/hypnopompic hallucinations, which would be suggestive of narcolepsy. He denied snoring loudly or waking up gasping for breath, and stated that his wife does not notice apneaic episodes. His current presentation, therefore, is not consistent with PLMs, narcolepsy, or sleep apnea. In addition, we have the data from Mr. Simpson's two sleep disorder center evaluations. This information is consistent with our clinical assessment. On PSG, there was no evidence of PLMs (repetitive myoclonic twitches that occur in association with frequent arousals) or narcolepsy (sleep onset REM sleep), and his sleep apnea appears to have been managed effectively with weight loss.

Not yet addressed is the possibility that DIMS complaints may arise from one of several circadian rhythm disorders. Although there are several syndromes that fall within this domain, the most commonly associated with the complaint of insomnia are referred to as *delayed sleep phase syndrome* and *advanced sleep phase syndrome*. These syndromes typically manifest as pure initial (sleep onset) or pure terminal (early morning awakening) insomnia, and are thought to represent a dysynchronization between the client's work/social schedules and his or her preferred sleep phase. One way to identify such phase disturbances is to determine if, when allowed to sleep ad libitum, the client continues to complain of insomnia. In practice, this is apparent by simply noting that the client sleeps during a significantly different time frame on weekends and days off ($+/- > 3$ h). Both phase disorders are thought to arise from dysregulation of the photosensitive circadian pacemaker located in the suprachiasmatic nuclei of the hypothalamus.

With respect to the possibility of a circadian component to Mr. Simpson's complaint, he endorses a relatively long sleep onset latency of 90 to 120 minutes and often sleeps late into the next day. This suggests the possibility that at least part of his sleep complaint may be related to a phase delay in his circadian rhythm. Interestingly, he first developed insomnia as a teenager/young adult, which is a developmental period when there is a normal phase delay in the circadian rhythm relative to other age groups. Mr. Simpson's insomnia, however, does not remit when he changes his sleep phase. For example, he continues to complain of sleep onset and maintenance trouble even on weekends when he stays up and sleeps late. This argues against the likelihood that the insomnia is due primarily to a delayed sleep phase. A more careful analysis of Mr. Simpson's sleep–wake diaries may help to further elucidate circadian and psychophysiologic dimensions of his insomnia complaint.

Behavioral Assessment

A behavioral analysis is crucial for both assessment and treatment, perhaps even more so than in other areas of behavioral medicine. As indicated previously, the primary method for acquiring data for the behavioral assessment is through prospective monitoring via daily sleep–wake diaries. Prospective assessment is important for (a) identifying the behaviors that maintain the insomnia, (b) determining to what extent circadian dysrhythmia is present, and (c) gathering the data needed to measure/guide treatment response. Self-report sleep–wake diaries require that the client code information pertaining to sleep quantity/quality and daytime function. The sleep measures, which are typically obtained over 1–2 weeks, include the following: time to bed, estimated sleep latency, number of nightly awakenings, time awake after sleep onset, total sleep time, and subjective sleep quality. The daytime measures typically include nap frequency and duration, fatigue ratings, stimulant consumption, and medication usage.

In Mr. Simpson's case, sleep diaries are important for several determinations. First, the diaries allow for a more reliable assessment of his night-to-night sleep quality and quantity and a more accurate assessment of the behaviors that may maintain and/or ameliorate his insomnia, including amount and timing of meals, substance use (i.e., caffeine and alcohol), the prophylactic value of ranitidine when used in the evening, and so on. Second, the diaries may be used to confirm that Mr. Simpson's sleep problems persist despite the phase of the 24-hour day in which he sleeps. Finally, the sleep diaries allow for the effects of the treatment prescriptions to be assessed and altered as needed.

Prioritization of Targets for Treatment

Analysis of the information from the intake interview and the daily sleep diaries suggests three interrelated and equally important targets for Mr. Simpson's treatment: (a) improve sleep efficiency/continuity, (b) decondition arousal associated with sleep-related stimuli and reassociate the bed/bedroom with sleep, and (c) establish a consistent sleep–wake schedule during the preferred sleep phase.

Improving sleep efficiency is essentially the goal of any approach to the treatment of insomnia. This is true because it is usually the case that patients with insomnia spend considerably more time in bed awake and therefore have low sleep efficiency. As a result, treatment involves both a reduction in sleep initiation or reinitiation times and the consolidation of sleep throughout the preferred sleep phase.

A second aim of treatment is to break the learned association of the bed and bedroom stimuli with sleep-interfering states of arousal and rumination. This aim is based on the behavioral/conditioning perspective of chronic insomnia, which holds that cognitive, somatic, and/or CNS arousal may be classically conditioned to the sleep environment. Conditioned arousal is extinguished by reassociating the bed and bedroom with sleep. This is done by ensuring that the client is sleepy or asleep when in the bedroom.

A third focus of treatment is to help Mr. Simpson establish a consistent sleep–wake schedule. This intervention targets Mr. Simpson's tendency to sleep late on mornings after a poor night's sleep.

Selection of Treatment Strategies

There are several empirically validated pharmacologic and nonpharmacologic treatments for insomnia. The most commonly used therapies for insomnia are benzodiazepine and the newer benzodiazepine-receptor agonists like zolpidem and zaleplon. For a discussion of pharmacologic treatment approaches, the reader is referred to Buysse and Perlis (1996). As for the clinical efficacy of the medical approach, it is clear that sedative hypnotics produce rapid results and about a 50% reduction in illness severity in the short-term (2–4 weeks) (Nowell et al., 1997). Hypnotics, however, are generally not recommend for long-term use due to concerns regarding tolerance, possible daytime side effects, and rebound insomnia when discontinued. Although some of these concerns are mitigated by the newer benzodiazepine-receptor agonists, no studies yet exist that demonstrate the long-term efficacy of these agents beyond 6 months or that treatment gains are maintained on withdrawal from the drug. Of the studies that are as long as 6 months, although the data are suggestive, none of the studies is placebo controlled and several do not use intent to treat–type statistical approaches.

The most common behavioral therapies for primary insomnia are: sleep hygiene education, stimulus control, relaxation training, and cognitive therapy. For a detailed explanation of each of these therapies, the reader is referred to *Insomnia: Psychological Assessment and Management* (Morin, 1993). As for the clinical efficacy of the behavioral approach, there is clear evidence that the treatment modality is effective (Murtagh & Greenwood, 1995), and that the clinical gains are comparable to those produced by hypnotics. Unlike hypnotics, behavioral interventions tend to produce long-term benefits after treatment is discontinued (McClusky, Milby, Switzer, Williams, & Wooten, 1991).

Because Mr. Simpson's insomnia is chronic in nature and medications are generally not recommended for long-term use, behavior therapy is the most appropriate treatment for his insomnia. Of all the available treatments, stimulus control therapy is the most well validated and is considered the gold standard for the behavioral treatment of insomnia. In practice, most clinicians adopt a multicomponent approach, which usually contains stimulus control and sleep restriction, and often has other components including relaxation training, sleep hygiene, and some form of cognitive therapy.

Priority of Treatment Strategies

Stimulus Control Therapy. Stimulus control therapy is considered to be the first-line behavioral treatment for chronic primary insomnia and therefore should be prioritized accordingly (Chesson, et al., 1999). Stimulus control instructions limit the amount of time clients spend awake in bed or the bedroom and are designed to decondition presleep arousal. Typical instructions include: (a) keep a fixed wake time 7 days per week, irrespective of how much sleep you obtained during the night; (b) avoid any behavior in the bed or bedroom other than sleep or sexual activity; (c) sleep only in the bedroom; (d) leave the bedroom when awake for approximately 15 to 20 minutes; and (e) return only when sleepy. The combination of these instruction reestablishes the bed and bedroom as strong cues for sleep, and entrains the circadian sleep–wake cycle to the desired phase.

Sleep Restriction. Sleep restriction therapy (SRT) requires clients to limit the amount of time they spend in bed to an amount equal to their average total sleep time. In order to accomplish this, the clinician works with the patient to (a) establish a fixed wake time and (b) decrease sleep opportunity by moving the client's bedtime to later into the night. Initially, the therapy results in a reduction in total sleep time, but over the course of several days, results in decreased sleep latency, and decreased wake time after sleep onset. As sleep efficiency increases, clients are instructed to gradually increase the amount of time they spend in bed. In our practice, patients "roll back" their bedtime in 15-minute increments, given sleep diary data that show that on the prior week the patient's sleep was efficient [85% or more of the time spent in bed was spent asleep (TST/TIB)]. This therapy is thought to be effective for two reasons: First, it prevents the patient from coping with their insomnia by extending sleep opportunity. This strategy, although increasing the opportunity to get more sleep, produces a form of sleep that is shallow and fragmented. Second, the initial sleep loss that occurs with SRT is thought to increase the "pressure for sleep," which in turn produces quicker sleep latencies, less wake after sleep onset, and more efficient sleep. It should be noted that the treatment has a paradoxical aspect to it. After all, clients who report being unable to sleep are in essence being told to sleep less. Such a prescription must be delivered with care, and compliance must be monitored. Sleep restriction is contraindicated in patients with histories of mania or seizure disorder because it may aggravate these conditions.

Sleep Hygiene. Sleep hygiene education addresses a variety of behaviors, such as use of stimulants, alcohol, exercise, etc., which may influence sleep quality and quantity. This therapy is most helpful when tailored to the behavioral analysis of the client's sleep–wake behaviors.

Relaxation Training. Different relaxation techniques target different physiological systems. Progressive muscle relaxation is used to diminish skeletal muscle tension. Diaphragmatic breathing is used to make breathing slower and shallower, and, interestingly, resembles the form of breathing that occurs naturally at sleep onset. Autogenics training focuses on increasing peripheral blood flow. Most practitioners select the optimal relaxation method based on what technique is easiest for the patient to learn, is most consistent with how the patient manifests arousal, and is not contraindicated by medical conditions (e.g., progressive muscle relaxation would not be an ideal choice for patients with neuromuscular disorders).

Phototherapy. There is substantial empirical evidence that bright light has antidepressant and sleep-promoting effects. The sleep-promoting effects of bright light may occur via several mechanisms, including shifting the circadian system; enhancement of the amplitude of the circadian pacemaker, promoting wakefulness during the day and sleep at night; or indirectly via its antidepressant effects. In practice, bright light (10,000 Lux) is used to shorten or lengthen the diurnal phase of the client's day. In cases where the client's insomnia has a phase-delay component (i.e., the patient prefers to go to bed late and wake up late), bright light exposure in the morning for a period of 30–60 minutes may enable them to feel sleepy at an earlier time in the evening. In cases in which the client's insomnia has a phase-advance component (i.e., the patient prefers to go to bed early and wake up early), bright light exposure in the afternoon for a period of 30–60 minutes may enable them to stay awake later. It is generally assumed that phototherapy has no significant side effects, but this is not always the case. Mania may be triggered by bright light, but rarely, if ever, in clients not previously diagnosed with bipolar mood disorder. Other side effects are hypomania, agitation, visual blurring, eye strain, and headaches. Light therapy should not be used in patients with certain eye diseases (e.g., diabetic retinopathy.)

Cognitive Therapy. Several forms of cognitive therapy for insomnia have been developed. Some have a didactic focus (Morin, 1993), some use paradoxical intention (Shoham-Salomon & Rosenthal, 1987), and some use a form of cognitive restructuring (Buysse & Perlis, 1996). Although the approaches differ in procedure, all are based on the observation that clients with insomnia have negative thoughts and beliefs about their condition and its consequences. Helping clients challenge the veracity of these beliefs is thought to decrease the anxiety and arousal associated with insomnia.

Therapeutic Regimen. The behavioral treatment of insomnia generally requires 4–8 weeks time with once-a-week face-to-face meetings with the clinical provider. Sessions range from 30 to 90 minutes, depending on the stage of treatment and degree of patient compliance. Intake sessions are usually 60 to 90 minutes in duration, during which the clinical history is obtained and the patient is instructed in the use of sleep diaries. No intervention is provided during the first week. This time frame is used to collect the baseline sleep–wake data that guide treatment for the balance of the therapy. The primary interventions (stimulus control, sleep restriction, and sleep hygiene) are deployed over the course of the next one or two to 60-minute sessions. Once these treatments are delivered, the client enters into a phase of treatment in which sleep opportunity is upwardly titrated over the course of the next two to five visits. These follow-up sessions require about 30 minutes unless additional interventions are being integrated into the treatment program. Adjunctive treatments may include relaxation training, bright light therapy, and or relapse prevention.

In Mr. Simpson's case, the standard clinical regimen is likely to be maximally effective. Relaxation training such as progressive muscle relation might be added to further help him manage presleep cognitive and somatic arousal. This procedure would best be practiced prior to bedtime or during an extended awaking in the middle of the night. Cognitive therapy may also be useful in Mr. Simpson's case to address his unrealistic concern about the negative consequences of a poor night's sleep and performance anxiety related to sleeping. Finally, phototherapy might be considered should his sleep-onset difficulties persist and/or if he has difficulty waking up at the prescribed time.

Dealing with Complicating Factors

Mr. Simpson's case points to a number of complicating factors that must be monitored and evaluated throughout the course of treatment, particularly if he fails to show expected clinical gains after 2–4 weeks of active treatment. The most common complicating factors are poor treatment compliance and issues related to comorbid psychiatric and medical disorders.

Treatment Compliance. The single most important complicating factor is poor treatment compliance. At the beginning of treatment, the therapist should address proactively the facts that prescriptions may seem counterintuitive and adhering to the treatment will be difficult. Providing the client with a complete and thoughtful rational for each aspect of the treatment, managing the client's expectations, and encouraging an active self-management approach are essential. Providing the rationale for treatment is likely to gain compliance in at least two ways. First, providing a rationale is less imperative and thereby makes the client an active partner in the treatment process and less resistant or reactive to the prescriptions. Second, a fluid, interesting, and compelling rationale supports and enhances the client's perception of the therapist as a competent authority. With respect to expectation, clients should not expect immediate treatment effects. In fact, clients should be cautioned that their sleep problem is likely to briefly get worse before it gets better. Sometimes an appeal to the research literature demonstrating that treatment gains are maintained and often continue to improve in the long term may help maintain their motivation despite the short-term difficulty adjusting to the procedures. With respect to active self-management, it is important to remember that the treatment alternative is medication, which requires very little in the way of lifestyle change. Thus, the therapist must spend a considerable amount of time persuading the client to "make and stay with the investment."

Comorbity of Mental and Medical Disorders. The therapist should monitor the client continually for both psychiatric and medical factors that often complicate treatment of insomnia. In the case of Mr. Simpson, he demonstrated mild, but significant symptoms of depression and anxiety. He also reported a degree of chronic and intermittent pain related to sport injuries. As indicated previously, there may also be a slight phase delay in his circadian rhythm, which would complicate treatment, and there is always the possibility of a redevelopment of sleep apnea. Throughout the course of treatment, any of these factors could become aggravated and require independent evaluation/interventions.

Role of Pharmacotherapy in the Case

In general, pharmacologic treatment for insomnia is generally not recommended as the treatment of choice for chronic primary insomnia. Chronic use of hypnotic medications, particularly benzodiazepines, is often associated with diminished effectiveness, hypnotic dependency, and rebound insomnia on discontinuation of the medication. Mr. Simpson also does not wish to use hypnotics on a regular basis.

Not yet addressed is the possibility of using sedative hypnotics acutely with behavioral treatment for insomnia (i.e., dual or combined therapy). This is an underinvestigated area of inquiry, but the initial results are mixed. The benefit of combined therapy is a more rapid reduction of symptoms. The risk of combining pharmacotherapy and behavioral treatment is that once a client begins using medications, he or she is less inclined to adopt or tolerate the behavioral interventions. Finally, for many clients who present to treatment for primary insomnia, the first task is often to work with their prescribing physician to wean them off medication before starting behavioral treatment. Delaying the weaning to a time after standard behavioral treatment has begun is likely to result in a relapse, thereby undermining the client's confidence in the behavioral regimen.

Managed Care Considerations

The behavioral treatment for insomnia, in many respects, could be considered an ideal treatment in a managed care environment that emphasizes short-term treatments with demonstrated efficacy, clear measurable treatment goals, and the potential of reducing overall costs on the medical system. Although effective behavioral treatment of insomnia is usually short term (Morin, Culbert, & Schwartz, 1994), it is nevertheless expensive (approximately $500 for a course of treatment). Research is only beginning to address the possible savings in decreasing psychiatric morbidity and health care utilization when clients with chronic insomnia are treated effectively. Despite being an ideal treatment for insomnia, many managed care organizations fail to reimburse for the behavioral treatment of insomnia. In instances in which reimbursement is possible, the benefit is usually covered under mental health, which often carries a higher copayment and a stigma that can be a barrier to treatment for many. Continued research and organized advocacy is necessary to reduce the barriers to care for clients with primary insomnia.

SUMMARY

Contrary to what many believe, insomnia is a significant and underrecognized public health problem. Between 5% and 35% of the population of the United States complain of sleep disturbance, and approximately 26 million persons, or 10% of the population, suffer from insomnia. The complaint of insomnia has been found to be associated with increased vulnerability for medical and psychiatric disorders, diminished work performance, increased absenteeism, increased risk for automobile accidents, and increased rates of health care utilization. Because insomnia may be both a symptom and a primary disorder, careful differential diagnosis and behavioral assessment is required. As a disorder, primary insomnia may be treated pharmacologically or with targeted cognitive–behavioral interventions.

REFERENCES

American Sleep Disorders Association (1990). *The international classification of sleep disorders: Diagnostic and coding manual.* Rochester, MN: Author.

Ancoli-Israel, S., & Roth, T. (1999). Characteristics of insomnia in the United States: Results of the 1991 National Sleep Foundation Survey. *Sleep, 22,* (Suppl 2), S347–S353.

Association of Professional Sleep Societies (1986). Guidelines for the Multiple Sleep Latency Test (MSLT): A standard measure of sleepiness. *Sleep, 9,* 519–524.

Beck, A. T., & Steer, R. A. (1990). *Manual for the Beck Anxiety Inventory.* San Antonio: Psychological Corporation.

Beck, A. T., Ward, C. H., Mendelson, M., Mock, J., & Erbaugh, J. (1961). An inventory for measuring depression. *Archives of General Psychiatry, 4,* 561–571.

Buysse, D. J., & Perlis, M. L. (1996). The evaluation and treatment of insomnia. *Journal of Practical Psychiatry and Behavioral Health, March,* 80–93.

Buysse, D. J., Reynolds, C. F., Monk, T. H., Berman, S. R., & Kupfer, D. J. (1989). The Pittsburgh Sleep Quality Index: A new instrument for psychiatric practice and research. *Psychiatry Research, 28,* 193–213.

Chesson, A. L. Jr., Anderson, W. M., Littner, M., Davila, D., Hartse, K., Johnson, S., Wise, M., & Rafecas, J. (1999). Practice parameters for the nonpharmacologic treatment of chronic insomnia. An American Academy of Sleep Medicine report. Standards of Practice Committee of the American Academy of Sleep Medicine. *Sleep, 22,* 1128–1133.

Ford, D. E., & Kamerow, D. B. (1989). Epidemiologic study of sleep disturbances and psychiatric disorders. An opportunity for prevention? *JAMA, 262,* 1479–1484.

Johns, M. W. (1991). A new method for measuring daytime sleepiness: The Epworth Sleepiness Scale. *Sleep, 14,* 540–545.

Kupperman, M., Lubeck, D. P., & Mazonson, P. D. (1995). Sleep problems and their correlates in a working population. *Journal of General Internal Medicine, 10,* 25–32.

McClusky, H. Y., Milby, J. B., Switzer, P. K., Williams, V., & Wooten, V. (1991). Efficacy of behavioral versus triazolam treatment in persistent sleep-onset insomnia [see comments]. *American Journal of Psychiatry, 148,* 121–126.

Morin, C. M. (1993). *Insomnia: Psychological Assessment and Management.* New York: Guilford Press.

Morin, C. M., Culbert, J. P., & Schwartz, S. M. (1994). Nonpharmacological interventions for insomnia: A meta-analysis of treatment efficacy. *American Journal of Psychiatry, 151,* 1172–1180.

Murtagh, D. R., & Greenwood, K. M. (1995). Identifying effective psychological treatments for insomnia: A meta-analysis. *Journal of Consulting & Clinical Psychology, 63,* 79–89.

Nicassio, P. M., Mendlowitz, D. R., Fussell, J. J., & Petras, L. (1985). The phenomenology of the pre-sleep state: The development of the pre-sleep arousal scale. *Behaviour Research & Therapy, 23,* 263–271.

Nowell, P. D., Mazumdar, S., Buysse, D. J., Dew, M. A., Reynolds, C. F. III, & Kupfer, D. J. (1997). Benzodiazepines and zolpidem for chronic insomnia: A meta-analysis of treatment efficacy. *JAMA, 278,* 2170–2177.

Perlis, M. L., & Youngstead, S. (2000). The diagnosis of primary insomnia and treatment alternatives. *Journal of Comprehensive Therapy, 26* (4), 298–306.

Perlis, M. L., Giles, D. E., Buysse, D. J., Tu, X., & Kupfer, D. J. (1997). Self-reported sleep disturbance as a prodromal symptom in recurrent depression. *Journal of Affective Disorders, 42,* 209–212.

Shoham-Salomon, V. & Rosenthal, R. (1987). Paradoxical interventions: A meta-analysis. *Journal of Consulting & Clinical Psychology, 55,* 22–28.

Spielman, A., Caruso, L., & Glovinsky, P. (1987). A behavioral perspective on insomnia treatment. *Psychiatric Clinics of North America, 10,* 541–553.

Spielman, A. J., & Glovinsky, P. (1991). The varied nature of insomnia. In: P. J. Hauri (Ed.), *Case studies in insomnia* (pp. 1–15). New York: Plenum Press.

World Health Organization (1992). *The ICD-10 Classification of Mental and Behavioural Disorders: Clinical descriptions and diagnostic guidelines.* Geneva: World Health Organization.

12

Bulimia Nervosa

David M. Garner
*River Centre Clinic, Bowling Green State University
and University of Toledo*

Cristina Magana
University of Toledo and the River Centre Clinic

DESCRIPTION OF THE DISORDER

Bulimia nervosa is characterized by morbid overconcern with weight and shape, leading to extreme and often dangerous weight-controlling behaviors. This eating disorder is generally conceptualized as a final common pathway, with the symptoms resulting from the interplay of biological, psychological, familial, and sociocultural etiologic factors. There are a variety of associated psychological symptoms, such as depression, anxiety, poor self-esteem, hostility, somatization, social maladjustment, confused sex-role identity, and borderline personality features, that may have etiologic significance in bulimia nervosa, but, in any case, contribute to the heterogeneity in the disorder on presentation. Finally, bulimia nervosa results in potentially serious physical and psychological sequelae that may not only perpetuate the eating disorder, but may also cloud the assessment picture.

The criteria for diagnosis of bulimia nervosa according to the *Diagnostic and Statistical Manual of Mental Disorders* (*DSM–IV*, American Psychiatric Association, 1994) are summarized as follows:

1. Recurrent episodes of binge eating (a sense of lack of control over eating a large amount of food in a discrete period of time, which would be considered unusual under similar circumstances).

2. Recurrent inappropriate compensatory behavior(s) in order to prevent weight gain (e.g., vomiting; abuse of laxatives, diuretics, or other medications; fasting or excessive exercise).

3. A minimum average of two episodes of binge eating and inappropriate compensatory behaviors per week for the previous 3 months.

4. Self-evaluation unduly influenced by body shape and weight.

5. The disturbance does not occur exclusively during episodes of anorexia nervosa.

Clients with bulimia nervosa are further divided into purging and nonpurging subtypes based on the regular use of self-induced vomiting, laxatives, or diuretics (*DSM–IV*, APA, 1994).

Although binge eating is considered the key symptom identifying bulimia nervosa, agreement has not been reached concerning the definition, measurement, or relative significance of this behavior in the disorder. There is relatively little empirical justification for the requirement that the episodes must be rapid and discrete. Similarly, specifying that binges must be large is inconsistent with research indicating that a significant proportion of binges reported by bulimia nervosa clients involve small amounts of food. There are many similarities in the clinical features of bulimia nervosa and the related disorder, anorexia nervosa; however, it is generally agreed that bulimia nervosa clients tend to have a more favorable response to treatment.

There are limitations to estimates of the incidence and prevalence of bulimia nervosa because most have been derived from methods that have not been well validated. However, it has been suggested that serious cases occur in as many as 4% of female high school and college students (APA, 2000). Suspected cases of clinical eating disorders or subclinical variants are even more common among groups exposed to heightened pressures to diet or maintain a thin shape, such as ballet students, professional dancers, wrestlers, swimmers, skaters, and gymnasts (Garner, Rosen, & Berry, 1998). Although there have been case reports of bulimia nervosa in young children and geriatric adults, the consensus is that it is rare in these age groups. Although it is less common in men than in women, it has a similar clinical picture.

METHODS TO DETERMINE DIAGNOSIS

Assessment should be considered integral to the ongoing treatment process. Various approaches to information gathering have been developed for eating disorders, including standard clinical interviews, semistructured interviews, behavioral observation, standardized self-report measures, symptom checklists, clinical rating scales, self-monitoring procedures, and standardized test means. There are three broad areas of focus in the assessment process (Garner,

Vitousek & Pike, 1997): (a) assessment of specific symptom areas that allow the diagnosis of the eating disorder, (b) measurement of other attitudes or behaviors characteristic of eating disorders, and (c) identification and measurement of associated psychological and personality features that are indicative of overall psychosocial functioning.

Assessment should include careful questioning about the duration and frequency of binge eating as well as extreme measures designed to control body weight, such as vomiting, abuse of laxatives, and excessive exercise. It should also cover weight-controlling behaviors, such as other drug or alcohol use to control appetite, chewing and spitting food out before swallowing, prolonged fasting, and vigorous exercise for the purpose of controlling body weight. Clients with diabetes or who take thyroid replacements may manipulate their dosages to control weight (APA, 2000).

Marked personality changes mimicking primary personality disorders may actually stem from prolonged undernutrition (Garner, 1997). The assessment should include a careful evaluation of premorbid personality features. Clients may recall being sociable and more confident prior to the onset of the disorder, and as the disorder progressed, they may have become more sullen and isolated from others. Other clients describe a passive, compliant, and reserved premorbid personality style. Formal personality testing may be useful in some cases; however, the confounding of primary and secondary symptoms is a concern (APA, 2000). When primary personality disturbance is identified, it usually means a longer and more difficult course of therapy. Adaptations are required for clients whose disorder is complicated by substance, physical, or sexual abuse.

ADDITIONAL ASSESSMENT REQUIRED

In many cases, standardized self-report measures can be efficient in gathering information about eating behavior and other symptoms common in clients with eating disorders. The Eating Disorder Inventory–2 (EDI–2; Garner, 1991) is a standardized, multiscale measure that adds three subscales to the original EDI. It is aimed specifically at assessing a range of psychological characteristics clinically relevant to eating disorders, and consists of three subscales (Drive for Thinness, Bulimia, Body Dissatisfaction), for tapping attitudes and behaviors relating to eating, weight, and shape in addition to eight subscales (Ineffectiveness, Perfection, Interpersonal Distrust, Interoceptive Awareness, Maturity Fears, Asceticism, Impulse Regulation, and Social Insecurity) assessing more general organizing constructs or psychological traits clinically relevant to eating disorders. In clinical settings, the EDI–2 is designed to provide information helpful in understanding the client, planning treatment, and assessing progress. In nonclinical settings, it is intended as an economical means of identifying individuals who have subclinical eating problems or who may be at risk for developing eating disorders.

CASE ILLUSTRATION

Presenting Complaint

Jane is a 24-year-old, full-time university student who is 5'4" tall and weighs 110 lbs. She was referred by her family physician, who had been aware of her eating disorder for the previous 3 years and had repeatedly attempted to refer Jane for treatment. She resisted these attempts at referral because she felt that acknowledging a psychiatric problem would be humiliating to her and her family.

At the time of the initial assessment, Jane typically binged and vomited between 1 and 10 times a day and had consciously attempted to restrict her food intake over the previous 6 years. She reported that she did not remember any days in the previous 6 months in which she had not binged and vomited at least once, and indicated that bingeing and vomiting episodes would often last for 3 hours or more. The types of foods consumed on a binge typically consisted of those foods prohibited from her diet, such as desserts and other sweet foods that were high in fat content; however, she would also binge eat other foods that were not proscribed from her daily diet. The eating behavior during a binge was often frenzied and with an experience of complete loss of control. A typical bout would involve impulsively purchasing 2–3 dozen doughnuts, eating the top icing layer and then throwing the remainder off of the balcony of her apartment in order to avoid consuming more. Eating binges were followed by intense guilt, depression, and self-induced vomiting.

Jane also reported abusing laxatives by taking between 5 and 10 Ex-Lax tablets several times a week. There was no reported history of diuretic, alcohol, or drug abuse. Although binge-eating episodes usually involved consuming more than 1000 calories of food before vomiting, she also described vomiting after eating small amounts because of feeling guilty or bloated. Her degree of disparagement and revulsion related to her body was striking, even for someone with a diagnosis of bulimia nervosa. She experienced her body as "disgustingly fat," and burst into tears several times during the initial interview because of thoughts about her body. Her distress about her shape and weight was compounded by marked cyclical edema related to vomiting and abuse of laxatives. Jane described feeling highly anxious about losing control over her eating, and experienced severe depression on most days. She had contemplated suicide many times but had not made any suicide attempts, and indicated that one of the major factors that had prohibited her committing suicide was that she could not tolerate others seeing her body, which she viewed as grotesque.

History of the Disorder

Jane described herself as being very concerned about her weight for as long as she could remember and stated that she was chubby as child and adolescent. Her weight concerns were intensified markedly when she gained approximately 15 lbs at a summer camp at the age of 16. Jane's mother became distressed at her daughter's weight gain and insisted that corrective action must be taken. Jane made diligent efforts to restrict her intake, gradually lost 25 lbs and reached a weight of about 90 lbs. However, she reported resenting her mother's hypervigilance at meal times and the intensity of the efforts to control food intake. She indicated that her episodic bingeing began when she was about 17 years old following this period of intense dieting. She described the bingeing as disturbing but at the same time satisfying because she felt that it allowed her to discharge anger that had been building toward her mother. Binge eating escalated over time, and her weight increased to between 110 and 120 lbs. Vomiting and laxative abuse began about 1 year later. At first, vomiting was infrequent, occurring usually less than once a month and following a particularly large binge-eating episode. It progressed over the following year to its current level of 1 to 10 times a day, with laxative abuse several times a week. Jane continued to maintain excellent academic standing, despite her depression and eating disorder.

Jane's highest adult weight was approximately 130 lbs at age 16. Her weight had fluctuated between 110 and 120 lbs since achieving her lowest adult weight of 90 lbs. When her weight fell below 105 lbs, she remembers that her menstrual periods ceased for approximately 6 months; thus, she met diagnostic criteria for anorexia nervosa at that time. The return of her periods, her current weight, and her binge-eating patterns give her a current diagnosis of bulimia nervosa.

Medical History

Jane denied any medical problems other than cyclical edema and gastrointestinal discomfort that resulted from her bingeing and purging. She did report erosion of dental enamel related to her purging behavior. She was referred back to her family physician in order to evaluate any further medical complications resulting from her eating disorder.

Sexual History

Jane's overconcern with her weight and shape interfered with her sexual relationship with her current boyfriend and her only sexual partner, whom she had dated for the previous 4 years. She reported having little interest in sex as she found her body disgusting. Her boyfriend had repeatedly tried to reassure her that he found her attractive; however, this only intensified her weight and shape concerns. Currently, she engaged in sexual activity infrequently and only as a way to please her boyfriend. She rarely found sexual activity enjoyable because it heightened her weight and shape sensitivity.

Family History

At the time of the initial assessment, Jane lived alone in an apartment near the university. Before enrolling in the university, Jane lived at home with her family. Her mother is a 46-year-old, full-time homemaker and her father is 52 years old and a prominent radiologist in the city. Jane has a 17-year-old brother who is currently living in the family home.

Jane described her early childhood in very positive terms. Until she reached adolescence, she indicated that her relationships with mother, father, and brother were extremely close and supportive. Although there had always been pressures for academic achievement in the family, Jane had been a model student and conformed to the expectations for superior performance without difficulties until she reached adolescence. She described her relationships with her parents as extraordinarily close and sometimes even smothering. Jane's mother and father were extremely concerned about diet and weight. Her father was described as highly obsessional and preoccupied with keeping detailed records of family events. He was concerned about diet and health; his concern was later determined to be related to his own father's death from heart disease at a young age. Jane's mother apparently had developed anorexia nervosa during her own adolescence, and, although her eating disorder improved without treatment, she remained extremely diet, fashion, and youth conscious.

Mental Status Examination

Jane arrived with her parents on time for the appointment. She was well groomed, although she appeared to be pale, sickly, and fatigued. She was tearful, anxious, and nervous during the interview. She appeared to be withdrawn, and spoke only to answer questions. Her mood was depressed and affect was appropriate. She was oriented to person, place, and time. Her immediate and remote memory and thought process appeared within normal range. Her speech quality and language were normal. Despite being quite intelligent, she exhibited poor insight, judgment, and impulse control regarding her eating disorder.

Prior Treatment

As indicated earlier, Jane had resisted repeated attempts by her family physician to refer her for counseling for her eating disorder. She revealed that she would sometimes minimize her symptoms because she was afraid that her physician would press her to seek counseling. Nevertheless, she did discuss her eating problems with the family physician on several occasions, and tried to implement his suggestion that she eat in a healthy way and try to avoid bingeing and vomiting. She felt like a failure because she was not able to follow his recommendations, and lied to him by telling him that the behavior had stopped.

CASE CONCEPTUALIZATION

Modeling and Learning

Jane's mother's own struggles with anorexia nervosa as an adolescent, her current concerns about weight, and her current strict control over her own eating provided an environment in which Jane built hypersensitivity to weight and shape. Furthermore, battles over food intake and peculiar eating habits were common in Jane's family, as discussed in the section entitled Behavioral Assessment.

Life Events

Jane's 15-lbs weight gain at the age of 16 while at summer camp prompted her parents' overconcern for her weight and shape. Although Jane had grown up in a household in which weight and shape were a focal issues, she did not actively engage in eating disorder symptoms until she returned from summer camp and her parents reacted with alarm to her weight gain. This was followed by Jane's diligent efforts to restrict her food intake and she gradually lost 25 lbs, reaching a weight of about 90 lbs.

Genetics and Temperament

As indicated earlier, Jane's mother reported having an eating disorder. Although there is evidence from genetic studies that eating disorders run in families, it is not clear whether the family transmission is genetic, environmental, or a combination of factors. As indicated earlier, Jane briefly met the diagnosis of anorexia nervosa also, there is evidence that genetic factors may play a direct role in the transmission of the disorder or an indirect linkage through temperamental predisposition, such as obsessionality (APA, 2000). Another possible genetic factor could be a predisposition to overweight or obesity, which would increase the risk of weight sensitivity. As mentioned, Jane gained weight quickly at summer camp, and this may reflect genetic factors. However, the specific genetic contribution to Jane's eating disorder remains purely speculative, and would not have any effect on treatment decisions.

Physical Conditions

As mentioned, the effects of weight loss on psychological functioning is extraordinary, and this fact is often underestimated by clinicians not familiar with the psychobiology of human starvation (Garner, 1997). Severe psychological symptoms, such as depression, mood swings, and apparent personality disturbances, ameliorate with stabilization of eating and body weight in clients with eating disorders; therefore, nutritional stabilization was a priority in Jane's treatment. Similarly, dietary chaos produces physical changes, such as low potassium levels, that can lead to psychological symptoms such as depression. The general assumption in the understanding and the treatment of eating disorders is that there is an interplay between physical and psychological symptoms. This assumption played a central role in the selection of Jane's treatment.

Drugs

Jane reported no history of drug use.

Socioeconomic Status and Cultural Factors

Jane's socioeconomic status was upper middle class. Eating disorders were once thought to be overrepresented in the upper social classes; however, more recent research indicates that they affect women across the socioeconomic spectrum (Garner, 1997). As described later in more detail, a major socioeconomic factor in the United States relates to the lack of adequate insurance coverage for many of those with eating disorders. Fortunately, Jane had sufficient insurance benefits and financial resources, and economic issues did not interfere with her treatment.

Overall Conceptualization

As is common with many other bulimia nervosa patients, Jane's disorder can be conceptualized as multidetermined, resulting from the interplay of familial, psychological, sociocultural, and biological factors. Each of these factors may or may not have etiologic significance in Jane's bulimia nervosa, but, in any case, contribute to or maintain it. Jane's sensitivity to weight and shape was heightened in her family of origin via her mother's unresolved eating disorder and her father's dread of physical illness. In addition, given her perfectionistic tendencies, it is difficult to differentiate these as primary from symptoms that are secondary to the eating disorder. Furthermore, there is evidence to believe that in Jane's case, her symptoms of depression, anxiety, and low self-esteem were exacerbated as a direct result of dieting and weight suppression. Despite

Jane's extreme concerns about weight and the pressures from others to control weight having been prominent for almost 10 years, it is important to exemplify the occurrence of this against the backdrop of a culture totally fixated on thinness as an ideal for feminine beauty, supported by a multibillion-dollar-a-year diet industry that profits on the insecurity that it breeds in women regarding their shape. This has been further reinforced by the strong and consistent messages from the health professions warning of the risks associated with obesity. In conceptualizing Jane's disorder, it is important to take into account the interplay of all of the aforementioned factors.

Diagnostic Assessment

As with other clients with eating disorder, Jane's initial and ongoing assessment may be divided into two broad areas. The first relates to attitudes toward weight and shape, as well as symptoms fundamental to the eating disorder. The second concerns the various psychological and social factors that are not specific to bulimia nervosa but that may predispose toward or maintain the eating disorder. Accordingly, the initial assessments covered several key areas, including (a) weight history; (b) attitudes toward weight and shape; (c) presence, frequency, and duration of bingeing and vomiting; (d) details of weight losing behaviors, such as dieting, exercise, abuse of laxatives, diuretics, and appetite suppressants; (e) complications (i.e., self-induced vomiting, purgative abuse, and resulting electrolyte disturbances may cause various symptoms or abnormalities, such as general weakness, muscle cramping, edema, swollen salivary glands, erosion of dental enamel, paresthesia, various neurologic abnormalities, kidney and cardiac disturbances, and finger clubbing or swelling), which should be evaluated by a physician familiar with the complications of eating disorders; (f) psychological state with particular reference to depression, anxiety, and personality features; (g) impulse-related behaviors; (h) social and family functioning; (i) reasons for seeking treatment; and (j) motivation for change. Clinicians should be familiar with specific questions or probes aimed at assessing symptoms of eating disorders (Garner et al., 1997).

The increasing recognition that eating disorders are heterogeneous along various psychological dimensions provides the rationale for the assessment of the typography, depth, and severity of associated symptomatology. The clinical features and background information that guide the approach to treatment are best derived from a clinical interview; however, psychometric evaluation with standardized psychological tests is also recommended. As part of the assessment process, Jane completed the EDI–2 and had markedly elevated subscale scores on Drive for Thinness, Body Dissatisfaction, Bulimia, Ineffectiveness and Perfectionism, Asceticism, and Social Insecurity. Other self-report instruments indicated that she was experiencing severe depression, anxiety, poor self-esteem, and interpersonal sensitivity. Personality testing indicated that she had an obsessional style with some evidence of poor impulse regulation, suggestive of a possible borderline personality disorder.

Behavioral Assessment

Much of the initial assessment interview with Jane was devoted to obtaining detailed information related to attitudes and behaviors pertaining to eating habits, dieting, and weight control practices outlined earlier. She spent most weekends with her family but would not eat in front of any family members. Her level of depression and possible suicide risk presented a serious concern. Through detailed questioning, it was determined that much of her depressive thought content emanated from a sense of hopelessness about her condition. She was reassured at learning that treatment for her condition had a good likelihood of success, and it was determined that the current suicidal risk was low. Arrangements were made for her to contact either the primary therapist or a crisis center if she felt like harming herself.

After Jane was interviewed alone, she, her brother, and her parents were interviewed together. Jane's mother was an attractive woman who appeared considerably younger than her stated age. She was tearful during the interview and blamed herself for her daughter's eating disorder. She described herself as extremely insecure, and avoided virtually all interpersonal contact outside of her family. She confirmed that she had anorexia nervosa as an adolescent and also admitted to marked concerns about her own weight as well as strict control over her own eating ever since. Battles over food intake were common in the family. Jane described her mother as continually trying to overfeed others in the family while restricting her own food intake. Her mother would provide others in the family with prodigious amounts of food at mealtime, and Jane would either try to surreptitiously dispose of food or would vomit after eating. Her father was highly involved in his professional life and tended to leave all family matters in the hands of his wife. He avoided eating foods served to the other family members by adhering rigidly to a cholesterol-reduced diet. Since his own father died of a heart attack (at age 46), Jane's father described being preoccupied with his own diet and health. He refused to confront his wife or daughter about their odd eating behavior because he basically accepted and shared their preoccupation about weight. Both parents had become quite concerned about Jane's weight gain in adolescence, and even suggested that she consider breast reduction surgery at the peak of her weight gain. Jane was unable to express any anger openly to her parents related to their concerns about her weight. She idealized both parents and believed that the family environment had little to do with her eating disorder. Her brother was shy and withdrawn in the interview. He stated that he did not understand his sister's eating disorder, and believed that it must be related to academic pressures.

Prioritization of Targets for Treatment

Challenging underlying assumptions related to dieting and obesity would be the primary focus early in treatment. Behaviorally, Jane would be able to have her eating symptoms under control with a significant decline in her bingeing and purging behavior. In addition, she would adhere to the following eating pattern: (a) increase her caloric intake to an appropriate nondieting level without anxiety, (b) space meals so that food was consumed throughout the day rather than just in the evening, (c) gradually incorporate "forbidden foods" into her diet, and (d) inhibit urges to diet or engage in weight-controlling behaviors. More emphasis would be placed on controlling dieting rather than controlling bingeing because the dieting efforts are conceptualized as the primary cause of the urge to binge eat (Garner, 1997). Simultaneously, the therapist would review the psychoeducational material regarding social pressures on women to diet, the biological resistance to weight change, the range of starvation symptoms (including binge eating) that result from weight loss (Garner, 1997; Garner & Wooley, 1991).

Later, more general themes would be explored related to family-of-origin relationships and how they related to self-definition, and feelings of insecurity in current relationships. She would be able to address her own negative feelings about obesity and recognize that her disparagement of her own shape was based on assumptions about obesity in general that were inaccurate and inconsistent with her other principles for viewing human worth. She would be able to express her feelings toward the fashion and dieting industries for promoting superficial standards for judging women's self-worth exclusively in terms of physical appearance and understand the untoward consequences of following such doctrine.

Selection of Treatment Strategies

The treatment chosen was individual cognitive–behavioral therapy for Jane in addition to separate cognitive family therapy meetings for Jane and her family. Treatment reviews indicate that cognitive therapy is particularly effective for bulimia nervosa (Fairburn, 1985). Many of the cognitive–behavioral techniques originally developed by Beck (1976) for the treatment of depressive and anxiety disorders are directly applicable to bulimia nervosa. However, other methods have been developed or adapted to address features, which distinguish eating disorders from other diagnostic groups (Garner & Bemis, 1982; Garner et al., 1997). For example, much of the behavior of clients with eating disorders can be understood as a direct consequence of the firm conviction that weight or body shape are of the utmost importance in their overall self-evaluation. Because cognitive–behavioral theory of eating disorders generally has not focused on early historical antecedents of symptomatic behavior, it has been described as a proximal or abbreviated model of pathogenesis (Garner & Bemis, 1982). The primary point of emphasis of the cognitive–behavioral view has been the analysis of functional relationships between current distorted beliefs and symptomatic behaviors related to eating, weight, and body shape.

Nevertheless, the cognitive–behavioral model is equally suited for examining other historical, developmental, or family-interactional themes identified with some eating disorder clients, and psychodynamic and family theorists best describe these themes such as fears of separation, engulfment, or abandonment; failures in the separation–individuation process; false-self adaptation; transference; overprotectiveness; enmeshment; conflict avoidance; inappropriate involvement of the child in parental conflicts; and symptoms as mediators of family stability all involve distorted meaning on the part of the individual, the family, or both. Although the language, style, and specific interpretations may differ sharply between the cognitive–behavioral model and the dynamic models that have generated these respective formulations, it is notable that both orientations are concerned specifically with meaning and meaning systems. Moreover, the respective therapies are aimed at identifying and correcting misconceptions presumed to have developmental antecedents (Garner & Bemis, 1985; Garner et al., 1997). The advantage of the cognitive–behavioral approach is that it allows the incorporation of developmental themes when they apply to a particular client, but does not compel all cases to fit into one restrictive explanatory system.

The cognitive–behavioral model of eating disorders also emphasizes the interplay between current cultural pressures on women to diet and the untoward consequences of dietary restraint. Given the current cultural pressures for thinness, it is not hard to understand how women, particularly women with persistent self-doubts, could arrive at the conclusion that personal failings are to some degree related to weight or that the attainment of slenderness would measurably improve self-estimation. It has been asserted that for some clients who develop eating disorders, the motivating factors do not seem to go beyond a literal or extreme interpretation of the prevailing cultural doctrine glorifying thinness (Garner, 1997; Garner & Wooley, 1991). However, for other clients the impetus is more complicated, with a range of psychological and interactional factors playing a role (Garner et al., 1997). There are a number of general treatment principles and issues considered central to this model, including: (a) giving special attention to the therapeutic relationship, (b) enhancing motivation for change, (c) using a directive style, (d) following a "two track approach" (track one pertains to issues related to weight, bingeing, and vomiting; track two addresses beliefs and thematic underlying assumptions that are relevant to the development and maintenance of the eating disorder), (e) recognizing and addressing ego-syntonic symptoms, (f) differentiating starvation symptoms from primary psychopathology, and (g) enlisting special strategies to normalize eating and weight. These factors have been described fully in previous publications (Fairburn, 1985; Garner, 1997; Garner et al., 1997) and are touched on here only to the extent that they pertain to the case material presented.

Priority of Treatment Strategies

Following a complete individual and family assessment in Jane's case, the therapist provided an initial formulation of possible psychological and family factors that may have contributed to the development and/or the maintenance of the eating disorder, and then reviewed psychoeducational material aimed at managing the eating disorder symptoms (Garner, 1997).

In cases in which there is such obvious family psychopathology, it is critical to recognize and counter any attempts to vilify family members as the cause of the eating disorder. In this case, the mother's unresolved eating disorder and the father's dread of physical illness must be addressed with the same sensitivity and compassion as Jane's eating disorder. Moreover, it is often difficult, particularly early in treatment, to differentiate primary psychopathology or family dysfunction from symptoms that are secondary to the eating disorder.

Therapist: [To family] It is important to emphasize that it would be wrong to blame anyone for Jane's eating disorder. Rather, it is the goal of treatment to understand the values, beliefs, underlying assumptions, and feelings of each member of the family so that Jane can overcome her eating problems and also to provide the opportunity for other people to address difficulties they may identify as sources of concern.

Mother: But I feel like my own eating disorder and my pressuring Jane about weight is the cause of her current problems.

Therapist: Clearly the concerns you and your husband have had about weight have had an impact, but I don't think that you planned to have an eating disorder yourself or that your husband had any malicious intent in his weight concerns. In fact, you have both suffered for many years without adequate help.

Therapist: [To Jane after family leaves the room] You and your family have been extremely helpful in giving me some idea of the evolution of your eating disorder. I think the factors that have probably contributed to your disorder can be divided into two broad areas. The first relates to things in your background that we've only touched on now or that haven't been discussed but need to be understood in order to help you recover from your eating disorder. Also, there may have been other things that have gone on in your past that may not even be related to your eating disorder, but turn out to be important issues to address in treatment. The second relates to the fact that there is good evidence that many eating-disorder symptoms are the direct result of dieting and weight suppression. Clearly, your extreme concerns about your weight and the pressure from others to control your weight have been prominent for almost ten years. This has occurred against the backdrop of a culture totally fixated on thinness as an ideal for feminine beauty, supported by a multibillion-dollar-a-year diet industry that profits on the insecurity it breeds in women regarding their shape. This has been further reinforced by the strong and consistent messages from the health professions warning of the risks associated with obesity. I want to take a few minutes to review some specific points.

The therapist then reviewed some of the psychoeducational material described in detail elsewhere regarding social pressures on women to diet, the biological resistance to weight change, and the range of starvation symptoms (including binge eating) that result from weight loss (Garner, 1997; Garner & Wooley, 1991). These points have to be covered carefully, with sensitivity to resistance or fear that they might generate. Periodic statements such as "Does this make sense so far?" or "How do you feel so far about what I have said?" and being attuned to nonverbal signs of anger, fear, anxiety, and withdrawal are particularly important in pacing the presentation of the educational material. If the client balks at any point, the source of concern should be identified and explored. It may be necessary to proceed more slowly or to curtail the educational mode of discussion temporarily while attempting to deal with emergent issues.

The use of an educational approach has several major advantages. First, there is intrinsic value in clarifying misunderstandings related to bodily functioning and weight control. Second, the suggestion that certain symptoms and behaviors may be derived logically from cultural pressures on women to diet and the biological reactions to dieting, rather being purely psychogenic in nature, may diminish potential untoward effects associated with psychiatric labeling. Third, educational material can provide the basis for testing and refining beliefs that drive symptomatic behavior. For example, Jane weighed herself at least 20 times each day and assumed that the dramatic daily shifts in her body weight reflected changes in actual body fat levels rather than changes in fluid retention due to edema. This created panic and resulted in drastic weight control methods when her weight would increase. By linking the weight changes to water rather than fat, it was possible to reduce Jane's panic and also convince her that weighing herself less often was justified. At the same time, it was helpful in illustrating how closely tied her intense affect was to numbers on the scale, irrespective of their true meaning. This was underscored in a simple experiment.

Therapist: When you step on the scale, how do you feel?

Jane: I feel extremely apprehensive beforehand, and then I completely panic when I step on the scale and find that my weight has gone up.

Therapist: Do you feel elated when your weight goes down?

Jane: Sometimes I feel good, but usually I feel upset because I know it will just go up later.

Therapist: What does it mean when the numbers go up?

Jane: It means that I've gained weight and I'm fat and disgusting.

Therapist: I wonder if the scale has become an independent barometer for your feelings regardless of what the numbers really mean? Let's try an experiment. We've discussed the issue of water balance and the scale. I'm going to ask you to stand on the scale while I gently step on the back and change the numbers. [This is done, and the numbers slowly increase while Jane is standing on the scale.] How do you feel as the numbers go up?

Jane: [Visibly distressed] I'm really frightened when I see the numbers go up.

Therapist: How do you feel about yourself when you look at the scale now? [Up 15 lbs from her actual weight]

Jane: I feel like a disgusting pig. I hate myself. I can't stand this.

Therapist: And this is true when you know that I am making the numbers increase on the scale. You can see that your feelings and what it means when the numbers go up have become almost automatic. The feedback is distressing and destructive even when you know that it has nothing to do with actual changes in body fat. This is why it would be good for you to avoid weighing yourself daily, and we can begin just weighing you once a week here to make sure that your weight is not out of control.

The more fundamental therapeutic issue in this case, as with virtually all eating disorder clients, relates to the degree to which weight or shape have become the sole or predominant yardstick for determining or modulating self-worth (Garner & Bemis, 1982). This key issue must be addressed repeatedly and from many different vantage points throughout the course of therapy with Jane and her family. In challenging this value system, particular care must be taken to guard against a frontal attack that could strip the individual or the family of the core marker for their identity in the absence of a replacement system for regulating self-concept. Initially, Jane's feelings about weight and her self-definition were so strong that simply saying the word fat would result in her bursting into tears. Later in therapy, her feelings about herself were tied more to relationships with others who she valued and doing certain things that she enjoyed rather than being driven strictly by performance and evaluation of outcome.

In summary, during initial sessions, Jane was encouraged to monitor her eating, bingeing, vomiting, laxative abuse, mood, circumstances surrounding eating, and eating symptoms (Fairburn, 1985). In session, the therapist challenged underlying assumptions related to dieting and obesity. Jane's mother was referred to another therapist for help with her own eating problems. The family meetings lasted for 2 months and focused on raising their consciousness regarding the prejudice that family members shared about obesity (Garner & Wooley, 1991). In family meetings, Jane was able to express her competitive feelings toward her mother and how the competition had extended to food and weight. The family meetings also allowed Jane's father to articulate his ongoing distress regarding his father's death and the family was able to support his attempts to challenge his unrealistic view of his heightened health risks. It also became evident that he suffered from chronic depression, and some time was spent in the family meetings focusing on cognitive–behavioral techniques to address his mood. In the course of family meetings, Jane's brother revealed that he was angry at the family for what he perceived as undue pressure to follow a program of studies that would lead to a career in medicine rather than follow his own interests in art.

Dealing with Complicating Factors

Jane was seen in therapy for about a year. Although many reports of cognitive–behavioral treatment for bulimia nervosa describe a relatively brief course of treatment, it is important to emphasize that there are patients who may be recalcitrant in the short term but who benefit with extended treatment. Jane's fears related to maintaining a normal body weight were extreme, and she required longer term treatment in order to consolidate her more accepting attitudes regarding her own body weight and decouple her self-esteem from her weight. She had numerous relapses that led to the reemergence of weight suppression attempts; however, she gradually became more consistent in resisting urges to diet with growing awareness of how it interfered with other life goals that she valued deeply. She was able to keep her competitive feelings toward her mother from translating into weight control; however, her mother's continued symptoms around eating and weight were a source of distress for Jane. She spent less time with her parents and focused increasing energy on her relationship with her boyfriend. She was able to see how her early family environment had provided a window through which cultural values toward weight and achievement had been magnified. At the 1-year follow-up, Jane reported no disturbed eating patterns, and the improvements in general psychological functioning had been maintained.

Role of Pharmacotherapy in the Case

Medication should be considered for clients with bulimia nervosa or binge-eating disorder who fail an initial trial of cognitive–behavioral therapy. There have been many well-controlled trials throughout the 1990s indicating the effectiveness of some antidepressant medications for bulimia nervosa. However, in reviewing the research in the field, Raymond, Mitchell, Fallon, and Katzman (1994) suggested that medication should not be "the primary mode of therapy with patients with bulimia nervosa" (p. 241). This conclusion is based on the following observations: (a) psychological interventions have been shown to be very effective, (b) there are high dropout rates reported in most medication studies, (c) there are risks of drug side effects, and (d) data suggest high relapse rates with drug discontinuation. Fluoxetine hydrochloride (Prozac) is currently the first choice for the treatment of bulimia nervosa (daily dosages of 60 mg were generally superior to 20 mg) and probably should be used at least as an adjunct to psychotherapy in many cases failing in a course of adequate psychological treatment (APA, 2000). Following the Raymond et al. (1994) suggestion, Jane responded positively to psychological treatment and did not necessitate pharmacologic intervention.

Managed Care Considerations

During the 1980s, there were extraordinary economic incentives for inpatient care, surging demands for clinical services, and widespread misinformation regarding optimal treatment. This led to the unnecessary hospitalization of many clients with eating disorders who could have been easily managed as outpatients or at a partial hospitalization level of care. Abuse of residential and inpatient treatment was followed by a backlash by the insurance industry, resulting in inappropriate denial of hospital coverage or absurd limitations of coverage for eating disorder clients. Unfortunately, this has put many eating disorder clients at unnecessary risk for chronic illness or death. Part of the problem has been a failure to articulate clearly the different objectives for correcting acute medical complications and comprehensive treatment of the eating disorders. Hospitalization is most appropriate for clients who are in acute medical danger and who require medical stabilization. When aimed at treating physical complications, hospitalization is a medical priority that does not require a commitment by the client to recover from his or her eating disorder. In contrast, treatments aimed at recovery from the eating disorder have the goals of nutritional rehabilitation, containment of eating disorder symptoms, and addressing the psychological problems that led to the development and the maintenance of the eating disorder. In most cases, this can be conducted in a cost-effective manner in a specialized eating disorder program at a partial hospitalization level of care. Partial hospitalization or intensive day-treatment programs provide the preferred alternative to inpatient care for most clients. These programs provide structure around mealtimes plus the possibility for intensive therapy without requiring the client to become totally disengaged from the supports and therapeutic challenges outside the hospital. Partial care programs offer the distinct advantage of being more economic than full hospitalization. They can also provide a useful bridge between inpatient and outpatient care. There are various models for day-treatment programs that generally share many features with inpatient programs. The major difference is that clients receive the therapeutic services but do not stay overnight. Again, inpatient treatment is still the preferred modality for clients who are seriously emaciated, require close medical monitoring, fail to progress in partial care, or are at serious risk of self-harm.

It is generally pointless to negotiate with clients or insurance carriers around the duration of partial hospitalization treatment required for weight restoration because the time needed is relatively straightforward and easy to calculate. It is the number of weeks or months required to reach at least 90% of expected weight, gaining at a rate of between 2 and 3 lbs a week and assuming optimal compliance with the treatment program. Even though this is a time-consuming and expensive process, it is an economic alternative if it leads to recovery because a chronic eating disorder inflicts heavy price in both monetary and emotional terms.

SUMMARY

Illustrating cognitive therapy for eating disorders using the case study format has the primary advantage of providing concrete examples of actual interventions, giving life to otherwise sterile theoretical accounts of treatment. Unfortunately, the case study format has a number of disadvantages that are particularly important in illustrating the treatment of eating disorders. It has been emphasized repeatedly that eating disorders are multidetermined and present with a myriad of associated forms of psychopathology. The case presented here demonstrates only one set of presenting problems, underlying assumptions, application of the method, format for delivery, duration of treatment, and resolution among a wide array of possibilities. Jane presented with other primary psychopathology in addition to her eating disorder, although much of her initial psychological distress was secondary to her chaotic eating patterns (Garner, 1997). There are many bulimia nervosa clients whose presentation and course are more straightforward and respond favorably to brief cognitive–behavioral or educational techniques outlined here and elsewhere.

The case illustration could unwittingly convey the impression that simply recognizing a flawed underlying assumption is sufficient for change, whereas in most instances, there is a tremendous amount of creative redundancy required to essentially relearn a more accurate or adaptive system of thinking. Effective cognitive interventions can be brief in some cases, but for others they assume a lengthy course. Individual, group, or family therapy formats each may be advantageous for certain patients or they may be combined in some instances. For some clients, even inpatient treatment may be necessary to normalize eating and weight, interrupt bingeing, vomiting or laxative abuse, treat complications, and occasionally disengage the family from destructive interactional patterns. Many of the nuances of treatment go well beyond the scope of the preceding case presentation but have described in detail elsewhere.

REFERENCES

American Psychiatric Association [APA]. (1994). *Diagnostic and statistical manual of mental disorders–4th ed.* Washington, DC: Author

American Psychiatric Association. (2000). Practice guidelines for eating disorders. *American Journal of Psychiatry, 157,* 1 (Suppl), 1–39.

Beck, A. T. (1976). Cognitive therapy and the emotional disorders. New York: International Universities Press.

Fairburn, C. G. (1985). Cognitive–behavioral treatment for bulimia. In: D. M. Garner & P. E. Garfinkel (Eds.), *Handbook of psychotherapy for anorexia nervosa and bulimia* (pp. 160–192). New York: Guilford Press.

Garner, D. M. (1991). *Eating Disorder Inventory–2 Professional Manual.* Odessa, FL: Psychological Assessment Resources.

Garner, D. M. (1997). Psychoeducational principles in treatment. In: D. M. Garner & P. E. Garfinkel (Eds.), *Handbook of treatment for eating disorders* (pp. 145–177), New York: Guilford Press.

Garner, D. M., & Bemis, K. M. (1982). A cognitive–behavioral approach to anorexia nervosa. *Cognitive Therapy and Research, 6,* 123–150.

Garner, D. M., Rosen, L., & Barry, D. (1998). Eating disorders in athletes. In: *Child and Adolescent Psychiatric Clinics of North America* (pp. 839–857). 7, New York: WB Saunders.

Garner, D. M., Vitousek, K., & Pike, K. (1997). Cognitive–behavioral therapy for anorexia nervosa. In: D. M. Garner & P. E. Garfinkel (Eds.), *Handbook of treatment for eating disorders* (pp. 94–144). New York: Guilford Press.

Garner, D. M., & Wooley, S. C. (1991). Confronting the failure of behavioral and dietary treatments for obesity. *Clinical Psychology Review, 11,* 1–52.

Raymond, N. C., Mitchell, J. E., Fallon, P., & Katzman, M. A. (1994). A collaborative approach to the use of medication. In: P. Fallon, M. Katzman & S. C. Wooley (Eds.). *Feminist Perspectives on Eating Disorders* (pp. 231–250). New York: Guilford Press.

13

Alcohol Use Disorders

Paul R. Stasiewicz and Clara M. Bradizza
Research Institute on Addictions

DESCRIPTION OF THE DISORDER

Alcohol use disorders can be classified according to the *Diagnostic and Statistical Manual of Mental Disorders–4th Ed.* (*DSM–IV*; American Psychiatric Association, 1994) as either alcohol abuse or alcohol dependence. *Alcohol abuse* is defined primarily by the occurrence of negative consequences that are the result of alcohol use. These can include recurrent problems with fulfilling responsibilities at work, school, or home; using substances in situations that may result in a physical harm (e.g., driving a car, operating large machinery); legal difficulties; and interpersonal conflicts. *Alcohol dependence* is usually considered a more severe disorder than alcohol abuse and is generally diagnosed when an individual experiences signs of tolerance, withdrawal, and difficulty controlling consumption. *Tolerance* occurs when an individual requires increasing amounts of alcohol to achieve the same level of physical or psychological effects. *Withdrawal* results when an individual stops drinking or greatly reduces alcohol intake after having consumed large amounts of alcohol over an extended period of time. Symptoms of alcohol withdrawal can include autonomic hyperactivity (e.g., sweating, racing pulse); hand tremor; insomnia; nausea/vomiting; visual, tactile, or auditory hallucinations; psychomotor agitation; anxiety; and grand mal seizures. Withdrawal usually begins fairly rapidly, within 4–12 hours after stopping alcohol consumption; however, it can start as late as 60 hours following abrupt cessation or reduction in alcohol use. Symptoms usually peak during the second day of abstinence. If a delirium develops in which the individual experiences significant memory deficits, disorientation, or language disturbance, it is likely that a serious medical condition may be present, such as liver failure, pneumonia, or gastrointestinal bleeding, and a medical evaluation is necessary.

Clients may present to treatment for a variety of reasons; it may be court mandated or court referred, in which case there may be legal consequences if alcohol use continues or if the client leaves treatment prematurely. Even clients who are not involved in the criminal justice system may be experiencing pressure from family members, employers, or friends. As a result, clients presenting for treatment may appear to be reluctant consumers of services. This reluctance is often expressed as an unwillingness to acknowledge the extent of negative consequences due to drinking, sporadic treatment attendance, or little enthusiasm for participation in the treatment sessions. These behaviors are often termed *denial* by alcoholism treatment providers. More recently, interventions have been developed to address these cognitive and behavioral barriers to change.

METHODS TO DETERMINE DIAGNOSIS

The *DSM–IV* is based on a medical model classification in which alcoholism is viewed as a disease process that is similar for all individuals. Although most clinicians determine a diagnosis based on an unstructured clinical interview, the most valid and reliable means of assessing whether an individual has an alcohol abuse or dependence diagnosis is by means of a structured diagnostic interview. The most frequently used instrument in clinical practice is the Structured Clinical Interview for *DSM–IV* (SCID–IV; First, Gibbon, Spitzer, & Williams, 1995). The patient version of this instrument (SCID–P) is reasonably brief and intended to gather only information directly relevant to making a diagnosis. The substance use disorders section of the SCID–P includes a separate diagnostic evaluation of alcohol abuse and alcohol dependence.

In instances in which administration of the SCID–P is not feasible, a symptom checklist (e.g., a brief screening interview) can be useful in structuring the interview to ensure that the clinician asks all questions that pertain to making a diagnosis.

ADDITIONAL ASSESSMENTS REQUIRED

Alcohol problems are determined by multiple factors that include both the individual and his or her environment. With regard to the assessment of alcohol-related problems, it is worth noting that many instruments have been developed and validated with male populations (Russell, Chan, & Mudar, 1997).

Therefore, knowledge of gender differences in the signs and symptoms of alcohol abuse can be helpful in identifying alcohol problems accurately in women. For example, compared to men, women are less likely to drive while intoxicated, and less likely to get into physical fights. However, women are more likely to feel guilty about their drinking and to have higher rates of psychiatric comorbidity. There are also gender differences in help-seeking patterns, risk factors for problem drinking, and relapse precipitants. Despite these differences between men and women, a comprehensive assessment that includes but is not limited to sociodemographics, motivation to change, drinking pattern, negative consequences of alcohol use, other drug use, and physical and mental status is essential.

As a starting point, the clinician should assess the quantity, frequency, and pattern of alcohol consumption. In order to confirm self-report of substance use, the clinician may obtain written consent to contact a close friend or family member who is familiar with the client's daily activities. This individual can be asked about the client's drinking behavior in order to gauge the accuracy of the client's reporting. In addition, a breath sample should be obtained at the beginning of each treatment session to ensure the client has not been drinking; if alcohol use is detected, the appointment should be rescheduled. A client's pattern of drinking is important, because a client who drinks daily may require a different treatment focus than someone who binges only on weekends. Information on the amount of alcohol consumed per drinking day and the number of drinking days per week provides an indication of total weekly consumption. This information can then be compared to national norms to determine how the client's drinking compares to other adults of the same sex. Although the risk for developing negative health consequences increases in proportion to alcohol intake, men who drink more than three drinks per day and women who drink more than two drinks per day are at increased risk for liver damage, cognitive impairment, cardiomyopathy, problems with immune and hormonal functioning, and many digestive cancers. All clients who have not had a physical examination in the previous year should be referred to a primary care physician to determine their current state of physical health.

In addition to these physical problems, prolonged periods of heavy drinking are more likely to lead to high physical dependence on alcohol. During the first interview, the clinician should determine the client's current level of alcohol dependence. If the client is still engaged in heavy drinking, the extent of physical dependence has implications for how detoxification from alcohol should proceed. Clients experiencing moderate to high dependence should be detoxified in consultation with a physician, who may decide to prescribe a benzodiazepine (e.g., Valium, Ativan) to manage alcohol withdrawal symptoms.

Motivation to change an alcohol problem can be viewed on a continuum in which clients with little or no motivation anchor the lower end and clients with very high motivation the upper end. Motivation should be assessed early in treatment because this can assist the clinician with the development of initial treatment goals. Generally, clients can be assessed on three dimensions: (a) ambivalence about drinking, (b) recognition of a problem, and (c) extent to which they have made significant changes in their alcohol consumption. Individuals who are ambivalent are likely to report both pros and cons related to changing their drinking behavior and are concerned about being labeled a problem drinker or an alcoholic. Clients who recognize they have a problem are willing to discuss the extent of their alcohol use and the resulting problems openly. These clients often have taken some steps to change their drinking habits prior to seeking treatment (i.e., reduced drinking). Clients who have made significant changes in their drinking behavior are often seeking treatment to gain support for their abstinence or deal with a recent relapse. In addition, they may be seeking help with marital, family, or employment problems that may have accumulated during their period of problem drinking.

Negative consequences of alcohol use are often the reason clients present for treatment. It is important to assess the entire range of possible negative consequences, including physical, interpersonal, emotional, psychological, vocational, legal, and social. Providing the client with feedback about the negative consequences can be a useful means of increasing motivation to change alcohol use and can also be helpful in setting treatment goals and monitoring outcomes. Assessing the negative consequences of alcohol use often is done in the context of asking the client about the perceived benefits and costs of alcohol consumption.

Frequently, there is overlap between alcohol and drug abuse. More recently, there has been an increase in the number of persons presenting for alcohol treatment who also meet diagnostic criteria for a drug use disorder. As a result, all clients presenting for alcohol treatment should be assessed for drug use. The clinician should determine extent of current and past drug use, date of last use, whether the client meets diagnostic criteria for a diagnosis of abuse or dependence, and any negative consequences of drug use. Assessing the interrelationship of alcohol and drug use is an important issue that has implications for treatment. For example, it is important to know the extent to which drug use may precipitate alcohol craving or alcohol use.

Clients diagnosed with alcohol abuse often have high rates of depression; therefore, all clients presenting for treatment should be assessed for depression and suicidality. Clinicians are often faced with determining which disorder came first: depression or alcoholism. Among some individuals, depression precedes alcohol abuse and can even precipitate increased drinking. Alternatively, chronic heavy alcohol use can result in biological changes and increases in negative consequences that lead to the onset of depression. Determining the primary disorder often can be difficult because the clinician is relying primarily on the client's self-report of information that may have occurred years ago. In addition, the benefits of determining which disorder came first are limited. Therefore, rather than attempting to determine the primary disorder, it is often more useful to address the issue more practically. The majority of clients who begin treatment with an alcohol problem and clinical depression are no longer clinically depressed following an extended period of abstinence from alcohol (i.e., 1 month). For clients who continue to experience significant depressive symptoms, the clinician should consider providing psychological treatment (e.g., cognitive–behavioral, interpersonal) or a referral for pharmacologic treatment (i.e., antidepressant medication).

CASE ILLUSTRATION

Presenting Complaints

John is a 41-year-old married White male who called the outpatient clinic seeking treatment for alcohol-related problems. During the assessment session, John reported that he was unable to reduce his drinking despite several recent attempts to cut down. He also reported missing several days at work because he was recovering from the previous night's drinking episode; there were also increased marital arguments and less time engaged in social activities that do not involve drinking.

History of the Disorder

John first began drinking at age 16 and experienced his first problem related to drinking at age 19. Since beginning drinking at age 16, his longest period of abstinence from alcohol was 4 months when he was 38 years old. For the previous 3 years, his longest period of abstinence was 2 weeks, with several shorter periods of abstinence occurring over this 3-year period. He never sought treatment for an alcohol problem, but did acknowledge attending several Alcoholics Anonymous (AA) meetings during the previous year.

Medical History

John's only surgery was when he was 6 years old and had his tonsils removed. He broke his arm while skiing when he was 21, and states that he had been drinking with friends on the day of the accident. His last physical exam was more than a year previously, and a review of those medical records indicated elevated levels of gamma-glutamyl transpeptidase (GGTP, a liver enzyme) and red blood cell size (mean corpuscular volume; MCV). Both of GGTP and MCV are reliable markers of recent heavy alcohol consumption.

Family History

John is the oldest of three children. His parents are still married and live in the same city as John and his two siblings, a 38-year-old sister and a 36-year-old brother. John reports that he gets along well with his parents and siblings, and described his father as a "heavy drinker." He remembers his father spending considerable time in the evenings and on weekends at a corner bar just down the street from the family home. Although his father no longer drinks, John admitted to several similarities between his father's drinking pattern and his own. For example, like his father, John drinks more heavily during the weekends and while watching sports programs on television. Neither his mother or sister drink, and John states that his brother has one or two drinks during holidays and other family celebrations. His paternal grandfather is considered by the family to have been an alcoholic. There was no other family history of substance abuse reported. John has two children of his own, a 15-year-old son and a 12-year-old daughter. He indicated that he spends less time with his family these days and that he and his wife have not had an evening out together in more than 6 months.

Sexual History

John's first sexual encounter occurred at age 17, and he had six different sexual partners prior to getting married at age 25. He indicated that he and his wife enjoyed a healthy sex life until approximately 3 years ago, when his wife began refusing to have sexual relations when John was intoxicated. During the previous 3 years, the frequency of sexual intercourse has decreased from two to three times per week to less than once per month. Although John is unhappy with their sex life, efforts to pursue more frequent sexual relations with his wife have been largely unsuccessful. Further complicating this issue, John reported two episodes of erectile failure during the previous 2 years. He admitted to feeling embarrassed about these events and worrying about future episodes. Furthermore, the worrisome thoughts have made him hesitant to initiate sexual relations with his wife. In order to cope with the anxiety surrounding his sexual performance, he drinks. However, when he drinks, his wife refuses his sexual advances.

Mental Status Examination

Although John appeared alert and oriented, his mood appeared depressed. This was confirmed by his score of 21 on the Beck Depression Inventory–II (BDI–II; Beck, Steer, & Brown, 1996), which places him in the moderate to severe range of clinical depression. Other than the intermittent periods of worry concerning his sexual performance, no problems with anxiety were reported. His memory for distant and recent events appeared normal, and there was no evidence of any cognitive disturbance.

Prior Treatment

Although John has made several recent attempts to reduce his drinking, he has never before sought formal treatment for an alcohol problem. During the previous year he attended one or two AA meetings, but states that he attended these meetings at the request of his wife and that he is uncomfortable discussing his problems in a group setting. He also did not think he belonged in AA because he "wasn't an alcoholic."

CASE CONCEPTUALIZATION

Modeling and Learning

Throughout his life, John has been exposed to models of heavy drinking. His father's drinking pattern and that of his father's friends stand out as salient examples of heavy drinking. As mentioned earlier, John noticed similarities between his father's drinking pattern and his own. For example, 3 to 4 evenings per week John has two or three beers with dinner and walks several blocks to a neighborhood pub and consumes five or six more drinks with several friends who are also heavy drinkers. On Saturday, he begins drinking earlier in the day and consumes 12 to 15 drinks. He also recalls his father drinking more heavily on weekends and holidays. Since college, John has had friends who drank as much or more than he does, and never considered his drinking a problem as long as he was drinking less than his friends. Finally, he also reports drinking to reduce stress or tension, and says that a few drinks make him more relaxed and elevate his mood, making it easier for him to socialize with others. More recently, alcohol has been used to cope with the increased marital distress.

Life Events

In general, John reports drinking more since he and his wife began experiencing increased marital problems 3 years ago. Specifically, he is more likely to drink following an argument with his wife. In fact, John's reason for seeking treatment at this time is that his wife has threatened to leave him unless he sought help for his "drinking problem." This upsets John because he doesn't believe that he is an "alcoholic" and he does not want to be separated from his two children.

Genetics and Temperament

It is frequently observed that drinking problems tend to run in families. However, a behavior such as alcohol consumption is best understood as a product of the interaction between a variety of genetic and environmental influences. Thus, an individual is more or less disposed to heavy drinking or to particular alcohol-related problems. This level of predisposition determines the probability of developing an alcohol-related problem. John's family history of alcohol problems (i.e., paternal grandfather and father) increases his personal risk for developing problems with alcohol. Although the exact reason for this higher risk is unknown, he may have inherited a higher tolerance for alcohol, or is in some way more sensitive to alcohol's effects (e.g., tension reduction).

Physical Conditions

Two episodes of erectile failure have resulted in worrisome thoughts regarding his sexual performance. Further assessment is required to determine whether the problem is due to a general medical condition (e.g., diabetes, peripheral vascular disease) or to the direct physiologic effects of a substance (e.g., medications, drugs of abuse). In order to rule out a general medical condition, John will be referred to his physician. A behavioral assessment of the two episodes of erectile failure will be conducted by the therapist to determine the antecedent events in both situations.

Drugs

John does not currently use drugs. He last smoked marijuana when he was 37 years old.

Socioeconomic and Cultural Factors

John is employed full-time as an assistant manager in the parts department of an automobile dealership, a job he has held for the previous 9 years. His wife works part-time, and together their annual income is approximately $45,000. Although they can afford to pay expenses, they have very little discretionary income. In fact, the amount of money that John spends on liquor per month is frequently a precipitant of marital arguments. On the Timeline Follow-back Interview (TLFB; Sobell & Sobell, 1992), it was estimated that John spends between $149 and $357 per month on alcohol; the actual dollar amount varies according to the number of drinks John consumes at home versus the bar in a given month. Cultural factors do not appear to be influential in John's drinking behavior.

Overall Conceptualization

Multiple factors have influenced the development and maintenance of John's drinking behavior. First, there is a positive family history for alcohol problems, which suggests that John may have inherited certain predisposing factors that increase the reinforcing effects of alcohol. Consistent with this notion is his report that alcohol reduces tension. Second, throughout his life, John has been exposed to heavy drinking models, and his current peer group is composed of several heavy drinking friends. In this regard, heavy drinking in certain contexts may seem normal to him. Finally, John receives both positive and negative reinforcement from drinking. He receives positive reinforcement from alcohol's pleasurable effects and from the social interaction that accompanies drinking with several friends at the bar. He also reports that drinking helps to elevate his mood. He receives negative reinforcement from alcohol's stress-reducing effect. For example, following an argument with his wife, he leaves home and walks to the neighborhood bar. In addition to alcohol's tension-reducing effects, drinking in the bar is also negatively reinforced because he has removed himself from the stressful home environment.

Diagnostic Assessment

John was administered the Substance Use Disorders section of the SCID–P during the second treatment session. He met criteria for alcohol dependence and endorsed a number of symptoms, including regularly drinking more than he intended, difficulty cutting down or stopping drinking, reduced social contact with family because of his alcohol use, and elevated liver enzymes due to prolonged periods of heavy drinking. He also met criteria for alcohol abuse: He endorsed experiencing recurrent problems meeting his family and work obligations, and continued alcohol use despite a knowledge that it was affecting his physical health. However, in keeping with *DSM–IV* principles, a diagnosis of alcohol dependence supercedes a diagnosis of alcohol abuse. The client also met criteria for a lifetime diagnosis of cannabis abuse. He indicated that he stopped smoking marijuana 4 years ago, but had regularly used it for 11 years prior to quitting. He admitted having used hallucinogens several times in college, but did not meet any other diagnostic criteria for substance abuse. The client endorsed several symptoms of depression, including feeling sad, difficulty sleeping, and a decreased interest in sex. Despite this symptomatology, John did not meet criteria for either a current or past diagnosis of major depression or dysthymia. He identified his current stressors as primarily the result of negative consequences resulting from his drinking behavior, particularly arguments with his wife.

Behavioral Assessment

A cognitive–behavioral model of alcohol use proposes that substance use occurs on a continuum from abstention to social drinking to alcoholism. This perspective primarily involves the evaluation of cognitions, drinking behavior, and high-risk situations. A behavioral assessment of alcohol use was conducted 1 week following admission to the outpatient clinic. The general approach to assessment involved a nonconfrontational style with the goal of minimizing resistance and increasing John's motivation to change his drinking behavior. The TLFB procedure was used to assess quantity and frequency of alcohol use during the 6-month period prior to his admission to the clinic. On the TLFB, John drank 4–5 days per week and consumed an average of 9 drinks per drinking day. His heavier drinking days were Friday and Saturday, and lighter drinking days were Monday through Thursday. He generally abstained from drinking on Sundays. John reported that his last drink occurred 3 days prior to his current admission. The client was administered the Short-form Alcohol Dependence Data Questionniare (SADD; Raistrick, Dunbar, & Davidson, 1983) in order to assess his current level of alcohol dependence. He obtained a score of 12, suggesting a medium level of alcohol dependence. John endorsed only a few items indicative of physical dependence, but a number of items suggesting he is experiencing psychological dependence. He reported experiencing few physical symptoms during periods of abstinence; therefore, no referral for detoxification was made. However, it had been more than 1 year since his last physical exam, and he was referred to his primary care physician for a medical evaluation.

John was administered the Drinker Inventory of Consequences (DRINC; Miller, Tonigan, & Longabaugh, 1995), a 50-item questionnaire assessing possible negative consequences of alcohol use. The items sample a number of domains of possible negative consequences, including physical (e.g., trouble sleeping, physical health), intrapersonal (e.g., guilt, negative personality changes), social responsibility (e.g., missed work, failure to meet expectations), interpersonal (e.g., problems with family or friends, damaged social life), and impulse control (e.g., drinking and driving, physical fights). His responses indicated that he has experienced a high level of interpersonal negative consequences, moderate levels of social responsibility and negative physical consequences, and low levels of impulse control and negative physical consequences.

In order to assess current level of motivation to change his alcohol use behavior, John was administered the Stages of Change and Treatment Eagerness Scale (SOCRATES; Miller & Tonigan, 1996). This instrument assesses motivation on three distinct factors: Ambivalence, Recognition, and Taking Steps. As compared with a large sample of outpatient alcoholics, John's responses on the Ambivalence scale items suggested some acknowledgment that he may drink too much and that his drinking may be hurting others. His responses on the Recognition scale items indicated a low level of Recognition of an alcohol problem. Although he acknowledged alcohol-related problems, he did not see himself as an alcoholic or a problem drinker. John's responses to the Taking Steps items indicated that he has made very few changes to his drinking behavior.

High-risk alcohol use situations were assessed using the Inventory of Drug-Taking Situations–Alcohol (Annis & Martin, 1985), which consists of 50 questions that assess the risk of drinking in a variety of situations that are then classified into one of eight categories, including Unpleasant Emotions, Physical Discomfort, Pleasant Emotions, Testing Personal Control, Urges/Temptations to Use, Conflict with Others, Social Pressure to Use, and Pleasant Times with Others. John's responses to this questionnaire indicated that his highest risk situations were those involving negative affect, conflict with others, and pleasant times with others. He indicated that he often drank when he was experiencing negative feelings such as depression, hopelessness, anger, and anxiety. He stated that his primary conflicts were with his wife and with a coworker he was supervising. John also identified watching sports events at the bar or at home as high-risk situations, and often watched these events with his drinking buddies.

An important component of behavioral assessment is a functional analysis, which is useful for isolating the antecedents and consequences of a behavior such as alcohol consumption. A functional analysis specifies the relevant events that are associated with both increases and decreases in alcohol use and can be useful in forming hypotheses about the nature of the relationships among variables, and can include cognitive, emotional, interpersonal, and environmental events. The consequences of alcohol use are also examined in order to determine the potential sources of reinforcement that maintain the alcohol use. The functional analysis assumes an idiographic (individualized) approach to understanding alcohol use behavior, and the information gathered during this assessment is used to inform the treatment planning process. A functional analysis was conducted with John to identify the factors that maintain his drinking in several high-risk alcohol use situations. Table 13.1 illustrates several situations he identified as posing the greatest risk for heavy drinking. With regard to the first situation, John reported that he and his wife often argue about his alcohol use and lack of time spent with the family. The second high-risk situation involves social pressure to drink, and the third situation is an example of a positive social situation. In all three situations, John reports low confidence in this ability to abstain from drinking and often drinks more than he intended.

As the three high-risk situations in Table 13.1 illustrate, both the immediate and delayed positive and negative consequences of alcohol use were assessed. In all three situations, John reported experiencing short-term positive consequences following alcohol use. Short-term consequences are often

TABLE 13.1
Functional Analysis of High-Risk Drinking Situations

Trigger	Thoughts	Feelings	Behavior	Consequences	
				Short Term	Long Term
Argument with wife	"She doesn't care about me" "She's trying to control me"	Depressed, frustrated	Drink	Reduces depression and stress	Expensive, increases marital stress
Friends pressure him to have a drink	"They won't stop until I have a drink" "Why won't they leave me alone?"	Pressured, anxious	Drink	Relief, has a good time	Hangover, missed work
Thanksgiving holiday	"I have four days off from work"	Excited	Drink	Enhances mood, socializes with family, passes out	Wife is angry

more salient than long-term consequences and can also exert a stronger influence on behavior. Although John reported delayed negative consequences from drinking, he often did not recall these when in a high-risk drinking situation.

Prioritization of Targets for Treatment

The comprehensive diagnostic and behavioral assessment revealed the following problems: (a) diagnosis of alcohol dependence, (b) ambivalence about changing his drinking behavior, (c) marital distress resulting from poor communication skills and very little positive reinforcement within the relationship, and (d) depressed mood. With regard to the last, the diagnostic interview revealed that John's alcohol problem preceded his depressed mood, indicating that the depressed mood may be a consequence of his extensive drinking history and alcohol-related problems. The functional analysis revealed that both negative and positive emotional states frequently preceded drinking. Thus, the behavioral assessment revealed an interdependence between John's emotional states and his use of alcohol. Finally, heavy drinking also was more likely to occur in social pressure situations involving his friends.

The behavioral assessment also revealed that the quantity and frequency of John's drinking resulted in a number of negative consequences (e.g., marital arguments, hangovers, missed work) and that continued drinking increased his risk for developing future harmful consequences (e.g., health problems).

However, on the readiness to change scale, John indicated ambivalence about changing his drinking. As mentioned earlier, he was seeking treatment at this time because his wife had threatened to leave him if he did not seek help for his drinking. In this regard, seeking treatment was externally motivated, and the first target of treatment is his ambivalence regarding changing his drinking behavior. Toward this end, motivational interviewing strategies are used to increase his motivation for change. Early on, it is important for John to state the reasons for change, as behavior change is more likely to occur when it is the client rather than the therapist who gives voice to concerns. Therefore, in the early stages of treatment the therapist must clarify John's goals (e.g., remain with his children, increase pleasurable time with his wife) and explore how his present behavior conflicts with those goals. By creating a discrepancy between where he is and where he wants to be, motivation for change should increase. Increasing John's internal motivation for change also paves the way for addressing the additional treatment targets described next.

One set of treatment targets involves the stressful marital interactions between John and his wife. As he reported, marital interactions are characterized by blaming, defensiveness, avoidance, and few positive exchanges. Another set of treatment targets include his negative thoughts and feelings. For example, John reports thoughts of hopelessness regarding his ability to communicate more effectively with his wife. These negative thoughts often lead to negative feelings that are also a trigger for drinking. Therefore, the treatment also focuses on teaching him more effective skills for coping with these negative thoughts and feelings. Finally, John reported other high-risk situations for heavy drinking (e.g., pleasurable times with others), and he may benefit from learning a set of behavioral coping skills to help him avoid alcohol use in these situations.

Selection of Treatment Strategies

Many individuals suffering from alcohol problems benefit from treatment. However, no single treatment approach has been demonstrated to work for everyone. Therefore, how does the clinician choose from among a variety of treatment options for clients who present with a wide range of problems, many of which may be interrelated with their drinking problem? One approach involves patient–treatment matching. However, the results from Project MATCH (a large clinical trial investigating patient–treatment matching for alcoholics) indicate that patient–treatment matching does not increase the overall efficacy of treatment substantially. Another approach involves the therapist engaging the client in a process of informed decision making to evaluate the range of available treatment options. As treatment approaches vary widely in their demonstrated efficacy, it may be useful to begin by reviewing empirically supported approaches. It is important that this process be viewed as a partnership between client and therapist. Client involvement in treatment selection and goal setting can increase treatment engagement and commitment to change. In John's case, the following empirically supported treatment strategies were chosen for their ability to initiate behavior change and reduce problematic alcohol consumption: (a) motivational interviewing (Miller & Rollnick, 1991) to increase John's motivation to change his drinking, (b) behavioral couples therapy targeted at improving communication and conflict resolution skills (O'Farrell & Rotunda, 1997), and (c) cognitive–behavioral coping skills training to teach new skills for coping with high-risk drinking situations (Kadden et al., 1992).

Relapse, or the return to substance use, is common among the substance use disorders. Hunt, Barnett, and Branch (1971) reported 65% to 75% relapse rates (defined as any use of the abused substance) in the year following treatment for smokers, alcoholics, and heroin addicts. Furthermore, about two thirds of all relapses occurred within the first 90 days following treatment. Because alcoholism is often conceptualized as a chronic relapsing disorder, relapse prevention strategies also will be incorporated into John's treatment plan. Relapse prevention not only teaches people how to prevent a relapse, it also teaches them how to cope with a relapse should it occur. Marlatt and Gordon (1985) distinguish between a *lapse* (or *slip*) and a *full-blown relapse*. Given the high rates of lapses, John will be taught cognitive–behavioral strategies to cope with and prevent a lapse from turning into a relapse. Although Marlatt and Gordon (1985) developed relapse prevention into a treatment in and of itself, many of the core elements included in relapse prevention (e.g., cognitive restructuring, skills training, identification of high-risk situations) are also included in cognitive–behavioral treatment programs for substance use disorders.

Priority of Treatment Strategies

The first step in treatment is to increase John's engagement in treatment and his motivation to change his drinking behavior. Throughout the 1990s, there has been a shift in thinking about the motivation of individuals with alcohol problems. Previously, treatment failures often were attributed to the client's lack of motivation. However, motivation is currently thought to be the result of an interaction between the problem drinker and the therapist. In addition, motivation is not something that one has; rather, it is viewed as something one does. For example, a client may be viewed as motivated to the extent that he or she engages in behaviors that are consistent with changing a problem behavior (e.g., problem recognition, help seeking). This view of motivation allows the therapist to intervene to increase the client's motivation for change. Motivational Interviewing (MI) is based on principles of motivational psychology and is designed to increase an individual's level of intrinsic motivation to change a problem behavior.

In John's case, MI techniques were used during an initial assessment and feedback session with the goal of increasing his awareness of alcohol-related problems as well as his risk for future problems (e.g., health problems). An initial step in this process was to clarify his reason(s) for seeking treatment and increase his level of internal motivation for change relative to his level of external motivation (i.e., pressure from wife). Miller and Rollnick (1991) described five basic motivational principles underlying this approach: express empathy, develop discrepancy, avoid argumentation, roll with resistance, and support self-efficacy. These principles were used by the therapist to minimize client resistance and to evoke from John statements of problem recognition and a need for change. Following a discussion of the assessment results, which were presented by the therapist in a nonconfrontational manner reflective of MI, John recognized that his drinking was often the cause of marital arguments and that his use of alcohol was impeding his ability to achieve his stated goals (e.g., resolve marital conflict, increased intimacy with his wife). After weighing the pros and cons of change, he decided that abstinence from alcohol would be his treatment goal. It is important to note that the choice of treatment goal was John's and not the therapist's. Although the therapist provided John with a rationale for abstaining from alcohol, to impose this goal would have been inconsistent with the general style of MI. John could have decided to reduce his drinking, and the therapist would have supported that goal choice as well.

Although John reported pressure from his wife to seek help, it was important to first meet with him alone to clarify his reasons for seeking treatment (i.e., internal motivation) and strengthen his commitment to treatment. Also, during the initial sessions the therapist was creating an atmosphere of trust by providing support for John's treatment goals. The next step was to involve John's wife in treatment. Although at first hesitant to involve his spouse, exploring the pros and cons associated with his wife's involvement in treatment helped him reach a decision. It is important to note that if John remained ambivalent about spousal involvement, then the therapist would have continued to see John in individual sessions. The goals for the initial conjoint session were to gauge the level of spousal support, observe the couple's interactions directly, and to further enhance the motivational process established during the individual therapy sessions. During this session it was clear that John's wife was willing to participate in treatment and was supportive of his efforts to seek help for his drinking problem.

A series of conjoint sessions were prescribed to address the marital problems identified by John and his wife. The conjoint sessions would be scheduled weekly for the first 4 weeks to develop and implement the couples therapy program, and then once every 3 weeks thereafter to monitor their progress. Additional conjoint sessions could be scheduled if needed. Behavioral couples therapy (BCT), which targets relationship factors that can help achieve and maintain abstinence, was indicated because of the functional relationship between marital arguments and John's drinking behavior. BCT assumes that family members can reward abstinence and that alcoholics with healthier relationships have a lower risk of relapse. A cornerstone of BCT is the daily Sobriety Contract, in which John expressed his intention not to drink on a given day, and his wife provided support for his effort to remain abstinent. His wife then recorded John's daily performance on a calendar. Other sessions focused on increasing positive feelings, shared activities, and communication skills. For example, the couple decided to spend a portion of the money saved by not drinking on dinner and a movie one night per month. The overall goal was to increase positive interaction and help John and his wife cope more effectively with the stressors in their relationship and in their lives.

In between the conjoint sessions, John met individually with the therapist. During these sessions, cognitive–behavioral coping skills treatment was implemented to teach him several basic skills for coping with high-risk drinking situations. To help him learn the skills, role-plays were conducted during the treatment sessions and homework exercises were given that allowed him to apply these skills in his natural environment. There were 7 core sessions and 3 elective sessions, for a total of 10 individual sessions. The core sessions included an introduction to coping skills training, coping with urges and craving to drink, managing thoughts about alcohol and drinking, problem solving, drink refusal skills, planning for emergencies/coping with a lapse, and coping with seemingly irrelevant decisions. The three elective sessions included awareness of negative thinking, managing negative thinking, and managing negative moods. These elective sessions were chosen to help John cope with situations involving negative affect—situations identified by the behavioral assessment as posing a risk for heavy drinking.

Three months after beginning treatment, John came to his scheduled individual therapy session and reported that he had consumed two beers on the weekend. The situation he described was consistent with the results of the behavioral assessment, which indicated that John was at risk for drinking in response to situations involving social pressure. He was driving past the neighborhood bar and he saw his friend's car parked outside. He had not seen his friend in some time, and athough John had intended only to say hello, he was caught off guard when his friend purchased a beer for him. However, after drinking two beers, John began thinking about the negative consequences of continued drinking. In particular, thoughts about feeling depressed and losing his wife's support provided the deterrent against continued drinking. John and the therapist were able to use the drinking episode as an opportunity to discuss the difference between a lapse and a full-blown relapse. In addition, it was a good opportunity for John to learn more about the kinds of seemingly irrelevant thoughts and behaviors that culminate in a high-risk drinking situation.

Complicating Factors

There were two additional factors that warranted attention. First, John reported to the therapist that he experienced two episodes of erectile failure during the previous 2 years and that he worried about experiencing future episodes. As a result, John now reported feeling anxious prior to engaging in sexual intercourse with his wife, and worrisome thoughts were distracting him from focusing on more pleasurable sexual cues, therefore diminishing his sexual response. An assessment of the two episodes revealed that John had been drinking heavily on those days, and after ruling out other potential causal factors (e.g., hypertension, diabetes, smoking, heart disease), both episodes of erectile failure were attributed to acute alcohol intoxication. In the conjoint sessions, his wife reported that on both occasions she had "given in" to his sexual advances but had not been "in the mood" because of his intoxicated state; however, she indicated her desire to improve their sexual relations. To reduce his concerns, John was given education about male sexual response and the kind of physical and psychological factors that could affect this response. For the next few times they were intimate, John and his wife were instructed to take the focus off the act of sexual intercourse and instead to focus on merely pleasing each other. On the second attempt at intimacy, they reported engaging in sexual intercourse and felt very close to each other. From this point forward, no subsequent sexual problems were reported.

A second complicating factor was John's depressed mood. His score on the BDI–II indicated a moderate to severe level of clinical depression. However, the results of the diagnostic interview revealed that John did not meet diagnostic criteria for current or past history of major depression or dysthymia. Therefore, to avoid potentially costly and unnecessary treatment, and because the potential for harmful consequences was low (e.g., low suicide risk), his mood was monitored weekly to assess changes in his level of depression. In the majority of similar cases, the depressed mood decreases to a nonclinical level following a period of abstinence from alcohol (Brown & Schukit, 1988). One month after the initiation of treatment, John's depressed mood had decreased to a nonclinical level and remained stable throughout the remainder of the treatment.

Role of Pharmacotherapy in the Case

The use of antidipsotropic and psychotropic medications can be considered as adjuncts to behavioral treatment. Disulfiram (Antabuse) has a long history of use as deterrent medication. When taken with alcohol, it produces nausea, vomiting, dizziness, difficulty breathing, headache, flushing, and rapid heartbeat. It is administered orally on a daily basis, and the client cannot drink for 4–7 days following discontinuation of the medication. This delay often provides the individual with time to reconsider the decision to begin drinking. Naltrexone (Revia) is an orally administered opioid antagonist that has more recently been found to be effective for the treatment of alcohol problems. It decreases the craving for alcohol and produces lower relapse rates when added to psychosocial treatment for alcoholism. Medication can be used in the context of behavioral marital treatment in which the client's spouse or partner supervises the daily ingestion of the medication, thus rebuilding trust in the relationship because the spouse knows that the client is very unlikely to consume alcohol during that day.

The option to add these medications to John's current behavioral treatment was considered, and he was encouraged to meet with his physician to discuss the use of disulfiram or naltrexone as a part of his treatment program. However, he refused, stating that he would reconsider medication if he was having difficulty obtaining abstinence from alcohol.

Managed Care Considerations

Throughout the 1990s, managed care resulted in many changes in the field of treatment for alcoholism. The goal of these changes has been to provide briefer and less expensive interventions that have demonstrated efficacy for treating individuals with alcohol problems. Studies assessing the efficacy of a variety of treatments for alcoholism have found that less expensive treatments, such as brief motivational interventions, coping skills training, behavioral self-control training, behavioral couples therapy, and the community reinforcement approach, are more effective than higher cost treatments, such as residential milieu, chemical aversion therapy, and insight-oriented psychotherapy. As a result, most managed care companies have begun asking clinicians to describe the type of treatment that will be provided to the client.

With regard to the present case, John was enrolled in a managed health care plan through his employer. After a brief preapproval process, the therapist requested and was given a total of 24 sessions in which to complete the treatment. Most important is the fact that the interventions used during the course of treatment were empirically demonstrated and effective interventions with clearly defined treatment objectives and goals. Following 6 months of treatment, an outcome assessment (composed of several measures from the pretreatment assessment) indicated that, with the exception of one lapse, John had maintained abstinence from alcohol, was experiencing fewer negative consequences due to drinking (e.g., GGTP and MCV returned to normal levels), and had begun to achieve a more balanced lifestyle that included more time spent with his wife and children.

SUMMARY

This case illustrates the multiple factors involved in the assessment and treatment of alcohol dependence. These factors include mental and physical health, family history, antecedents and consequences of drinking, quantity and frequency of alcohol and other drug use, important relationships, and personal and social resources (e.g., coping skills, social support). These and other factors also account for the heterogeneity observed among individuals with alcohol dependence. Although the selection of a particular treatment strategy or set of strategies depends on the results of a comprehensive assessment, this case also demonstrated how a behavioral assessment can help simplify and organize complex clinical data in a meaningful way. For example, the assessment of antecedents and consequences of John's drinking behavior helped identify the functional relationship between negative affect and his drinking. Finally, this case also demonstrates the importance of conducting an assessment of the client's motivation to change. Clients entering treatment often express ambivalence about changing their drinking behavior, and this ambivalence may need to be explored before treatment options are discussed. Therapists who help their clients explore this ambivalence rather than immediately prescribing treatment are creating a more engaging treatment environment in which meaningful change is possible.

ACKNOWLEDGMENTS

Preparation of this manuscript was supported in part by Grant DA00311 from the National Institute on Drug Abuse and Grant AA12033 from the National Institute on Alcohol Abuse and Alcoholism.

REFERENCES

American Psychiatric Association. (1994). *Diagnostic and statistical manual of mental disorders–4th Ed.* Washington, DC: Author.

Annis, H. M., & Martin, G. (1985). *Inventory of drug-taking situations.* Toronto: Addiction Research Foundation of Ontario.

Beck, A. T., Steer, R. A., & Brown, G. K. (1996). *Beck Depression Inventory* (2nd ed.). San Antonio: Psychological Corp.

Brown, S. A., & Schuckit, M. A. (1988). Changes in depression among abstinent alcoholics. *Journal of Studies on Alcohol, 49,* 412–417.

First, M. B., Gibbon, M., Spitzer, R. L., & Williams, J. B. W. (1995). *User's guide for the structured clinical interview for DSM–IV Axis I disorders.* New York: Biometrics Research.

Hunt, W. A., Barnett, L. W., & Branch, L. G. (1971). Relapse rates in addiction programs. *Journal of Clinical Psychology, 27,* 455–456.

Kadden, R., Carroll, K., Donovan, D., Cooney, N., Monti, P., Abrams, D., Litt, M., & Hester, R. (1992). *Cognitive–behavioral coping skills therapy manual.* NIAAA Project MATCH monograph series. Washington, DC: Government Printing Office.

Marlatt, G. A., & Gordon, J. R. (1985). *Relapse prevention: Maintenance strategies in the treatment of addictive behaviors.* New York: Guilford Press.

Miller, W. R., & Rollnick, S. (1991). *Motivational interviewing.* New York: Guilford Press.

Miller, W. R., & Tonigan, S. (1996). Assessing drinkers' motivation for change: The Stages of Change Readiness and Treatment Eagerness Scale (SOCRATES). *Psychology of Addictive Behaviors, 10,* 81–89.

Miller, W. R., Tonigan, S., & Longabaugh R. (1995). *The Drinker Inventory of Consequences (DrinC): An instrument for assessing adverse consequences of alcohol abuse.* NIAAA Project MATCH monograph series. Washington, DC: Government Printing Office.

O'Farrell, T. J., & Fals-Stewart, W. (2000). Behavioral couples therapy for alcoholism and drug abuse. *Journal of Substance Abuse Treatment, 18,* 51–54.

O'Farrell, T. J., & Rotundo, R. J. (1997). Couples interventions and alcohol abuse. In: H. W. Kim, H. J. Markman (Eds.), *Couples interventions and alcohol abuse.* Chichester, England UK: John Wiley & Sons, Inc.

Raistrick, D., Dunbar, G., & Davidson, R. (1983). Development of a questionnaire to measure alcohol dependence. *British Journal of Addiction, 78,* 89–95.

Russell, M., Chan, A. K., & Mudar, P. (1997). Gender and screening for alcohol-related problems. In: R. W. Wilsnack & S. C. Wilsnack (Eds.), *Gender and alcohol: Individual and social perspectives* (pp. 417–444). New Brunswick, NJ: Rutgers Center of Alcohol Studies.

Sobell, L., & Sobell, M. (1992). Timeline Follow-back: A technique for assessing self-reported ethanol consumption. In: J. A. Allen & R. Z. Litten (Eds.), *Measuring alcohol consumption: Psychosocial and biological methods* (pp. 41–72). Totowa, NJ: Humana Press.

14

Sexual Dysfunction

Neil McConaghy
Visiting Professor, School of Psychiatry
University of New South Wales

DESCRIPTION OF THE DISORDER

The Diagnostic and Statistical Manual of Mental Disorders–4th Ed. (*DSM–IV*; American Psychiatric Association, 1994) describes *sexual dysfunctions* as being characterized by disturbance in sexual desire and the psychophysiological changes that characterize the sexual response cycle, causing marked distress and interpersonal difficulty. It presents criteria for seven categories. Sexual Desire Disorders include *Hypoactive Sexual Desire Disorder*, which is defined as deficient (or absent) sexual fantasies and desire for sexual activity; and *Sexual Aversion Disorder*, which is defined as extreme aversion to and avoidance of all (or almost all) genital sexual contact with a partner. Interpreted literally, this *DSM–IV* diagnosis could not be used for the condition of women who accept genital contact but have an aversion to their breasts being fondled or touching their partner's genitals. Sexual Arousal Disorders include *Female Sexual Arousal Disorder*, which is defined as the inability to attain or maintain an adequate genital lubrication–swelling response of sexual excitement until completion of the sexual activity; and *Male Erectile Disorder*, which is defined as the inability to attain or maintain an adequate erection until completion of the sexual activity.

Orgasmic Disorders include Female and Male Orgasmic Disorders and Premature Ejaculation. *Female Orgasmic Disorder* is delay or absence of orgasm following a normal sexual excitement phase. The diagnostic criteria point out that women vary widely in the type or intensity of stimulation that triggers orgasm, and that the diagnosis should be based on the clinician's judgment that the woman's orgasmic capacity is less than would be reasonable for her age, sexual experience, and the adequacy of sexual stimulation she receives. *Male Orgasmic Disorder* is delay or absence of orgasm following a normal sexual excitement phase during sexual activity, which the clinician, when taking into account the person's age, judges to be adequate in focus, intensity, and duration. Orgasmic disorder in men is commonly an inability to reach orgasm by ejaculation in the vagina, orgasm being possible with other types of stimulation. The *DSM–IV* criteria for *Premature Ejaculation* include ejaculation with minimal sexual stimulation before, on, or shortly after penetration and before the person wishes it. The clinician must take into account factors that affect duration of the excitement phase, such as age, novelty of the sexual partner or situation, and recent frequency of sexual activity. The fourth category of dysfunctions, Sexual Pain Disorders, includes *Dyspareunia*, genital pain associated with sexual intercourse in either a male or a female; and *Vaginismus*, involuntary spasm of the musculature of the outer third of the vagina that interferes with sexual intercourse. Vaginismus usually prevents penetration of any object greater than a certain size into the vagina, including the subject's finger or a tampon. If intercourse is attempted, vaginismus is commonly accompanied by spasm of the adductor muscles of the thighs, preventing their separation; however, it does not prevent women experiencing sexual arousal and orgasm with activities other than coitus.

To receive the diagnosis of sexual dysfuntion, the *DSM–IV* Criterion A requires that the condition is recurrent or persistent, and Criterion B requires that the disturbance cause marked distress or interpersonal difficulty. Criterion B presumably allows absence of orgasmic capacity to be considered not a dysfunction in at least some of the people who report that they enjoyed intercourse very much, although they did not reach orgasm. This has been investigated and commonly found in surveys of women (McConaghy, 1993). Its occurrence in men has attracted less interest, presumably reflecting general acceptance that males reach orgasm readily in sexual activity. In a large representative British population sample age 16–59, 50% of women and 35% of men disagreed with the statement that sex without orgasm or climax cannot be really satisfying. An earlier study of a representative U.S. adolescent sample found that of those who reported having masturbated in the previous month, 74% of girls and 21% of boys had done so without orgasm. It was not reported how many if any were distressed concerning this.

Criterion C for sexual dysfunction is that it does not occur exclusively during or is not better accounted for by another Axis 1 disorder and is not due exclusively to the direct physiological effect of a substance or a general medical condition. These dysfunctions are classified separately. Diseases associated with pain or that result in debility, anxiety, or depression may impair sexual desire, arousal, and orgasm, as may a wide range of medications and drugs of abuse. These include antihypertensive agents, diuretics, vasodilators, and psychiatric and anticonvulsant drugs (Schiavi & Segraves, 1995). The effects of neurologic and vascular disease on women's sexuality are more poorly documented than the effects on men. The final category, *Sexual Dysfunction Not Otherwise Specified*, includes substantially diminished or no subjective erotic feelings despite otherwise normal arousal and orgasm, and sexual dysfunctions that the clinician cannot determine are primary, due to a general medical condition, or are substance induced.

Apart from the issues left to the judgment of the clinician specified by the *DSM–IV* criteria for the three orgasmic disorders, it is pointed out that diagnosis of sexual arousal disorders is not appropriate in women or men if the problems in arousal are due to sexual stimulation that is not adequate in focus, intensity, and duration. It is also stated that older males may require more stimulation or take longer to achieve a full erection. As no operationally defined criteria are provided for the clinician's judgment of these issues, reliability of the diagnoses made by different clinicians using *DSM–IV* definitions is unlikely to be high. Lack of such criteria is probably the major reason *DSM* diagnoses are rarely used in studies of sexual dysfunctions. Some researchers have developed individual criteria (McConaghy, 1996). Anorgasmia was diagnosed in women if they report that orgasm resulted from 5% or less of all sexual activities with their partners, and premature ejaculation was diagnosed in men who estimated ejaculation latencies of 2 min or less on at least 50% of intercourse occasions as well as perceiving a lack of control over the onset of orgasm.

A further limitation of the *DSM–IV* descriptions of sexual dysfunction results from their derivation from the medical model. They ignore sexual difficulties shown in both surveys of healthy couples and persons presenting with lack of sexual satisfaction to be more common and more strongly related to lack of such satisfaction than *DSM–IV*-defined dysfunctions (McConaghy, 1993). In women, these difficulties included inability to relax, too little foreplay before intercourse, and disinterest; in men, the difficulties were more likely to be attraction to persons other than their spouses, too little foreplay before intercourse, and too little tenderness after intercourse; and both sexes reported the partner choosing an inconvenient time, the partner's lack of response to sexual requests, and frequency of intercourse being too low. The nature of sexual difficulties suggests that they result mainly from couples' poor communication or in appropriate resolution of conflict concerning their sexual wishes and needs.

METHODS TO DETERMINE DIAGNOSIS

The major method to determine diagnosis of sexual dysfunctions and difficulties remains the unstructured interview. Its flexibility, lacking in the structured interview, provides several advantages. It enables the therapist to frame questions so that they are understandable and acceptable to the clients, taking into account their education, value systems, and personalities. If, when investigating the presenting sexual problem, the therapist gains the impression that it is secondary to more generalized emotional and relationship difficulties, these can be explored as they may require priority in treatment. The unstructured interview allows for the specific inquiries necessary to establish the presence of sexual dysfunctions and difficulties in clients who do not report them spontaneously. Several studies established that such clients make up the majority of clients with these conditions (McConaghy, 1993). Their reluctance to report their sexual dysfunctions is (it is hoped unconsciously) conspired with by many therapists. A 1990 report of the Department of Health and Human Services cited studies indicating that only 11–37% of primary care physicians took a sexual history routinely from new clients. It was considered that many psychiatrists (and presumably psychologists) were ill at ease with taking an explicit sexual history (McConaghy, 1998). If clients show signs of guilt, embarrassment, or reluctance to talk when particular topics are introduced, as of course is common with the investigation of their sexual attitudes and behaviors, in an unstructured interview the therapist can respond with encouragement and support, and so elicit crucial information that may not be obtained using more structured assessments. Clients are unlikely to reveal such information unless the therapist establishes a relationship of trust so that they are confident that this information will not be disclosed, deliberately or inadvertently, without their permission. The flexibility of the unstructured interview is virtually essential when assessing clients with some degree of impairment, such as developmental delay, schizophrenia, depression, or brain damage, conditions that can render them unmotivated or unable to complete self-rating scales or questionnaires.

The unstructured interview also allows investigation of the possible presence of personality disorders in clients, identification of which is of major importance in determining the outcome of therapy of sexual disorders (McConaghy, 1993). Such disorders as psychopathy, borderline personality, and dependency markedly influence clients' ability or willingness to provide accurate information, motivation to change their behaviors, or the nature of the relationship they attempt to establish with the therapist. If this relationship is handled inappropriately, lack of compliance with or major disruption of the treatment plan can result, so that the client is not helped or may even be harmed, and the therapist may also suffer considerable distress. Less experienced therapists must monitor their own responses to the client, in particular for indications of overinvolvement and loss of objectivity produced by the client's unconscious manipulation. This could result, for example, from the client combining a recital of tragic life events with expression of intense admiration and gratitude, possibly tinged with sexual seductiveness, at the uniqueness of the therapist's interest and concern, which the client claims enables the therapist to elicit information never divulged previously.

When clients are in a relationship, one client usually identifies as the person seeking treatment. If so, he or she is interviewed initially without the partner, but with the expectation that the partner will be interviewed subsequently both alone and with the client. It may be necessary to emphasize the value of this procedure if the presenting client or the partner resists it on the grounds that the presenting client is the only one with a problem. It may eventuate that the partner who does not identify as needing help is the one most in need, although of course, he or she may not accept this. Only after assessing a woman's interaction with her partner may it become apparent her complaint of failing to reach orgasm during intercourse does not reflect her dissatisfaction, but that of her partner. At times, partners present as having a joint problem. It is then my practice to interview them jointly initially, although it is likely that at some stage it becomes appropriate to interview them singly as well. When it is suspected that clients not in a relationship have a significant personality disorder, it is essential that attempts be made to corroborate their history by interviewing relatives and contacts. Psychopathic and borderline clients may try to prevent this, saying, for example, that they dislike their relatives too much to allow any contact. If it appears sufficiently relevant, it may be necessary to make treatment conditional on their giving permission for such interviews.

Therapists usually initiate the interview by asking clients why they have sought help, and then adopt a nondirective listening approach, asking a minimum of questions and responding only as much as is necessary to maintain the flow of information within reasonable limits of relevance. This gives clients the opportunity to take charge of the interview temporarily, so that such aspects of client's personality as their confidence, verbal ability, assertiveness, and dominance can be assessed. This stage of the interview provides the initial information for determining why they want help and the likelihood of their cooperating with treatment. Once these assessments are made, the therapist then becomes more directive in questioning to obtain the additional information necessary to establish the global diagnosis of the client's condition. Therapists more strongly influenced by traditional behavioral assessment seek detailed information concerning the nature of the client's problematic behaviors and the specific stimulus situations in which they occur. Therapists trained in traditional psychiatric assessment enquire concerning any history of similar problems, other illnesses, previous treatment, childhood and adolescent relationships with parents and siblings, social and sexual relationships, and practices, including coercive sexual acts carried out or experienced; history of contraceptive use (where appropriate); sexual fantasies; educational and work history; and current domestic, social, sexual, and occupational situations. The nature and extent of recreational interests and activities and use of recreational drugs, including alcohol and tobacco, and medications, is determined. The possibility of memory or intellectual impairment may require specific investigation. Severity of depression requires assessment if there is evidence of this affect, which include reduced enjoyment of life events or of appetite or sleep disturbance.

Assessment of the presenting client and partner's relationship is commonly made from observation of the couple's interaction in the joint interview, interpreted in the light of both partners' account of their present and previous relationships. In addition to verbal expressions indicative of affection or hostility, or indeed of both, the couple's body language, including supportive touching, usually gives the interviewer insight into the nature of their relationship. In view of the importance of couples' communication of their sexual interest and needs, they should be questioned concerning this. Establishing the likelihood of accuracy of the information obtained in an unstructured clinical interview is dependent on the therapist's ability to assess correctly to what extent the client's self-report can be accepted without modification and to what extent it should be regarded as distorted and in need of further confirmation. Assessment of the client's personality is of value in this regard. The attention-seeking client is likely to exaggerate and the psychopathic client is likely to lie concerning their symptoms, whereas the depressed client or the client with high ethical standards commonly associated with obsessional features may present their symptoms in a manner reflecting poorly on themselves.

Because it provides the clients' final impression, the nature of the termination of the initial interview is of major importance in establishing their acceptance of the therapist's understanding and ability; therefore, it requires careful planning, and adequate time must be set aside for this. Clients should not leave feeling they have been asked a lot of questions or been allowed to talk freely but have been given no answers. It is my practice at this stage to present the client with either a treatment plan or an explanation as to why I require further information or laboratory investigations before this can be done. When a treatment plan is proposed, the therapist should ensure that clients are fully aware of what it entails, including its likely cost, and why it has been chosen over other treatments. Any reservations clients have concerning the plan should be dealt with fully, so that following its discussion they can commit themselves either to accepting the plan or to making a decision concerning this in the near future, possibly in consultation with the person who referred them.

ADDITIONAL ASSESSMENTS REQUIRED

Structured interviews, behavioral inventories, and questionnaires or dairies completed by the client are widely used in research studies because they can provide specific and extensive information collected in the same manner at minimal cost. Wincze and Carey (1991) pointed out that they are used infrequently in clinical practice, as in this situation they are time consuming, inconvenient, and of limited clinical utility because many of the available procedures were developed for specific purposes in research studies. Nevertheless, they reported that in assessing patients with sexual dysfunctions they used a number of self-report questionnaires, including the Sexual Interaction Inventory and the Derogatis Sexual Functioning Index, and suggested sources of other measures that could be useful. (One of these, the compendium of Davis et al., 1998, was recently updated.) A detailed criticism of the methodology, reliability, and validity of the research use of these assessments for sexual dysfunctions is provided elsewhere (McConaghy, 1998).

Observation of clients' nonverbal behaviors is an important component in assessment by unstructured clinical interview. LoPiccolo (1990) pointed out that observations of sexual behaviors, either directly or by videotape (including the *sexological exam*, in which sex therapists stimulated the breasts and genitals of the opposite sex partner to assess and demonstrate physiological responsiveness), were briefly popular in the more permissive climate of the 1970s. LoPiccolo argued against the use of such procedures, considering that the effect of observation would make it unlikely that the subjects' observed behaviors would be similar to their private behaviors, that the procedure would be unacceptable to the majority of couples, and that it allowed the exploitation of clients by therapists. It would seem possible to provide adequate ethical safeguards to investigate the value of videotaped observational assessment of couples' sexual interactions, and with the use of preliminary sessions to allow the couples to adjust to the procedure, their observed behavior could be sufficiently related to their private behavior to provide information of value. This is accepted to be the case with the observational assessment of nonsexual behaviors such as phobias; however, in the current climate of opinion, use of such assessment remains unlikely. Determination by surrogate sex therapists of the sexual activity, including erectile function of clients, particularly of value in single clients with distorted perceptions of their sexual ability, is also no longer possible with the current rejection of surrogate therapy. Observational and physical determination of erectile adequancy remains acceptable as part of the much more expensive nocturnal penile tumescence assessment and the examination of the erection produced by intracavernosal injection of prostaglandin E1 or other substances (McConaghy, 1998).

Erectile disorder, hypoactive sexual desire, and sexual pain disorders are the sexual dysfunctions for which possible organic causes are sought by physical examination and laboratory assessments. They are required for men with hypoactive sexual desire and in men whose erectile disorder is not situational. *Situational erectile disorder* is that occurring with some but not other partners, or with all partners but not in private masturbation, where no pressure to produce an erection is experienced. Physical examination is indicated to exclude certain physical conditions, such as hypertension, Peyronie disease, and hypogonadism; and blood and urine screening is used to exclude hyperlipidemia, diabetes, hyperprolactinemia (raised level of the pituitary hormone prolactin), and thyroid dysfunction. The level of testosterone to maintain erectile function is markedly below that necessary to maintain sexual interest (McConaghy, 1993), consistent with the finding that levels in men with erectile dysfunction younger than age 50 years are almost invariably in the normal range in the absence of signs of hypogonadism. These signs include loss of libido, physical signs of regression of male hair pattern, gynecomastia (increased breast development), or small, soft testes. Although reduction of bioavailable testosterone was found in about 40% of men older than 50, there was no relation between the reduction and erectile disorder (McConaghy, 1998). Nevertheless, determination of testosterone levels is usually recommended in men with nonsituational erectile disorder and hypoactive sexual desire who do not show physical signs of hypogonadism.

Of the more expensive laboratory investigations, assessment of clients' nocturnal penile tumescence (NPT) has received most attention by sex therapists. Wincze and Carey (1991), state that it has been considered the gold standard of differential diagnosis in erectile dysfunction. At the same time, they point out it is well beyond the financial means of most clients, and there are much more affordable and perhaps more valid psychophysiologic measures. Its use was justified mainly on the basis that it could distinguish psychogenic from organic impotence, although studies in which the two conditions were diagnosed by criteria independent of the NPT measurements to support this belief were never carried out. Extensive evidence of its failure to accurately make the distinction has been advanced. Also, it seems likely different neurophysiologic mechanisms may be involved in the production of NPT and erections in sexual situations (McConaghy, 1998). The current acceptance that erectile dysfunction usually results from an interaction of both psychogenic and organic factors (Althof & Seftel, 1995) may reduce interest in the assessment; however, it is likely to remain a requirement for legal purposes in clients complaining of erectile disorder secondary to compensatable accidents or injuries.

In men who fail to maintain an erection adequate for penetration when under no pressure to perform (i.e., during private masturbation or on awakening), adequacy of penile blood flow requires assessment. This is probably still most commonly done by determination of the penile–brachial index (PBI), the ratio of the blood pressure in the penile arteries, originally measured by Doppler ultrasound probe, and conventionally measured blood pressure in the brachial artery in the arm. It is generally stated that arterial insufficiency is very likely to be the cause of the impotence of subjects with a PBI of less than 0.6, but that a higher ratio does not exclude the possibility, although a PBI of greater than 0.9 should indicate sufficient perfusion to maintain erection. Increasingly, the pharmacologic erection test is used to assess the penile vascular supply. Vasodilating chemicals (papaverine, alone or with phentolamine, prostaglandin E1 alone, or a mixture of all three) are injected into one of the cavernous sinuses of the client's penis. Development of a rigid, well-sustained erection within

10 minutes suggests no major vascular abnormality exists. Development of the erection may be recorded using a Rigiscan; a slow onset suggests the presence of some degree of arterial disease, and rapid detumescence suggests a venous leak. If the client does not develop an adequate erection following the injection, he may with masturbation or viewing an erotic video. Of course, his acceptance of these procedures must be established. Other men who find the test situation stressful may develop a full erection after leaving it. Many men with erectile dysfunction who are in otherwise good health may be prescribed sildenafil citrate (Viagra) by their general practitioner and maintained on it if they develop a satisfactory erection with its use without undergoing further investigation or psychological assessment.

When the pharmacologic erection test indicates the presence of significant vascular pathology, further investigation is required if determination of its nature is necessary. Althof and Seftel (1995) considered these investigations would be reserved for subjects in whom vascular reconstructive surgery was being considered or who wished to further understand the cause of their dysfunction. These investigations include duplex Doppler color ultrasonography and penile cavernosography. As the introduction and continuing development of such tests requires increasingly expensive equipment and considerable experience in interpretation, the investigation of vascular causes for impotence is being taken over by urologists with an interest in the treatment of erectile disorder.

Neurogenic impotence is usually recognized from the client's history and physical examination. Diabetes, pelvic pathology, radical prostatectomy, the absence of the cremasteric or bulbocavernosal reflex, and reduced lower limb reflexes are major indicators. Simple screening with a vibratory biothesiometer is considered useful, but not necessarily the more complex procedures developed to investigate impairment of nerve transmission, such as the latency of bulbocavernous reflex and the latency and form of cerebral potentials evoked by stimulation of the glans penis and the peroneal nerve. These procedures assess the afferent somatic pathway of the pudendal nerve, but do not evaluate the autonomic control of penile tumescence.

Physical and laboratory examination of women with sexual dysfunctions are more rarely carried out, although as in men, the possibility that illness, medication, or a substance is responsible for producing reduced sexual interest or ability to reach orgasm must be excluded. Gynecologic investigation is indicated when dyspareunia is present. Vaginal lesions, dermatitis, or infections are likely to be associated with pain on penetration, and inflammation or disease of the pelvic organs is associated with pain on deep penile thrusting. Hormone studies are rarely included in the routine investigation of sexually dysfunctional women in the absence of indications of hormonal imbalance, such as excessive hirsutism. The nature and significance of the influence of hormonal factors on the sexual interest and activity of women remains unestablished (McConaghy,

1993). There appears to be general agreement that the menopausal symptoms, including hot flashes and atrophic vaginitis that follow oophorectomy, are accompanied by reduced sexual interest and activity. Evidence is inconclusive concerning whether reduction is due to direct effects of hormones on the central nervous system or is secondary to the hot flashes and atrophic vaginitis. The severity of the latter both in these and menopausal and postmenopausal women requires investigation. Women's physiological arousal to erotic stimuli continues to be studied by assessment of vaginal, clitoral, or labial blood flow changes, measured either by the associated temperature changes using a thermistor or vaginal color changes using a photoplethysmograph. Clitoral responses have also been measured by use of a strain gauge. Clinical use of these assessments has been limited due to lack of consistent findings differentiating sexually functional and dysfunctional women (McConaghy, 1996).

CASE ILLUSTRATION

Presenting Complaint

Mr. B. D., age 44 years, reported he "was worried about the sexual side of getting into a relationship."

History of the Disorder

Mr. D.'s sexual disorder commenced when he was age 15, with reluctance to have any physical contact with any girlfriends because severe acne affecting his back made him feel dirty. When it improved in his early 20s, his attempts at intercourse were associated with feelings of inadequacy in relation to sexual technique and premature ejaculation. These problems persisted and were associated with the belief that in sexual activity, his aim should be to give pleasure to a partner rather than to himself. As a result, he continued to avoid intimate sexual activity. Three years prior to his seeing me, he attempted suicide by taking sleeping tablets with a bottle of wine, but woke the next morning.

Medical History

Mr. D. reported his physical health was good and was reviewed regularly by his general practitioner. His current alcohol intake was (on average) 750 ml of light beer and 750 ml of wine per day. I pointed out that this was a level likely to damage his physical and/or mental health and inquired whether he had recently had his liver function tested. He had not and agreed to the procedure. He was currently taking 375 mg of venlafaxine every morning, but did not think this medication had any effect on his sexual interest or ability.

Family History

Mr. D.'s mother, age 78, was in good physical health and continued to play tennis. His father, age 82, had a cardiac bypass operation 3 months previously but recovered well. They lived overseas, but he visited them regularly. He had two sisters, 3 and 7 years older. They were both well physically and were married with children. They lived outside the city where he lived, but came with their families to stay in his house frequently. He considered that his childhood was happy, and felt loved by his parents but not really close to them. They were emotionally nondemonstrative, and he did not feel that he could discuss his emotional problems with either of his parents or his sisters.

Sexual History

During his teenage years, Mr. D failed to commence any physical sexual activity with girlfriends, believing that they would find contact with the acne on his back disgusting. He used to commence friendly relationships with some girls who he felt were interested in being involved with him. When he did not commence any physical activity, he believed the girls soon lost interest in him. Following improvement in the acne, when he was 20 he attempted to have sex with a girl he considered sexually experienced, but felt sexually inadequate with her because he ejaculated prematurely, and she became angry because she had wanted him to withdraw prior to ejaculation. Following this, he would not allow relationships with women to develop sexually. If they showed signs of doing so, he would withdraw from them because he felt he was inexperienced sexually and "would be useless." His alcohol consumption increased over time, and occasionally while under its influence he had intercourse with women with whom he had had developed a friendly relationship. He believed that he "did not know what he was doing," and that neither his partner nor he enjoyed the experience. He believed he had no control over ejaculation, which would occur "in a minute, if that." He was aware that he was anxious about his performance on the few occasions he attempted intercourse. In answer to specific questions, he thought the time the average man took to ejaculate was 10 to 15 minutes. In private masturbation he would ejaculate in 1 to 5 minutes, and at times his erection would not be adequate for penetration. He added it would be firmest when he woke during the night or in the morning.

Asked about any relationships in which he felt strongly involved, he reported one several years previously. He said he had become very friendly with a woman for a few months and became "really fond of her." They had intercourse, but after a few days she told him she had subsequently had intercourse with an ex-boyfriend. He is still friendly with her, adding that she was now married with two children. His last relationship apart from the commercial ones (discussed later) was the longest. It lasted 3 years, until 3 years previously. It was with a married woman whom he said pursued him where he worked. He slept with her a number of times, and added that he was not very good at intercourse; either he lost his erection before penetration or ejaculated too quickly, and she seemed to satisfy herself by rubbing against him. This was the only relationship in which he talked to his partner about his concerns regarding his sexual ability. She would always say he was an adequate lover. He added that he knew she had quite a high libido and was in a domestic violence situation, and he felt she reassured him about his sexual ability in the hope of marriage. He never enjoyed the sex, "and it was adultery." At the end of the relationship they were meeting only every 6 months. She subsequently remarried and he remained friendly with her and her present husband. His suicide attempt took place a few months after the last sexual encounter with the married woman, but he did not consider the events related. Some months following the suicide attempt, he attempted to improve his sexual competence by having sex with a prostitute. He found he did not enjoy the sex, but did enjoy talking to her. He continued to visit her at least three times a week, not having sex after the first week. This continued for about 6 months, during which time he paid more than $30,000. He added that he was lonely and she helped him through a bad time. She was currently overseas and they corresponded by email. In the previous year he had visited other prostitutes. The encounters usually ended with him talking to them, without having sex. He added, "It feels as if you're forcing yourself on someone." He had also been to sex workers who gave massage followed by masturbation, but "at the end of the day you still feel dirty and guilty." Asked about these feelings, he said they resulted from his paying for the sex and not the sex itself. He said that currently there was not any woman with whom he had any involvement, but later in the interview he said he had recently met a girl who was interested in him, but that on a physical level she did not "ring any bells." He added that he would rather not get involved because if he decided not to continue the relationship, he would be upset at rejecting her. He had not kissed her, even on the cheek, and had not kissed anyone in a long time.

Asked about his level of sexual interest, he said he believed that he had a high libido. Frequency of his masturbation varied from two to three times a day to once every 3 weeks. It had been about four times a week in the previous few months. He did not use any erotic material, but fantasized about foreplay and penetrative sex with women. In reply to questioning, he stated he had never had sexual fantasies or experiences with males and did not believe he had any feelings of sexual attraction toward males. Asked about his enjoyment of sexual activity, he said he enjoyed foreplay and giving oral sex, adding, "I enjoy giving the woman pleasure rather than myself."

Mental Status Examination

In the light of Mr. D.'s academic and employment record and his verbal ability in recounting his history, it was apparent that he had no memory impairment and was of superior intelligence. There was no evidence of thought disorder. His low self-esteem was apparent from his history, but during the interview his affect was at a normal level and he expressed amusement appropriately. It was not considered necessary to conduct a more specific mental state examination.

Prior Treatment

Mr. D. had not sought treatment prior to his suicide attempt 3 years previously. When he informed his general practitioner of the attempt, he was referred to a psychiatrist who was recently qualified. He related to her well, but after several visits she said she felt she was not sufficiently experienced to help with his problem and referred him to a second (male) psychiatrist to whom he could not relate, and after a few consultations he ceased attending. Eighteen months previously he commenced attending a third (male) psychiatrist who prescribed antidepressant medication, initially nefazodone and currently venlafaxine. More recently, the psychiatrist had recommended that he seek a partner by placing an entry in a personal column in a magazine. He received about 50 replies, but after meeting 3 women whom he did not find attractive, he felt too distressed at rejecting them to contact any more. The psychiatrist then referred him to me for assistance in dealing with his sexual problem. In the referring letter, the psychiatrist stated that he believed the major problems to be an anxious and avoidant personality, excessive intake of alcohol, and that "Mr. D.'s ambition is to settle down into a relationship and have children. It is around this issue that his anxiety becomes particularly manifest." He added that Mr. D. still had recurrent thoughts of suicide.

CASE CONCEPTUALIZATION

Modeling and Learning

Mr. D.'s belief in adolescence that he was sexually unattractive due to the presence of severe acne resulted at least in part from his learned incorporation of the prevalent social model of attractiveness. This model is enhanced by advertisements directed at adolescents about the need for treatment of such conditions as acne if they are to be successful in their social and sexual relationships. Modeling of his family's lack of communication concerning emotional problems is likely to have contributed to his failure to reveal his concerns about his unattractiveness, and so obtain help for these.

Life Events

Mr. D. reported that at school he was large for his age and was captain of the rugby team. Consistent with this, he was socially confident and mixed well with his fellow pupils at his all-boy school. However, he mentioned that his acne led to his being embarrassed when there was blood on his jersey following playing rugby and when it could be seen when he wore a singlet while rowing. This indicated the strength of the effect of his acne in that it prevented any generalization of his social confidence to enhance his confidence in sexual relationships. Subsequently, Mr. D. attended the university and obtained a degree in law. He believed that he did not enjoy his studies but "treated them as a job." Even though he continued sports and did well at rugby, he believed he was never "one of the boys" and did not have any close friends, reflecting the persistence of his inability to communicate emotional feelings. After leaving the university, he traveled overseas and for 5 years was involved in professional rugby. Through his connections in this sport, he obtained a position in the financial market involving continuous buying and selling of money. This work was exciting and well paid but highly stressful, commencing at 5 or 6 AM and finishing at 8 or 9 PM. Following work, he would go out drinking with work colleagues. When he returned to Australia, he maintained this work and drinking pattern until 3 years previously, when he traveled overseas for a few months. After returning, he worked part-time until 2 years previously, when he ceased working. At the time he commenced treatment, he was completing a higher degree in environmental law, which involved studying and writing papers 10 hours daily, including weekends. He added that he had people, friends, or family staying with him in his house for 6 months or more, suggesting that he was not socially isolated. Yet he said he often felt lonely even when these people were staying. He maintained a good exercise regime, running and going to a gym three times a week. He had reduced his alcohol intake significantly, but it was still at a level that could be potentially harmful. He ceased smoking tobacco at age 32 and did not use illicit substances.

Genetics and Temperament

The major contributions of genetics and temperament would appear to be to Mr. D.'s inability to analyze and communicate his feelings and value his own needs in comparison to the needs of other people. He considered his failure to value his needs applied only to potential sexual partners, not to friends and relatives. He did not feel they exploited his generosity in accepting the use of his house for prolonged periods. This might require exploration at a later stage.

Physical Conditions

The major effect of his acne in adolescence on Mr. D.'s psychological development has been discussed previously. His experience early in his sexual development of a partner responding angrily to his premature ejaculation, believed to commonly have a physical basis (McConaghy, 1993), was another major influence, as was his subsequent erectile difficulty, which requires investigation to determine if there is a physical contribution to its etiology.

Drugs

Mr. D.'s previous excessive alcohol intake allowed him to avoid developing meaningful sexual relationships while reducing his distress concerning this avoidance. His attempts at sexual activity made under its influence were not only emotionally unsatisfying, they were also not associated with any discussion of his anxiety about such activity with his partner. Such discussion might have enabled him to overcome this anxiety. He was currently taking venlafaxine, which was effective in reducing his depression. Increase in ejaculatory latency has been reported regularly following intake of clomipramine and sertraline, a response attributed to their inhibiting the reuptake of serotonin. This property is shared by venlafaxine, so this drug may also increase ejaculatory latency, although so far this has not been reported consistently. Mr. D. had not attempted intercourse since he commenced the drug, and had not noticed any change in latency with masturbation.

Socioeconomic and Cultural Factors

The increasing emphasis that women should enjoy sexual activity that has accompanied acceptance of feminist ideology may have contributed to Mr. D.'s focus on giving pleasure to his partner rather than himself in sexual activity. His middle-class upbringing may also have been a factor, because (at least in the past) membership in the middle class as opposed to the working class has been associated with greater emphasis on the fact that men should give pleasure to women in sexual activity, and particularly in foreplay.

Overall Conceptualization

Mr. D.'s inability to value his emotional needs as equivalent to the needs of others in the area of sexual acitivity, and possibly more generally, was seen as the major source of his failure to establish a satisfying sexual relationship. This failure appeared to be the source of his depression leading to his earlier suicidal attempt. Achievement of such a relationship was seen as the major goal of therapy.

Diagnostic Assessment

Mr. D.'s referring psychiatrist believed that the major problem was his anxious and avoidant personality, raising the issue of whether his avoidance of sexual activity was due to this personality disorder. If this were the case, anxiety and avoidance should be apparent in other areas of his life. His educational and work history, involvement in sports, and his social activities indicate that this was not the case. Premature ejaculation and erectile disorder were appropriate diagnoses in view of the persistence and distress caused by both conditions. His intake of alcohol was above the range generally recommended, the upper limit of which is usually four standard drinks a day. The diagnosis of alcohol abuse is therefore appropriate. His suicidal attempt and periodic wishes to repeat the attempt despite his taking antidepressant medication indicated the persistence of an affective disorder. However, what appeared to be the problem central to his inability to form a sexual relationship, the complaint that appeared responsible for his depression and for which he sought treatment, was his inability to accept that meeting his own needs should be given equal value with meeting the needs of his sexual partner. This has not, to my knowledge, attracted a diagnostic label.

Behavioral Assessment

The only behavioral assessment was that of observing Mr. D.'s style of verbal and nonverbal communication in the nonstructured interview. He presented as confident and able to discuss all issues raised without anxiety or embarrassment and with a warm affect.

Prioritization of Targets for Treatment

As Mr. D.'s inability to value his own needs in relation to those of a potential sexual partner was seen as resulting in his inability to establish a relationship (his primary complaint), this inability was awarded the highest priority in treatment. His sexual dysfunctions of premature ejaculation and erectile dysfunction would require investigation and treatment either once he commenced a relationship or prior to this if his concerns about these conditions appeared to be inhibiting him from initiating a relationship that could result in him and his partner having sexual intercourse. Reduction of his alcohol intake to an acceptable level would require attention throughout treatment, as would monitoring the level of his depression. Such monitoring would aim at determining whether the nature and level of antidepressant medication was appropriate, and if it required augmentation with a cognitive–behavioral approach directed specifically at depression.

Selection of Treatment Strategies

A variety of cognitive–behavioral techniques would be used to change Mr. D.'s beliefs and attitudes and treat his sexual dysfunctions, as well as his depression if it did not remit with improvement in his ability to form pleasurable sexual relationships. If his sexual dysfunctions prevented him from forming a sexual relationship and investigation shows an organic determinant for the erectile dysfunction, use of sildenafil citrate (Viagra), intracavernosal injection of prostaglandin E1 or other substances, or an external vacuum device could be recommended. Alternatively, if considered appropriate, a penile implant or vascular surgery could be considered. In the absence of a demonstrated significant organic cause, if his erectile dysfunction failed to respond to cognitive–behavioral techniques, a trial of sildenafil citrate or intracavernous injections would be indicated. Failure of his premature ejaculation to respond to cognitive–behavioral techniques would be an indication to consider use of clomipramine or sertraline, either as alternatives to venlafaxine if he were still taking it, or prior to sexual activity if he was not. As discussed earlier, both medications have been consistently reported to increase ejaculatory latency. In reporting this response to clomipramine, Althof (1995) considered the drug was as effective if taken 4 hours before intercourse as if it were taken regularly. He found its effect did not persist following cessation, but pointed out that it had not been used for a prolonged period, so that the men treated may have had insufficient time to have learned control without the medication.

Priority of Treatment Strategies

Priority would be given to changing the value Mr. D gave to his needs in relation to those of a sexual partner, both by cognitive correction in interviews and by bibliotherapy. The latter would involve his reading a book such as *Men and Sex* (Zilbergeld, 1995) to correct his beliefs about men's sexual performance and women's expectations concerning these. Directly encouraging him to increase the value he gave to his own needs relative to the needs of his partner might be less effective than leading him to realize that his behavior did not reflect a true evaluation of his partner's needs. This could be done using a Socratic approach, so that he would be led to put forward as his own ideas the beliefs that the therapist wished him to accept. In relation to his method of dealing in adolescence with his potential partner's responses to the acne on his back by withdrawal from physical relations, he would be asked about the appropriateness and acceptability of this withdrawal. If the nature and affect of his response seemed to be nonthreatening, he would be challenged as to whether he was really respecting his partner's needs by denying her the opportunity to decide for herself what her behavior would be. Again, if it seemed appropriate, he would be asked how he might have given her this opportunity. The aim would be to lead him to put forward as his own idea that he had put his own needs ahead of hers by allowing his embarrassment at telling her he had acne to prevent him telling her about the problem and allowing her to exercise choice as to her response. If it also seemed appropriate, it would be pointed out that he did report that a number of girls were interested in forming a relationship with him, so they must have been attracted to him and liked him as a person. He would be asked what it indicated about his opinion of women that he believed that none of them valued a relationship with him sufficiently that they would allow a problem such as acne to prevent them continuing to express their affection or love for him. He would then be asked if he saw a parallel with his subsequent situation when he continued to withdraw from sexual activity in a relationship because he felt he was not sexually competent and what this revealed about his beliefs about the women who more recently showed an interest in forming a relationship with him. The aim of this educational procedure would be to encourage him to consider whether he had really been putting his partner's interests before his or whether he had denied them the opportunity to show their affection or love from him—in short, to encourage him to accept that in future relationships, by valuing his own needs he would also be valuing the needs of his partner.

During this stage of attempting to increase his motivation to form a relationship in which he would be sexually active, his anxiety about doing so would be dealt with by desensitization in imagination. An audiotape would be made of a session in which he was initially trained to relax, and then while relaxed visualize being in a sexual situation appropriate to the stage of his treatment. In the first such session, he would visualize being in a relationship in which kissing and petting occurred and he felt it was appropriate to introduce genital contact. He would then visualize telling his partner that he had some problem with more intimate sexual activity for which he was being treated, and he had been advised to take this stage more slowly, and then allow her to express her views about this. He would visualize her accepting this willingly and their sexual activity proceeding to genital fondling, resulting in their reaching orgasm without attempting intercourse. In their lovemaking, he would surrender control of his behavior to his own feelings, realizing that in doing so he was exciting his partner, increasing her enjoyment while encouraging her to surrender to her feelings in the same way. Concurrently with listening to this tape three or four times a week, he would be instructed to use Semans' stop–start technique when he masturbated (McConaghy, 1996) to determine whether this would result in increasing the time he took to ejaculate. If he continued to show episodes of erectile dysfunction during masturbation, he would be referred to a physician to determine if there was a possible organic cause.

When he felt his anxiety about forming a relationship that could include sexual activity was sufficiently reduced, he would be encouraged to commence such a relationship, while correcting any expectation he had that either he or his partner should expect initially that the relationship would be permanent. This would entail discussion both of the belief that a relationship without this expectation is exploitative of the partner and whether he would feel most comfortable about the issue if he discussed it with the partner. If desensitization of this discussion was necessary, it would be done making another audiotape. His establishing a relationship would then be monitored, with emphasis that initially sexual activity would not proceed to intercourse until during sexual activity he was consistently maintaining an erection and taking some minutes of masturbation before he ejaculated. Then, if he ejaculated prematurely during sexual intercourse, he would be recommended in future attempts at intercourse that if he felt about to ejaculate prematurely to temporarily cease movement, or if necessary to withdraw and use the penile squeeze technique (McConaghy, 1993).

Dealing with Complicating Factors

During all interviews, Mr. D.'s alcohol intake would be monitored. If the liver function test carried out after the initial interview showed impairment, this would be used to point out that his alcohol intake was already damaging his body to a significant extent. If it did not, it would be pointed out from time to time that a level of more than four standard drinks a day would be highly likely in the future to produce damage to his liver or other organs, including his brain, as well as being a possible factor in his erectile dysfunction.

The level of his depression would also be monitored constantly in interviews, with the expectation that with improvement in his ability to form a sexual relationship, the depression would improve as well, and a trial of reduction in venlafaxine could be made.

Role of Pharmacotherapy in the Case

The use of the antidepressant venlafaxine for Mr. D.'s depression would be maintained while necessary. If his premature ejaculation did not respond to the stop–start or penile squeeze techniques and he was still taking venlafaxine, a trial of clomipramine as an alternative would be made. If his erectile dysfunction persisted, the possible value of sildenafil would be investigated, even in the absence of evidence that an organic factor was involved.

Managed Care Considerations

In Australia, a government-funded Medicare system pays fees for all psychiatric consultations as well as investigatory procedures, the fee varying according to the length of the consultation or the nature of the procedure. The fees for consultations are halved if the consultations continue weekly or more for more than a year without the frequency being justified. Psychiatrists and procedural investigators can charge fees additional to the Medicare payment. In deciding whether to do so (and if so, how much to add), most clinicians take into account the financial situation of the patient. Mr. D.'s treatment was expected not to involve more than 20 consultations at most, the cost of which (along with that of possible investigations) he would have no difficulty meeting.

SUMMARY

Descriptions are provided of the sexual dysfunctions and methods for their diagnosis, including additional assessments, are discussed. A case illustration is given of a 44-year-old man with a lifelong inability to form sexual relationships that he believed resulted from his erectile disorder, premature ejaculation, inadequate sexual technique, and his belief that his partner would not enjoy sexual activity with him. He had commenced drinking alcohol excessively in early adulthood, and his intake was still at a level likely to lead to health problems. His inability to form a sexual relationship led to his becoming depressed and attempting suicide, and he was currently taking antidepressant medication. Investigation of possible organic factors contributing to his sexual dysfunctions are discussed and a treatment program involving cognitive–behavior therapy and possible pharmacotherapy is outlined.

REFERENCES

Althof, S. E. (1995). Pharmacologic treatment of rapid ejacultation. *Psychiatric Clinics of North America, 18*, 85–94.

Althof, S. E., & Seftel, A. D. (1995). The evaluation and management of erectile dysfunction. *Psychiatric Clinics of North America, 18*, 171–192.

American Psychiatric Association (1994). *Diagnostic and statistical manual of mental disorders–4th Ed.* Washington, DC: Author.

Davis, C. M., Yarber, W. L., Bauserman, R., Scheer, G., & Davis. S. L. (1998). *Handbook of Sexuality-Related Measures*. Thousand Oaks, Sage Publications, California.

LoPiccolo, J. (1990). Sexual dysfunction. In A. S. Bellack, M. Hersen & A. E. Kazdin (Eds.), *International handbook of behavior therapy and modification*. Second Edition (pp. 547–564). New York: Plenum Press.

McConaghy, N. (1993). *Sexual behavior, problems and management*. New York: Plenum Press.

McConaghy, N. (1996). Treatment of sexual dysfunctions. In V. B. Van Hasselt & M. Hersen (Eds.), *Sourcebook of psychological treatment manuals for adult disorders* (pp. 333–373). New York: Plenum Press.

McConaghy, N. (1998). Assessment of sexual dysfunction and deviation. In A. S. Bellack and M. Hersen (Eds.), *Behavioral assessment: A practical handbook*. Fourth Edition (pp. 315–341). Needham Heights: Allyn and Bacon.

Schiavi, R. C., & Segraves, R. T. (1995). The biology of sexual function. *Psychiatric Clinics of North America, 18*, 7–23.

Wincze, J. P., & Carey, M. P. (1991). *Sexual dysfunction*. New York: Guilford Press.

Zilbergeld, B. (1995). *Men and sex*. London: Harper Collins.

15

Marital Dysfunction

Gary R. Birchler
University of California, San Diego

William S. Fals-Stewart
Research Institute on Addictions

DESCRIPTION OF THE DISORDER

The *Diagnostic and Statistical Manual of Mental Disorders–4th Ed. (DSM–IV)* categories for relational problems, as defined by the American Psychiatric Association, include v61.1, *Partner Relational Problem*: "when the focus of clinical attention is a pattern of interaction between spouses or partners characterized by negative communication (e.g., criticisms), distorted communication (e.g., unrealistic expectations), or noncommunication (e.g., withdrawal) that is associated with clinically significant impairment in individual or family functioning or the development of symptoms in one or both partners" (APA, 1994, p. 681).

Typically, individuals displaying such symptoms have an *Adjustment Disorder*, which, according to the *DSM–IV*, is "the development of emotional or behavioral symptoms in response to an identifiable psychosocial stressor(s) occurring within three months of the onset of the stressor(s)" (APA, 1994, p. 623). For couples, the unnamed stressor may be marital conflict. The *DSM–IV* further codifies adjustment disorders according to specific types of symptom expression (e.g., adjustment disorder with depressed mood, anxiety, disturbed emotions, or conduct). In addition, certain couples may experience other *DSM–IV*-identified problems related to abuse; for example, physical abuse of adult or sexual abuse of adult. Within marriage, the former is exemplified by spouse beating and the latter by sexual coercion or rape (APA, 1994, p. 682).

Moreover, there is no doubt that, in addition to adjustment disorders, marital distress can be either the cause or the result of any number of major psychological disorders experienced by partners or other family members. These problems include but are not limited to depression, anxiety, substance abuse, personality disorders, and chronic medical problems.

Unfortunately, to the extent that divorce outcomes in the United States implicate marital dysfunction, the disorder is prevalent among the population. Nationwide, the divorce rate for first marriages exceeds 50%; for second marriages, it is even higher. Also, for those couples who remain married, marital stability guarantees neither healthy marital function nor partner satisfaction. A significant amount of dysfunction, as defined by the APA criteria listed previously, exists among long-term married couples. In the United States, relational problems are among the most common complaints among adults seeking mental health services.

METHODS TO DETERMINE DIAGNOSIS

Ideally, one day there will be a single standardized "diagnostic system" for marital dyads. Such a system would also indicate the most appropriate method of treatment for a given couple. Currently, such a standardized diagnostic system is far from reality, even though the field of marital therapy is increasingly embracing integrationist and couple-oriented perspectives. Nevertheless, given the practical challenge of being clinically competent in the practice of all types of approaches, most therapists end up learning well one or possibly two basic approaches.

In practice, what is assessed and how it is assessed tend to be heavily influenced by the interviewer's theoretical orientation and the couple's presenting problems. For example, marital therapists who are more traditional, psychodynamically oriented, or emotion focused may rely exclusively on the interview method for history-taking assessment information. In comparison, behaviorists as well as certain strategic family therapists may deemphasize history taking and instead focus on here-and-now interactions. Moreover, so-called brief treatment family therapists may use only a short, problem-focused assessment interview and then proceed with strategic interventions within the first hour of contact.

This chapter offers what the authors believe to be a basic, broadly endorsed, empirically validated, and behaviorally oriented clinical approach for assessing and treating marital dyads. In contrast to psychodynamic, strategic family systems and other approaches, many behaviorally oriented therapists engage the couple in a distinct assessment phase that is completed before formal treatment begins. In this approach, the clinical interview is a necessary but not sufficient tool for accomplishing a thorough assessment of the dysfunctional marital dyad. Typically, differential diagnosis of marital dysfunction is accomplished using both individual and conjoint interviews, supplemented by a battery of marriage assessment inventories and observation of an in vivo sample of the couple's marital conflict communication skills. Comprehensive diagnostic information obtained from these multiple assessment methods may then be used to develop specific treatment goals and strategies for intervention.

ADDITIONAL ASSESSMENTS REQUIRED

Broadly speaking, beyond the basic relationship assessments described previously, there may be additional assessments required for two reasons. First, even though the couple is presenting for marital dysfunction, one or both partners may be suffering sufficiently from individual problems such that additional assessments regarding these problems may be indicated. Examples of individual problems include substance abuse, significant affective or anxiety disorders, dementia, psychosis, disabling medical problems, and posttraumatic stress disorders. When present, these clients may need specialized psychodiagnostic testing or mental status examinations performed by the couple therapist or by way of referral to another clinician. Second, certain problems identified in the form of couple problems may require additional assessments beyond the typical and standard evaluation procedures. Common examples here include the presentation of domestic violence issues, in which safety and behavior control assessments must be made; the assessment of children, when parenting conflicts or child behavior problem issues are primary; and evaluation of sexual dysfunction, when complex sexual problems are encountered. For a given couple, problem-specific inventories and additional interview-based diagnostic sessions may be required to complete a comprehensive diagnosis of marital dysfunction.

CASE ILLUSTRATION

Presenting Complaints

Mariana and Jim were referred for marital therapy by a clinic psychiatric resident who had conducted an individual intake with Mariana, who presented to the resident for the treatment of depression but also reported significant marital conflict. In the first couple session, Mariana complained that Jim was being inattentive as a husband and father; was going out too frequently and drinking excessively with his friends; was coming home from work stressed out and in a bad mood; and was irritated, argumentative, and verbally abusive when she wanted to discuss relationship problems. For his part, Jim complained that Mariana was totally unhappy and uncomfortable being a mother, that she "ambushed" him with emotional problems when he came home from a stressful job, and that she resented any time that he spent with his lifelong friends. He said that despite being a full-time mother, she would not prepare any meals and she was always harping at him to take care of their 5-month-old baby. Both professed loving their child and reported no neglect or abuse, even though both admitted to having some adjustment problems regarding the demands and roles of parenthood. Basically, the partners were very unhappy with one another, and Mariana stated that if Jim did not change, she would seek a divorce. Jim denied the desire to divorce, but stated Mariana was depressed, angry, and impossible to live with.

History of the Disorder

Jim was a formerly married 36-year-old attractive white male who worked 9–12 hour days as a venture capitalist seeking and coordinating new investments. He made an income in the six figure range, but due to the nature of the business, he was often under considerable stress. Mariana, an attractive 34-year-old unemployed Hispanic female, was single before marriage to Jim. They met in a singles bar and were partying with friends, dating frequently, and enjoying an exciting sexual relationship for about 2 months when Mariana got pregnant. The couple decided to get married and had a healthy female baby, Nicole. The couple lived in Jim's expensive but small condo at the time of presentation. At couple intake, they had been married and living together for about 13 months. They claimed that the relationship problems described previously began on the honeymoon and had only continued to get worse over the course of a year. Both spouses noted that Mariana had stopped drinking (and partying) when she became pregnant, and this in turn led to reduced relationship camaraderie. In addition, when she also stopped taking Prozac due to pregnancy, her symptoms of mood instability and depression increased. Mariana also may have experienced postpartum depression. Due to the increased financial demands of providing for a child and the need for a larger residence, Jim experienced more pressure to produce a steady income. He was also reluctant to give up his singles lifestyle if it meant too little contact with his friends.

Medical History

At their ages, neither partner experienced major medical problems. Jim was being monitored for high blood pressure but he was not yet being treated with antihypertensive medication. He had no major surgeries or past medical history other than a couple of broken bones from sports injuries as a young man. Mariana had no current major medical problems. Her history included frequent childhood illnesses and several psychiatric issues (described later).

Family History

Mariana and Jim had quite divergent family histories. Mariana came from a very affluent family. Her parents were both of Hispanic origin, and in fact, during her early childhood she lived in Spain. During the children's formative years, the family, including a sister and two brothers, was supported by maids and a nanny to care for the children. They did not want for material things, but she described her parents as very disengaged from one another. After moving to the United States, marital conflict increased and her parents were divorced when Mariana was 13 years old. Her mother now lives primarily in Spain; the father and her three siblings live in Southern California. According to Mariana, the constant acrimony, destructive parent–child alliances, and the adversarial process associated with the parents' divorce had a significant negative impact on the adolescent children, from which they have yet to recover. Nevertheless, Mariana and her siblings continue to be supported by the family wealth as adults. Mariana, in particular, is still receiving a monthly stipend for personal use from her father. The continued monetary support is seen as a mixed blessing by the couple.

Jim grew up as an only child and had quite a different upbringing from Mariana. He claimed that his family had enough money, but nothing extra. His father was a hard worker in various wage-class jobs and his mother worked infrequently at odd jobs. Jim's father was described as at least a problem drinker, if not an alcoholic; he remains distant and disengaged from both Jim and Jim's mother. His parents are still married and live in the same town as the couple. Jim was average in school, but managed to get a partial football scholarship to a local university. Subsequently, by working during college, he graduated with a business degree and eventually progressed from a stockbroker to venture capitalist. The socioeconomic status represented by this position was far greater than that of any members of his family of origin.

Sexual History

Jim is a big, tall, and handsome man. He played high school and college sports, was in a fraternity, and dated girls and partied accordingly. His first sexual intercourse experience occurred when he was 17 with a girlfriend of 3 months. Subsequently, he had several casual sexual relationships before he married his first wife soon after college at age 23. Sex in that relationship was an initial attraction, but soon fell victim to marital conflict. The couple divorced after 3 years; the last 2 years were "lousy," according to Jim. He had no children by his first marriage and he remained single for about 10 years before meeting Mariana. Over that decade he had a few heavy dating relationships, including an active sex life, but none of these women was "marrying material." Jim reported that sex with Mariana was "great" until the second trimester of her pregnancy.

Mariana had her first sexual intercourse experience at age 15 with her second steady boyfriend after she moved from Spain to California. She reported having dozens of casual sexual experiences after this initial sexual relationship. She said she never really trusted men, but she could "wrap them around my finger" using her sexual attractiveness. Before her marriage to Jim at age 32, Mariana reported leading a promiscuous single lifestyle of being taken care of by men and in which mutual use and abuse was the prevailing pattern of interaction. Of course, during periods of depression and episodic outbreaks of an eating disorder (see Prior Treatment), she was less active and interested in sexual interaction. Mariana agreed that sex was the big attraction between her and Jim, and that it is still good when they are not fighting. More, recently, they are most likely to have sex when making up after a big fight.

Mental Status Examination

Formal mental status examinations typically are not part of conjoint marital evaluations. However, as mentioned previously, many cases, especially in a managed care environment, are referred for couple therapy after one of the partners has sought care for an individual problem. Alternatively, mental status exams may be required to assess one or both partners' individual psychological functioning when individual dysfunction is encountered during the assessment of the marital dysfunction. In this case, a mental status exam (MSE) had been conducted with Mariana during her clinic intake for depression. Jim had not received a MSE, nor did he require one. The clinician who conducted Mariana's MSE found her attitude and behavior to be cooperative and polite. She was oriented to person, place, and time, with evidence of sound intellectual and cognitive functioning. She had adequate memory and recall and a coherent thinking process, with adequate insight and judgment intact. The concern for Mariana was with regard to mood and affect. Her mood was dysphoric, and she expressed hopelessness and sadness marked by tearfulness during the personal intake session. Her affect was variable and labile, featuring irritation and anger (at her life circumstance and at her husband), sadness and self-deprecation, and humor (in a sarcastic manner) was expressed toward the interviewer and the health care system (HMO). As a result of the findings at intake, the psychiatry resident restarted Prozac for the treatment of depression and noted the possibility of restarting Ritalin for Attention Deficit/Hyperactivity Disorder (see Prior Treatment). The resident also made a note to rule out Borderline Personality Disorder, based on her personal history of parental and personal relationships.

Prior Treatment

Mariana had an extensive psychiatric history and related treatments. Although the details were vague to her, during her childhood in Spain, she may have been diagnosed with some type of attention deficit disorder. She believes she was prescribed Ritalin as a child. As a late teenager, she received outpatient treatment for more than 2 years for bulimia. Since age 15, she had been treated as an outpatient off and on for major depression, including suicidal ideation. She received psychotherapy primarily, but in her 20s she tried some Prozac given to her by her mother and then briefly obtained her own prescriptions. When she presented for couple therapy, she had been participating in long-term individual psychotherapy for 3 years at the rate of once or twice each month.

CASE CONCEPTUALIZATION

Modeling and Learning

There are several important aspects of modeling that each partner learned within their families of origin. Moreover, these differences between partners' developmental histories contributed to their core conflicts. Mariana grew up in a household in which money was plentiful but parental emotional validation of children was virtually absent. She learned that self-worth was somehow related to getting what she wanted in a material sense. Presents and material goods were used by her parents, who were otherwise disengaged from the children, as a reward for being good and behaving as the parents wished. Mariana interpreted withholding of material goods and privileges as a sign of not being loved. However, she was never made or taught to do much work. Everything was provided. For example, she did not learn how to shop for food, cook, keep house, or care for children. In addition, the parents engaged in marital conflict frequently, and Mariana witnessed many episodes of escalating negative affect, verbal abuse, and the threat of physical violence. She described her father as having a "scary" mean streak and her mother as being a "nasty manipulator" of everyone around her; she got what she wanted. Finally, worth noting is that during her time of living in the original home in Spain, her father and uncles periodically would drink heavily. She learned that alcohol served both as a bad influence and a convenient way of avoiding responsibilities and emotional connections with others. In sum, she learned that money and material goods were equated with self-worth, that she should not have to work or be responsible for herself, that spouses do not have positive emotional intimacy, that guilt induction and manipulation of others can get you what you want, and that alcohol use is bad for families.

In stark contrast to Mariana, Jim grew up as a single child in a lower-middle working class family. He learned from his upbringing that whatever extra money or privileges he would get would have to come from his own hard work. Indeed, for Jim, money also was related to self-worth, but he always felt insecure about having enough and protective about conserving what he had.

Similar to the experience of Mariana, Jim's parents did not express much affection to one another or to him, but the basic style of parental interaction was very different from Mariana's parents. Jim's parents were conflict-avoidant; they managed problems by mutual withdrawal and silent disengagement. Although Jim's father was reportedly an alcoholic, his behavior while intoxicated was neither mean nor disruptive; it was quiet and withdrawn. The mother, possibly dysthymic herself, was described as an adequate mother, but not very affectionate or assertive. In summary, what Jim learned from his developmental experience was that money is difficult to come by and should be spent conservatively, that one must work hard under stressful conditions to acquire the better things in life, that spouses do not experience much real intimacy, that conflict is managed by avoidance and withdrawal, and that using alcohol can be a crutch, but it is not a dangerous habit (nor does it keep one from functioning, at least at work).

Life Events

Mariana and Jim both had been single for a number of years of their adult lives. After his first marriage ended, Jim maintained professional positions and purchased his own condominium. He had a number of single male friends with whom he engaged in numerous sports activities. He felt "burned" by the experience with his first wife. Mistrustful of women and his ability to be intimate, for years he participated in casual, uncommitted relationships. At the time he met Mariana, he was leading a reasonably affluent and active lifestyle, drinking fairly heavily and partying frequently on the weekends with numerous friends.

Mariana also engaged in an active lifestyle when she met Jim. Her father was providing her with a nice apartment and a monthly stipend for spending money. Her mother visited from Spain two or three times each year. These visits were conflicted but obligatory. Previous relationships with men had been sometimes promiscuous, sometimes mutually verbally abusive, often manipulative, and ultimately unsatisfactory. She was attracted to strong, emotionally volatile Latin men who fit the fiery, machismo stereotype, but fundamentally she felt unloved and unlovable. Getting in and out of these relationships was often traumatic, at times resulting in major depression, vague suicidal ideation, and exacerbation of her lifelong eating disorder.

The common life event that changed the course of these two people's lives forever was the unplanned pregnancy. It occurred 2 months after they began dating out of the singles bar scene. Poor timing notwithstanding, Jim and Mariana decided to get married and have the child.

Genetics and Temperament

To the extent that genetics and temperament can be determined and described for Mariana and Jim, they demonstrated remarkably different if stereotypical gender characteristics. Jim is the strong, silent type. He is uncomfortable identifying and disclosing his emotions, positive or negative; he is very uncomfortable in the presence of Mariana's often-intense negative emotions. He avoids fights unless cornered, and then he blows up and becomes verbally abusive. In contrast, Mariana is hot-tempered and accustomed to men and women expressing strong emotions in an uninhibited and unconditional manner. In the context of marital conflict, Jim's natural avoidance and withdrawal was interpreted by Mariana as him not caring, thus his distant stance frustrated her all the more. Although it is clear that Jim's size, good looks, and calm demeanor attracted her to him and that Mariana's good looks and sexual and emotional vivaciousness attracted him to her, in the area of conflict resolution, these styles are virtually incompatible. These personality variables, to the extent that they are products of genetics and temperament, are presumably less amenable to change. Despite the attractions, these emotional styles of expression clearly provided the couple with mixed blessings.

Physical Conditions

As mentioned previously, with the possible exceptions of Mariana's low-grade, lifelong eating disorder and Jim's borderline hypertension possibly related to his hard-driving Type A personality, these people were physically quite healthy. Mariana had the usual morning sickness during her first trimester of pregnancy, but this was not a factor when the couple presented for marital therapy.

Drugs

At the time of couple intake, both partners were using drugs that affected their psychological well-being. Jim's drug of choice was alcohol, and he made a habit of drinking several beers or glasses of wine each night. Stresses related to his high-finance job and possibly the marital conflict were contributing to his need to reduce stress by using alcohol. At least once a week he would go out with his male friends and have more than a few drinks. This activity was causing overt conflict between him and Mariana. For her part, Mariana, previous to her pregnancy, had benefited from the prescription drug Prozac for depression management. Once pregnant, she stopped taking the medication and, unfortunately, her depressive symptoms worsened. One week before couple intake, she had restarted the Prozac regime. The couple denied the use of any other drugs or street substances.

Socioeconomic and Cultural Factors

The socioeconomic and cultural factors have been described previously. To summarize here, Mariana came from a very wealthy binational Hispanic family. She was raised nominally in the Catholic religion; she and three siblings were raised to be bilingual in Spanish and English. Prior to marriage, her primary source of support was from her father, who lives nearby. Her parents are divorced. Her mother lives in Spain, but she visits fairly frequently. Jim's white parents are of Protestant religion, and they have been (unhappily) married for more than 40 years. Jim's upbringing was lower-middle working class; the family had enough money to get by, but little discretionary income. His parents live nearby. Contact by three of the four grandparents with Nicole, the sole grandchild, has caused some conflict for the couple. Only visits with the divorced maternal grandfather are without problems.

Overall Conceptualization

Regarding the conceptualization of marital dysfunction in general, Birchler and associates developed a model called *The Seven C's* (cf., Birchler, Doumas, & Fals-Stewart, 1999). For a couple seeking marital evaluation and treatment, most of the ingredients important to a long-term intimate relationship can be accounted for by an analysis of the Seven C's: Character, Cultural and ethnic factors, Contract, Commitment, Caring, Communication, and Conflict resolution. For many couples, these domains of function constitute strengths to build on or goals to strive for:

1. Socially compatible personal values and healthy personalities (i.e., character)
2. Strong family traditions and compatible or stimulating cultural and ethnic backgrounds
3. A marital contract that offers ongoing adaptations and viable matches between partners' expectations and their experiences
4. Loyalty to the marriage with a long-term perspective and the will to work out the inevitable problems (i.e., commitment)
5. Love, sex, and affection; emotional support; and an optimal balance of individually and mutually rewarding activities (i.e., caring)
6. Open and effective communication
7. Problem solving, anger management, and conflict resolution skills

The sections that follow describe in more detail how the Seven C's conceptual model provides a useful framework for both diagnosing and treating the marital dysfunction experienced by Jim and Mariana.

Diagnostic Assessment

In an effort to diagnose couples' problems, there is no standard nosology beyond the possibility of the *DSM–IV* general categories of partner relational problem and primary sexual dysfunctions. Different theoretical approaches to marital dysfunction assess cases and categorize the problems according to certain content and process concerns. The content areas are represented by couples' complaints (i.e., spousal inattention; time together; and sexual, parenting, financial, in-law, and infidelity problems). The process issues are made up of dyadic interaction problems, such as dysfunctional communication patterns and maladaptive styles of marital conflict. In addition, as discussed previously, the individual partners also may be diagnosed with other *DSM–IV* disorders (refer to the types and criteria described throughout this book).

The behaviorally oriented Seven C's conceptualization scheme was applied to Jim and Mariana, and the following vulnerabilities were noted:

Character features: Jim has a problem misusing alcohol as well as a hard-driving personality vulnerable to stress and irritability. In addition, he had poor parental models regarding the establishment of adult intimacy and parenting skills. Mariana suffers from extreme emotional volatility and episodes of major depression, and she also had poor parental models for adult intimacy and parenting skills.

Cultural and ethnic factors: Jim and Mariana had significantly different and conflicted cultural and family backgrounds regarding the expression of emotions, the meaning of money, and core family values.

Contract: The original short-term physical and social attractions between them were soon contradicted by the long-term demands of parenting, working, and establishing true couple and family intimacy. If the notion of contract has to do with the goodness-of-fit between one's expectations and one's actual experience, Mariana and Jim were at a disadvantage. Their expectations were likely based on dysfunctional parental models; their individual ways of being close were so different from one another that their experiences were unsatisfactory.

Commitment: Mariana has threatened divorce seriously on numerous occasions. Jim reports his level of commitment to be higher, but the quality has a negative feel to it because it is influenced by the failure of his first marriage, financial threat, and the potential loss of the family image. For Mariana, lifestyle comparisons, loss of family image, and the prospect of personal failure influence her level of commitment to the marriage.

Caring: As a result of the abrupt change in contract, each partner sometimes questions whether they are loved or even liked by the other. Support and understanding between them is variable. Physical attraction remains intact, but the sexual connection has been weakened. Because the singles lifestyle is no longer something they share, they have failed to develop alternative couple and family activities.

Communication: The couple's interaction pattern is dysfunctional. Jim's style reflects a typical male stereotype: He has little interest in affiliative conversation, tends to minimize and avoid the discussion of relationship maintenance issues, and when confronted, he resorts to instrumental problem solving or withdrawal instead of providing emotional support through good listening and validation skills. In contrast, Mariana's style also contributes to their communication problems. She carries certain expectations about how Jim should attend to her needs, and when he is perceived to be inconsiderate or unknowing, she interprets his behavior as uncaring and abusive. She admits that she tends to store up resentments until she cannot tolerate the situation any longer then reacts intensely, with her negative emotions out of proportion to the problem at hand.

Conflict resolution: The communication styles noted previously set the couple up for a maladaptive style of marital conflict resolution. Virtually in collusion, they reflect a classic demand–withdraw or pursuer–distancer pattern of miscommunication. One partner seeks closeness, eventually by demanding that it occur; the other partner, experiencing the demand for closeness as aversive, withdraws, seeking relief through increased distance. Each partner's behavior elicits the undesired behavior from his or her mate. Mariana and Jim alternate between conflict avoidance and the build up of resentments, followed eventually by high-intensity and destructive arguments that feature blaming, character assassination, verbal abuse, and threats of separation and divorce.

In summary, the Seven C's analysis provides a framework to accomplish a differential diagnosis of couple problems. Some couples experience no problems in some of the Seven C's and their dyadic interaction in these areas reflects certain strengths for the couple relationship. Individualized couple treatment plans are designed to reflect differential findings. Unfortunately, Jim and Mariana are experiencing some degree of difficulty in all seven areas of relationship function. Some of these problems were further identified and quantified using behavioral assessment procedures.

Behavioral Assessment

Behavioral assessment procedures in couple therapy are composed of three types: the administration of various paper-and-pencil questionnaires, clinic-based observation of the couples' abilities to resolve a marital problem (called a *communication sample*), and self- or spouse-observation in the home environment. However, the last procedure tends to be used more frequently during the intervention phase of couple's therapy, in which partners are asked to keep track of certain targeted interactional behaviors.

Many behaviorally oriented therapists use standardized individual and relationship-oriented paper-and-pencil questionnaires to help them assess various levels of dissatisfaction and dysfunction and ascertain the marital system's assets and strengths (e.g., the Dyadic Adjustment Scale, Spanier, 1976; the Marital Satisfaction Inventory, Snyder, 1979). We use a number of such instruments in a package called the Marital Relationship Assessment Battery (Birchler, 1983). Although the specifics are beyond the scope of this chapter, essentially, the partners are asked to complete independently several behaviorally oriented questionnaires, a task that takes them approximately $1\frac{1}{2}$–2 hours to complete. Quantifiable and descriptive information is obtained regarding couple demographics, global marital satisfaction, steps toward separation and divorce, areas of desired relationship change, conflict management, and time allocation to individual and mutually rewarding activities. In addition, measures of individual function that assess levels of depression, anxiety, and physical symptoms are included.

Outside of behaviorally oriented treatment programs, the formal in vivo observation of a sample of marital conflict communication directed by the therapist may be rare. During diagnostic interviews, clinicians may or may not ask or allow the partners to discuss some topic with one another in order to observe how they are able to engage in problem solving. However, easily obtained, the communication sample has been a component of the behavioral assessment of distressed couples since the early 1970s. Observing how partners attempt to solve a typical marital conflict often provides unique and important diagnostic information about relationship-enhancing skills.

Basically, at the start of the session (and it is hoped before any other conflict-laden material is introduced) the couple is asked to provide a 10-minute sample of their communication. The therapist helps them identify a current, relevant, unresolved, and moderately intense issue about which the partners disagree. Typical topics selected are management of finances, the lack of quality time together, or conflict involving a child, in-law, or other adult. The couple is asked to spend about 10 minutes attempting to resolve the problem. The therapist may leave the room and observe from behind a one-way mirror or on a video monitor, or may simply push back the chair and ask the couple to proceed as if the therapist were not present. The observed communication sample demonstrates a variety of performance or skill deficits regarding the partners' relative abilities to assert themselves, maintain focus on the issue at hand, listen to one another, propose solutions to the problem, and generally engage in constructive (versus destructive) interaction.

With respect to the findings based on the behavioral assessment procedures conducted with Mariana and Jim, the paper-and-pencil instruments indicated that both partners scored in the maritally dissatisfied range, with Mariana significantly more unhappy than Jim. On a scale of 14 steps to separation, Mariana had taken 7 steps and Jim 4 steps, constituting a serious threat to marital stability. Their total conflict potential score for areas of desired change was 34; distressed couples entering the clinic average a score of 28. The conflict management scale indicated that these partners were engaging in high levels of both passive and active responses to conflict (e.g., yelling and screaming in 75% of their fights; crying or sulking in more than 50% of their fights). Reported time allocated to both couple-alone and family-together activities were very low due to work and child-rearing demands. Both spouses also reported low frequencies of individually rewarding activities, especially Mariana, who cared for the infant all day and resented this role. Finally, on the measures assessing individual function, Jim had elevated levels of tension and anxiety and Mariana's scores were elevated on measures of depression and physical symptoms (e.g., migraine headaches, stomach problems). On paper-and-pencil self-report of relationship problems, Jim complained primarily about Mariana's mood swings (between depression and anger) and she complained primarily about his excessive drinking with his friends and business associates.

The communication sample illustrated their significant difficulties with problem solving. The topic to be discussed was an issue raised by Mariana: spending more quality time together as a couple. Approximately 30 seconds into the discussion, they began arguing about Jim's drinking, his inattention to the baby, and about Mariana spending money without consulting Jim. The argument soon became heated, featuring blaming, cross-complaining and verbal attacks, highly defensive responses, and little evidence of the hallmarks of good couple communication; for example, "I" statements, listening, and validation. Both partners became very upset and failed to make any progress toward resolution of the original problem identified. Unfortunately, when the couple was debriefed after the discussion, they indicated that this very frustrating interaction pattern was typical for them.

Taken together, the behavioral assessments supplemented the information gathered through the clinical interview process to complete an analysis of the Seven C's outlined previously.

Prioritization of Targets for Treatment

Thus far, the initial evaluation consists of semistructured clinical interviews (Birchler & Schwarze, 1994), the completion of questionnaires, and an observed sample of communication. Our program features a feedback session at the end of the evaluation phase in which the therapist (with assistance from the couple, when possible) integrates all of the multimodal assessment information, formulates the various problems, and coconstructs the treatment plan. This meeting is designed strategically to influence and motivate the couple to enter treatment, if conjoint intervention is appropriate. Couples have been very responsive to an analysis of their relationships' strengths and vulnerabilities according to the Seven C's. In addition, targets for intervention can be categorized in terms of identified problems (i.e., content issues) and dysfunctional interaction skills and patterns (i.e., interpersonal processes). Based on this presentation, all parties discuss the findings and then decide whether to enter into the formal intervention phase of marital therapy and the proposed length of treatment. Sometimes the nature of the problems or levels of motivation are such that engaging in marital therapy is not advised. In such cases, one or both partners may be referred for individual or group therapy to work on personal issues.

Jim and Mariana realized that the most urgent component of their distress was in the interactional process areas of communication and conflict resolution; in particular, their frequent, high-intensity, and destructive arguments. The problematic content areas were multiple: Jim's drinking and response to work-related stress, Mariana's mood swings, sharing the child-rearing burdens and attending to the attachment needs of the infant, the amount and quality of couple-alone and family time, and dealing with in-laws. In this context, the couple also needed to make adjustments in their relationship contract (i.e., improving over time the congruence between each spouse's expectations and experiences) and consequently strengthen their commitment to the marriage and family. With encouragement from the therapists, the couple agreed to work initially on three areas: (a) Reducing destructive episodes of conflict; (b) improving couple contact, caring activities, and communication; and (c) each person gaining better control over moods (i.e., Jim's moods were influenced by his work stress and drinking habits; Mariana's moods were affected by her depression, frustration, and discomfort related to being a stay-at-home mother). Once basic skills related to effective couple communication, conflict resolution, and caring behaviors were improved, they would be better able to address contract issues, cultural and ethnic conflicts related to in-laws and family-of-origin traditions, and any remaining unresolved problems.

Selection of Treatment Strategies

The research literature suggests that among the various approaches applied to marital dysfunction, behavioral couple therapy has the most research validating its efficacy (Baucom, Shoham, Mueser, Daiuto, & Stickle, 1998) and is currently the only approach listed by the American Psychological Association as meeting the criteria of an "empirically validated treatment." Behavioral couples therapy (BCT), formerly called *behavioral marital therapy* (BMT), has a long tradition since the late 1960s of being offered to couples in distress. The primary treatment components are training in communication and problem-solving skills and behavior exchange interventions. Treatment strategies are based on interventions derived from social learning theory that feature a straightforward psychoeducational format. Therapists use a variety of cognitive–behavioral techniques to facilitate the acquisition of interpersonal skills and positive behavior changes for the couple: modeling, skill acquisition, behavioral rehearsal, coaching and feedback, videotape playback, extensive homework assignments, bibliotherapy, and post-treatment planning to guard against relapse.

For example, therapist modeling or using videotaped examples of appropriate ways of communicating is an effective strategy to help partners learn new interpersonal skills. Similarly, behavioral rehearsal, combined with coaching, feedback, and videotape playback of the couples' improving interactions, facilitates new learning. Finally, homework assignments help couples generalize their new skills and behavior change negotiations into the natural environment, and bibliotherapy is used to broaden partners' knowledge base about positive marriages. For example, therapists may assign readings from communication training manuals that offer exercises to be done at home (e.g., Notarius & Markman, 1993).

Priority of Treatment Strategies

Typically, the BCT approach combines in-session work with intersession homework assignments to achieve the desired goals. Most couples seem to benefit from the following combination and progression of treatment strategies: In the early stages of treatment, couples are helped to strengthen their relationship foundation by introducing basic communication skills training and the graduated exchange of caring behaviors at home. Midtreatment, with basic communication skills, collaborative motivation, and commitment to the relationship enhanced, the couple is helped to address interactional deficits in problem solving and conflict management while working progressively to resolve previously identified problems. If possible, the least difficult issues are addressed first and success is reinforced until the possibly more incompatible issues are confronted. Finally, in the end stage of therapy, couples learn to review the gains made and the associated strategies that were used to achieve them, understand the contractual nature of their relationship strengths and vulnerabilities, and be mindful of the executive actions necessary to prevent treatment gains from deteriorating over time.

Because Mariana and Jim were experiencing multilevel problems, clearly they needed assistance to learn new interaction skills and effective ways to achieve desired behavior changes in the home environment. More specifically, they needed to learn more effective communication skills, better conflict-resolution skills, more effective daily problem-solving skills, better behavior change negotiation skills, more effective stress-reduction skills, and better co-parenting skills. Consistent with the progressive approach noted previously but mindful of the need for this particular couple to reduce unusually destructive fighting immediately, training in conflict management skills would be introduced first. Reduction in fighting would be followed by additional areas targeted for treatment: basic communication skills training, enhancement of caring behaviors, daily problem-solving training, and then working on the remaining specific issues that confront this couple and threaten their relationship.

Dealing with Complicating Factors

When conceptualizing the problems that couples bring to therapy and in formulating their treatment plans, most of the complicating factors can be understood within the Seven C's framework. First, under Character features, if either partner's level of individual psychopathology is too severe to be managed or treated in conjoint therapy, there will be complications. For example, certain personality disorders [e.g., antisocial personality disorder (ASPD)] may include a predisposition and learning history regarding the use of physical violence to gain or maintain control of someone (conflict resolution). Cases featuring domestic violence and individuals with ASPD often present complicating factors.

In addition, one or the other partner may have a hidden agenda that is incompatible with relationship improvement. For example, the husband may desire to maintain an affair or the wife already may have a private plan to separate and divorce. Indeed, spouses may be willing to go to great lengths to maintain a relationship contract that requires their partners to be sick or remain inadequate so that they can feel more adequate. In some cases, significant complications come from outside the couple (cultural and ethnic factors); that is, parents, siblings, children, or stepchildren may have sufficient influence to interfere with the couple's prognosis and progress in marital therapy.

Finally, there are two complicating factors related to change in therapy. First, for some couples, change in well-practiced and familiar patterns, no matter how unsatisfying and destructive, can be very difficult to achieve. Because of more rigid personality styles or because of years of building up resentments and negative reciprocal interaction patterns, some individuals offer significant resistance to the concept of change itself. Therapeutic progress is more complicated for these people. Second, often the types of changes that partners seem to demand from their partners or the basic changes desired in the nature of the relationship itself are simply improbable if not impossible to accomplish. For example, one partner's core personality style may seem incompatible with the other's basic style, or partners may have totally unrealistic expectations for certain needs being met within the relationship. In situations in which significant incompatibilities exist, unless the therapy can facilitate an increase in partners' acceptance of one another, then progress is complicated.

For the sake of illustration given the case at hand, the marital therapist might anticipate a number of potential complicating factors. For example, if Jim's drinking problem turns out to be alcohol abuse or dependency, then he will likely need individualized or concurrent treatment for substance abuse before couple therapy will succeed. Similarly, if Mariana's depression is severe enough and is not or cannot be managed with individualized therapy or antidepressant medication, this will be a complicating factor for the marital therapy. In addition, it is known that Mariana has a very close relationship with her father: He is still providing her with a sizable personal stipend for spending money even after she has been married to Jim for more than a year. It is conceivable that jealousy or resentments could arise between the two men in her life that would amount to a significant complicating factor in the marital therapy.

Finally, there would be a complicating factor in this therapy to the extent that each partner is looking for a type of (personality) change in his or her partner that is unlikely to occur. Jim's quiet, steady, hard-working and hard-playing personality style attracted Mariana to him initially. Her vibrant, highly volatile, and stimulating personality style attracted Jim to Mariana. However, as can be all too typical for distressed couples, these partners now seem to be weary of and irritated by the other's style of emotional expression and associated emotional needs. They seem to be asking for someone who emotes and acts more like themselves. Of course, although not totally immutable, there are limits in how much people can (or will choose to) modify these core personality features. Without an appropriate balance of acceptance (where necessary) and change (where possible), progress in improving marital satisfaction is limited.

Role of Pharmacotherapy in the Case

In many community mental health outpatient settings, it is not unusual for one or both partners to be taking psychoactive medications. In particular, the comorbidity of major depression and marital distress is known to be about 50% (Beach & O'Leary, 1992). When psychiatric disorders are present in relationship partners, the failure to manage associated symptoms of the disorders can certainly affect the prognosis and course of couple therapy. In the present case, Mariana had been prescribed Prozac for depression both before and after her pregnancy. The couple reported that her moods seem to be more variable and severe when she is not taking the medication (given the recent experience during her pregnancy). In addition, she has taken Ritalin on and off for several years in an attempt to improve her attention and concentration abilities. When taking these medications, Mariana admits that both the little annoyances and the big problems affect her mood much less than when she is off the medications. Although pregnancy introduced a complication in taking the prescribed medications, clearly the couple does better when she is medicated. Our experience is that in certain cases, psychotherapeutic medications can play an important role in cognitive rehabilitation and mood management.

Pharmacotherapy should be considered when psychiatric symptoms are distressing individuals and affecting the couple relationship.

Managed Care Considerations

Behavioral couple therapy and related approaches to marital dysfunction are fairly well suited to a brief treatment model (i.e., 12–20 sessions). If managed care plans cover this amount of work, then couple evaluations can be fairly comprehensive and outcomes usually are positive. Typically, some requirement for meeting a "medical necessity" for care is involved in managed care plans and this may require that one partner meet criteria for a *DSM–IV* Axis I diagnosis. Although meeting these criteria may open the door for limited couple therapy, it also suggests that at least one of the partners is suffering from a major mental illness or psychiatric disorder. As discussed previously, such a condition may complicate and extend the need for couple treatment while also requiring individual therapy or psychotropic medications. Many practitioners believe that this somewhat restrictive system is workable, as long as 8–12 or more conjoint sessions are approved. However, many managed care plans either do not cover conjoint therapy at all or they cover as few as just three sessions. Attempting to evaluate and remediate usually long-standing marital dysfunction in three sessions requires more skill and magic than most therapists possess. Interestingly, Bagarozzi (1996) proposed a model for providing assessment and treatment for distressed couples in 3–6 sessions. However, the approach seems to require procedures that focus on a single salient problem (i.e., symptom), and lasting success would require tremendous motivation and readiness to change on the part of the couple. To complete the necessary work, most couples have to pay extra for extended services or seek couple therapy outside the plan.

SUMMARY

This chapter offers considerations for diagnosis, conceptualization, and treatment planning for marital dysfunction. The empirically validated approach for relationship distress referred to as *Behavioral Couple Therapy* (BCT) forms the basis for the discussion; however, the BCT model is complemented by the authors' presentation of the Seven C's framework for case conceptualization and treatment planning. When evaluating a couple for conjoint therapy, the Seven C's model takes into account individual factors, relationship factors, communication and problem-solving processes and skill deficits, and cultural and ethnic factors. Several diagnostic methods comprise the BCT approach, including semistructured interviews, paper-and-pencil instruments, and behavioral observations of marital conflict interactions. A case example is included throughout the discussion to illustrate the approach.

REFERENCES

American Psychiatric Association (1994). *Diagnostic and statistical manual of mental disorders—4th Ed.* Washington, DC: Author.

Bagarozzi, D. A. (1996). *The couple and family in managed care: Assessment, evaluation, and treatment.* New York: Brunner/Mazel.

Baucom, D. H., Shoham, V., Mueser, K. T., Daiuto, A. D., & Stickle, T. R. (1998). Empirically supported couple and family interventions for marital distress and adult mental health problems. *Journal of Consulting and Clinical Psychology, 66,* 53–88.

Beach, S. R. H., & O'Leary, D. K. (1992). Treating depression in the context of marital discord: Outcome and predictors of response for marital therapy vs. cognitive therapy. *Behavior Therapy, 23,* 507–528.

Birchler, G. R. (1983). Marital dysfunction. In: M. Hersen (Ed.), *Outpatient behavioral therapy: A clinical guide* (pp. 229–269). New York: Grune & Stratton.

Birchler, G. R., Doumas, D. M., & Fals-Stewart, W. (1999). The seven C's: A behavioral-systems framework for evaluating marital distress. *The Family Journal, 7,* 253–264.

Birchler, G. R., & Schwartz, L. (1994). Marital dyads. In: M. Hersen & S. M. Turner (Eds.), *Diagnostic interviewing, 2nd ed.* (pp. 277–304). New York: Plenum Press.

Notarius, C. I., & Markman, H. (1993). *We can work it out: Making sense of marital conflict.* New York: Putnam's Sons.

Snyder, D. K. (1979). Multidimensional assessment of marital satisfaction. *Journal of Marriage and the Family, 41,* 813–823.

Spanier, G. B. (1976). Measuring dyadic adjustment: New scales for assessing the quality of marriage and similar dyads. *Journal of Marriage and the Family, 38,* 15–28.

Author Index

Subject Index

S

U

Y

Milton Keynes UK
Ingram Content Group UK Ltd.
UKHW030903141024
449569UK00032B/1855